POPULATION AND REPRODUCTIVE HEALTH IN INDIA

POPULATION AND REPRODUCTIVE HEALTH IN INDIA

AN ASSESSMENT OF THE CURRENT SITUATION AND FUTURE NEEDS

SHIREEN J. JEJEEBHOY
P.M. KULKARNI
K.G. SANTHYA
FIROZA MEHROTRA

OXFORD
UNIVERSITY PRESS

OXFORD
UNIVERSITY PRESS

Oxford University Press is a department of the University of Oxford.
It furthers the University's objective of excellence in research, scholarship,
and education by publishing worldwide. Oxford is a registered trademark of
Oxford University Press in the UK and in certain other countries

Published in India by
Oxford University Press
YMCA Library Building, 1 Jai Singh Road, New Delhi 110 001, India

First Edition published in 2014

ISBN-13: 978-0-19-809623-8
ISBN-10: 0-19-809623-2

Typeset in Adobe Garamond Pro 11/13
by MAP Systems, Bengaluru 560 082, India
Printed in India by Akash Press, New Delhi 110 020

Contents

Foreword

Reproductive health care is vital for improving well-being and achieving other social and development goals. As India is witnessing a change in population dynamics there has also been a significant shift in the way reproductive health problems are conceptualized. The population programme now aims to provide family planning within a broad framework of maternal and child health care, with emphasis on voluntarism and informed choice.

Universal access to quality reproductive health services not only enhances the capacity of a couple in planning and limiting the family size but also enables them with the right to be free of many risks like unintended pregnancies and health related complications due to repeated pregnancies. This also helps in reducing high maternal mortality rate (MMR) and infant mortality rate (IMR). The reproductive health programme encompasses services for all sections and all people. Women's ability to choose the number of children they bear and the time intervals between births is the key to empowering women as individuals, mothers, and citizens.

In the XIIth Five Year Plan (2012–17) there will be increasing commitment at the national level towards population and reproductive health. India will need more evidences that influence the current policies and programmes so as to achieve better health for every section of society. Successful health programmes are built on a strong research foundation. This compilation, *Population and Reproductive Health in India: An Assessment of the Current Situation and Future Needs*, will, I trust, direct our actions towards the essential steps needed to achieve better health. We need a better understanding of population and reproductive health issues if we are to close the gaps and overcome the obstacles encountered in the past.

Keshav Desiraju
Secretary, Department of Health and Family Welfare
Ministry of Health and Family Welfare

Preface

India has experienced defining demographic changes in the past decade. With 1.2 billion people as per Census 2011, India is the world's second most populous country, and accounts for about one-fifth of the world's population. For the first time since Independence, its population has added fewer persons in absolute numbers from 2001–11 compared to the previous decade. Annual exponential growth fell from less than 2 per cent in 1991–2001 to 1.6 per cent in 2001–11. Despite this decline, the population will continue to rise, due to the momentum, as young people constitute nearly a third of the current population.

The demographic transition and changing age structure mean that the growth rate of the working age population is higher than overall and dependent growth rates, resulting in a demographic dividend. Whether India realizes its demographic dividend, and achieves the Millennium Development Goals, depends on the investments we make in reproductive and sexual health needs of young people. Subsequently, the growth rate of population over 60 will increase, posing challenges for coping with an ageing population. It is interesting to note that this transition is not unfolding uniformly across India as states are at different stages of the demographic transition. Additionally, we have witnessed another trend with far-reaching consequences: India's population is becoming more masculine, as the child sex ratio has fallen from 945 girls for 1,000 boys in 1991 to 914 girls for 1,000 boys in 2011. The study points to other emerging issues such as urbanization and migration that need to be factored into policies to address population needs.

To understand the interlinkages between these demographic changes, population trends, and the reproductive health needs of people, especially of women and young people, the United Nations Population Fund (UNFPA) commissioned a population needs assessment study in 2011. The study offers a comprehensive view of demographic trends and reproductive health indicators, combining data and information on youth, gender, reproductive health, and population from various sources. UNFPA has used insights from the study to design its eighth five-year country programme of assistance to India (2013–17).

This book presents findings which would be of interest to academics, policy makers, and development experts. Evidence-based policy making is key to achieving the goals of the ICPD plan of Action and the Millennium Declaration, and plays an even greater role in defining future development goals. UNFPA is happy to have contributed to this body of work on population issues to help direct efforts where they are needed the most.

I am grateful to the authors of this book for presenting the study to a wider audience. UNFPA India staff provided feedback at various stages; in particular, I thank my colleagues Ms Ena Singh, Assistant Representative, and Dr Sanjay Kumar, National Programme Officer, for coordinating the study.

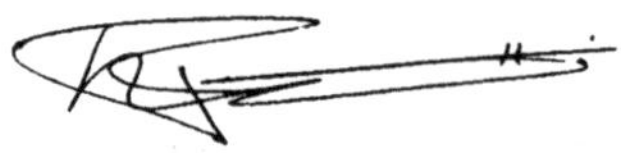

Frederika Meijer
UNFPA Representative, India/Bhutan

Acknowledgements

This volume provides a comprehensive review of the various dimensions of the health and population situation in India, including the changing population structure, the population and development scenario, the reproductive health situation, the situation and needs of adolescents and youth, women's empowerment and gender equity, and the role of development partners. It also describes the shifts in the policy and programme environment, and the growing stress upon the exercise of rights and informed choice.

India has witnessed major changes in the context of health and population over the past two decades. Some changes have been positive: notable declines in mortality, especially early childhood mortality, fertility, and unmet need for family planning. Many others are disturbing, such as persistence of gender imbalances, and the emergence of pre-natal sex selection. There is a need to assimilate the progress made in improving the health and population situation in India and to outline the gaps or obstacles that may have impeded progress. Currently, evidence is somewhat scattered and it is difficult to measure the significance of the change that has occurred or the obstacles that persist. This volume attempts to synthesize available evidence and provide a composite assessment of the situation that will provide indications for future strategies and programme directions for government and donor agencies.

This assessment would have been impossible without the insights, cooperation, and support of many. First and foremost, we would like to extend our deep gratitude to the UNFPA for envisioning the need for this assessment, and for supporting authors to conduct it. We would also like to acknowledge with thanks the initial feedback provided by staff members of UNFPA, India who attended two UNFPA sponsored consultations conducted in 2011, namely, the Consultative meeting with UNFPA staff and the National Consultation for Civil Society Organization on the Draft UNFPA Strategy in Country Programme 8. Each chapter has benefitted from the comments and suggestions made by a number of anonymous reviewers, and we are thankful to each of them for their insightful suggestions. We are especially grateful to the UNFPA team—Ena Singh, Sanjay Kumar, Venkatesh Srinivasan, K.M. Satyanarayana, Dinesh Agarwal, and Jaya—for their support and insights during the assessment as well as during the work on this volume. We also express our gratitude to the team at Oxford University Press and the anonymous reviewers appointed by the Press for their comments and insights. The careful reviews and helpful suggestions offered by all of these reviewers have helped shape the focus of the assessment and enriched the contributions.

Support from the John D. and Catherine T. MacArthur Foundation, the Ford Foundation, the Hewlett Foundation, and the UK Government's Department for International Development to the Population Council enabled Council editors to coordinate the task of turning a report into a book and is gratefully acknowledged.

A number of individuals have supported us in both the technical and administrative aspects of this study. We are grateful to Ramesh Chellan, Jawaharlal Nehru University. At the Population Council, we are grateful to A.J. Francis Zavier for his support with the analysis of data included in the volume, to M.A. Jose for his support in accessing literature, and to Komal Saxena for identifying and clarifying inconsistencies, preparing references, and taking on the responsibility for preparing the manuscript for publication. Their contributions in ensuring the quality of this volume are gratefully acknowledged.

We would like to end by expressing our appreciation to the several organizations that have made this volume possible: the UNFPA Oxford University Press, and our own organizations, namely, the Population Council and Jawaharlal Nehru University.

Shireen J. Jejeebhoy, Population Council, New Delhi
P.M. Kulkarni, Jawaharlal Nehru University, New Delhi
K. G. Santhya, Population Council, New Delhi
Firoza Mehrotra, Independent Consultant, New Delhi

Tables and Figures

Tables

Figures

Abbreviations

AIDS	Acquired Immune Deficiency Syndrome
ANC	Antenatal Care
ANM	Auxiliary Nurse Midwife
ARSH	Adolescent Reproductive and Sexual Health
ART	Assisted Reproductive Techniques
ARV	Anti-retroviral
ASHA	Accredited Social Health Activist
AWW	Anganwadi Worker
AYUSH	Ayurveda, Yoga and Naturopathy, Unani, Siddha, and Homoeopathy
CHC	Community Health Centre
EAG	Empowered Action Group
EMOC	Emergency Obstetric Care
FRU	First Referral Unit
GDP	Gross Domestic Product
HIV	Human Immunodeficiency Virus
ICDS	Integrated Child Development Services
ICPD	International Conference on Population and Development
ICTC	Integrated Counselling and Testing Centre
IEC	Information, Education and Communication
IFA	Iron and Folic Acid
IMR	Infant Mortality Rate
IUCD	Intrauterine Contraceptive Device
IUD	Intra-uterine Devices
JRM	Joint Review Mission

KSY	Kishori Shakti Yojana
MA	Medical Abortion
MNGO	Mother Non-government Organization
MO	Medical Officer
MOHFW	Ministry of Health and Family Welfare
MPW	Multipurpose Health Worker
MTP	Medical Termination of Pregnancy
MVA	Manual Vacuum Aspiration
NACO	National AIDS Control Organisation
NACP	National AIDS Control Programme
NCC	National Cadet Corps
NCERT	National Council of Educational Research and Training
NFHS	National Family Health Survey
NIOS	National Institute of Open Schooling
NPP	National Population Policy
NRHM	National Rural Health Mission
NSS	National Service Scheme
NYKS	Nehru Yuva Kendra Sangathan
ORS	Oral Rehydration Solution
PCPNDT	Pre-conception and Pre-natal Diagnostic Techniques
PHC	Primary Health Centre
PLHA	People Living with HIV/AIDS
PNDT	Pre-natal Diagnostic Technique
PPTCT	Prevention of Parent to Child Transmission
PRB	Population Reference Bureau
RCH	Reproductive and Child Health
RGSEAG	The Rajiv Gandhi Scheme for Empowerment of Adolescent Girls
RTI	Reproductive Tract Infections
SRH	Sexual and Reproductive Health
STD	Sexually Transmitted Disease
STI	Sexually Transmitted Infections
TFR	Total Fertility Rate
U5MR	Under-5Mortality Rate
VHND	Village Health Nutrition Day
VHSC	Village Health and Sanitation Committees
WHO	World Health Organization

1

Setting the Stage

K.G. Santhya

Shireen J. Jejeebhoy

Objectives

India's population scenario has undergone momentous and multi-dimensional changes in the last decade. Its population has now reached 1.21 billion, decadal growth rate has registered its sharpest decline since independence, and significant declines in the growth rate were observed even in the Empowered Action Group (EAG) states after years of stagnation (Office of the Registrar General and Census Commissioner, India 2013). The age structure of the population has, moreover, placed India in the advantageous position of being able to reap the demographic dividend, and the window of opportunity it offers for accelerated economic growth (Chandrashekhar, Ghosh, and Roychowdhury 2006). The nation's literacy rate has increased and the gender gap in literacy has narrowed impressively (Office of the Registrar General and Census Commissioner, India 2013). In the area of sexual and reproductive health, infant mortality has recorded notable declines, access to skilled attendance at delivery has expanded, and unmet need for contraception has fallen (International Institute for Population Sciences and Macro International 2007; UNICEF 2010). Moreover, over the last two decades, India has made many significant national and international commitments to improving the health and rights of its population. The National Population Policy (2000), the National Policy for the Empowerment of Women 2001, the National AIDS Prevention and Control Policy 2002, the National Youth Policy 2003, the Xth and XIth Five Year Plans (2002–07, 2007–12), and programmes such as the Reproductive and Child Health Programme and its National Rural Health Mission (NRHM), the Skill Development Initiative, and the The Rajiv Gandhi Scheme for Empowerment of Adolescent Girls (RGSEAG) (SABLA)/Kishori Shakti Yojana, are examples of the nation's commitment to improving the quality of life on multiple fronts. At the international level, India has reinforced these commitments by signing the International Conference on Population and Development (ICPD) Declaration (1994), the Convention on the Rights of the Child (1989), the Convention on the Elimination of All Forms of Discrimination against Women (1979) and, of course, the Millennium Development Goals (MDGs), articulating in many ways its commitment to meeting the multiple needs and rights of its people.

Despite these national commitments and progress on many indicators, improvements in population indicators have been slow. India lags behind many developing countries in terms of the key dimensions of human development (United Nations Development Programme 2012), and has failed to meet many health and development goals set to be achieved in the first decade of this century. For example, the child sex ratio, already adverse in 2001, has recorded a further decline over the last decade (Office of the Registrar General and Census Commissioner, India 2013), maternal mortality and even infant mortality levels have declined far too modestly, and wide gender imbalances and limited exercise of reproductive rights persist. The decade has seen the absorption and in some cases, misuse, of new technologies in everyday sexual and reproductive life, such as the misuse of pre-natal diagnostic techniques for sex selection, and increasing and poorly regulated access to assisted reproductive techniques (ARTs). In addition, over the course of this decade, concerns have arisen about the unique sexual and reproductive health needs of the young, a group whose needs continue to remain poorly understood and served (International Institute for Population Sciences and Population Council 2010). Finally, while the need for a rights-based approach has been recognized, deep-rooted gender inequities prevail, poverty levels remain unacceptable, and the socially and economically excluded remain alienated from the fruits of development. In short, despite the strides made on several fronts, India continues to face a situation of considerable sexual and reproductive ill health and lack of informed choice.

The failure to translate commitments into reality calls for efforts to better understand the population and reproductive health scenarios, and the lessons learned from programme experience, and to identify both the achievements in, and obstacles to, improving the wellbeing of India's population. While over the course of the last two decades several studies have addressed these issues, there remains a need to assimilate the lessons learned, identify achievements and obstacles, and outline strategies and actions to enhance the population and reproductive health situation. In this endeavour, a first step is the compilation of a profile on the current situation and an assessment of the needs in India in this sector.

The objective of this volume is to provide a synthesis of available evidence pertaining to the current situation and progress made in improving the population and reproductive health situation, and realizing rights in India, highlight gaps or obstacles that may have impeded progress, and outline priority areas for action. The volume addresses multiple dimensions of the population situation: its size and structure, its overall development, sexual and reproductive health situation and the exercise of reproductive rights, progress made in empowering women and achieving gender equity, and the situation and needs of its young people. It highlights major programmatic challenges and provides indications for future strategies and programme directions for the government and other development partners.

A review of India's population and sexual and reproductive health situation in 2012–13 is timely for many reasons. India has made national and international commitments to reach a significant number of goals and targets in the second decade of this century, and it is important to assimilate the evidence that will inform policies and programmes about the progress made and the obstacles encountered in achieving these goals and targets. For example, it has been more than a decade since the National Population Policy was introduced that set a number of goals for the nation to be achieved by 2010. Likewise, the year 2012 marks the completion of India's XIth Five Year Plan period and the initiation of its XIIth Plan, and as such, there is a need to reflect on the extent to which targets set have been met over the course of the XIth Plan, and underscore the outstanding issues that will confront the implementation of the XIIth Plan. At the same time, it has been 18 years since India signed the ICPD Declaration, and as ICPD+20 approaches, it is an appropriate time to take stock of the progress made and the outstanding challenges. Finally, India made a commitment to meet the MDGs by 2015, with Goals 2–6 heavily dependent on the population scenario, the sexual and reproductive health situation, and progress made in narrowing gender gaps.

This introductory chapter describes the approach and methodology adopted in this volume, and provides the background in which population issues, and sexual and reproductive health and choice, are experienced in India. The chapter describes the range of policies and laws affecting population and sexual and reproductive health in India, the goals and targets set in various policies, and a brief description of the extent to which these goals and targets have been achieved.

Approach and Methodology

This synthesis relies on a wide range of secondary sources of information, including census and survey reports, and further analysis of available data, policies and laws, and programme documents relevant to India's population and sexual and reproductive health situation. In order to understand the situation, evidence is presented from the census, the Sample Registration System, National Sample Surveys, National Family Health Surveys, the Coverage Evaluation Survey, and the Youth in India: Situation and Needs study, a sub-national study of young people in six states (hereafter referred to as the Youth Study). The review also encompasses findings from extensive searches of published and unpublished, qualitative and quantitative studies that refer to the population situation in India, and that were undertaken over the last decade or so. We acknowledge that evidence continues to be incomplete and patchy in some areas: for example, while evidence on the patterns of contraceptive use is not only comprehensive but also available at national and sub-national levels, evidence on other topics–infertility and RTIs, to name a few–comes from smaller case studies, perhaps raising questions about their applicability to the population at large.

Relevant policies were also reviewed, notably those that address the broad themes of population and development, sexual and reproductive health, young people's health and development, and gender issues. The policies reviewed were the National Population Policy 2000, the National Youth Policy 2003, the draft Youth Policy 2012, the National Health Policy 2002, the National AIDS Prevention and Control Policy 2002, the National Policy for the Empowerment of Women 2001, the National Policy on Education 1986 (as modified in 1992) and the National Skill Development Policy. Additionally, legislative measures in the area of sexual and reproductive health, youth, and gender issues have been addressed, such as the Prohibition of Child Marriage Act 2006, the Protection of Women from Domestic Violence Act 2005, the amended Medical Termination of Pregnancy (MTP) Act (2002), the Pre-Natal Diagnostic Techniques (Regulation and Prevention of Misuse) Act, 1994, and the Pre-Natal Diagnostic Techniques (Regulation and Prevention of Misuse) Amendment Act 2002, the Immoral Traffic (Prevention) Amendment Bill 2006, and the proposed Bill for the Protection of Women from Sexual Harassment in the Workplace. We also reviewed various Five Year Plan documents, notably the Eleventh Five-Year Plan (2007–12).

At the programme level, we reviewed various programme and strategy documents, including the NRHM (2005–12), the Reproductive and Child Health Programme, the *Janani Suraksha Yojana* (or JSY, launched in 2005), the National Adolescent Reproductive and Sexual Health Strategy, and the National AIDS Control Programme Phase 3 (NACP-III) Strategy and Implementation Plan. In assessing programme achievements, we have perused the annual reports and other printed and web-based materials provided by various ministries, including the ministries of Health and Family Welfare, Youth Affairs and Sports, Human Resource Development, and Women and Child Development, as well as various Joint Review Mission and Common Review Mission reports relating to progress made on population issues. We also reviewed selected adolescent and youth initiatives undertaken by civil society organizations.

Policy Context

The way population and reproductive health issues were conceptualized in India underwent a significant shift during the 1990s. New policies to address the needs of underserved population groups and previously neglected issues, and to bring both gender and rights perspectives to population and sexual and reproductive health issues, have been introduced in the last one-and-half decade. Additionally, several path breaking legislative measures that have implications for population and reproductive health issues have been introduced during this period. We provide a broad overview of the main policies and laws that have a bearing on population and sexual and reproductive health issues. While not described in this volume, we note that India is a signatory to a number of conventions and international commitments that have a bearing on its population and sexual and reproductive health situation, including the Convention on the Rights of the Child (CRC), 1989, the Convention on the Elimination of All Forms of Discrimination Against Women (CEDAW), 1979, the ICPD declaration, 1994, and the MDGs.

Key policies

Key policies that have a bearing on population and sexual and reproductive health issues included the National Population Policy (2000), the National AIDS Prevention and Control Policy (2002), the National Health Policy (2002), the National Youth Policy (2003), and the National Policy for the Empowerment of Women (2001). In the subsections below, we describe in detail these five key policies. Given the focus of this book on issues related to population, sexual and reproductive health, and youth and women's empowerment, we focus on policy prescriptions that directly address these topics, although these policies have addressed a range of topics. At the same time, we note that many other policies formulated in the recent past have also contained discussions of these topics, particularly of youth issues, and these policies are also described, although briefly, in the subsections below.

National Population Policy 2000 The National Population Policy, adopted in February 2000, legitimized the paradigm shift toward greater client centeredness. It provided a policy framework for achieving the twin objectives of population stabilization and promoting reproductive health within the wider context of sustainable development. Its immediate objectives were to address the unmet need for contraception, strengthen health care infrastructure, build capacity of health personnel, and provide integrated service delivery for basic reproductive and child health care (Ministry of Health and Family Welfare 2000). Specific targets were to achieve infant mortality rates below 30 per 1,000 live births, a maternal mortality ratio below 100 per 100,000 live births, 100 percent deliveries by trained personnel, and a total fertility rate of 2.1 by 2010; goals that are yet to be realized.

Twelve strategic themes were delineated to achieve these objectives, including decentralized planning and implementation, convergence of service delivery at the grassroots, empowering women and encouraging male involvement, meeting the unmet need for family welfare services, addressing the needs of disadvantaged and under-served population groups, and forging public-private partnerships. It recognized, for the first time, that adolescents constitute an under-served group with special sexual and reproductive health needs, and advocated special programmatic attention to addressing this population. It recommended the need to ensure for adolescents access to sexual and reproductive health information, counselling and services that are affordable and accessible, and to 'strengthen primary health centres and sub-centres to provide counselling, both to adolescents and also to newly-weds' (Ministry of Health and Family Welfare 2000). Its strategies for empowering women called for an enabling environment for women and children, establishment of child care centres in rural areas to encourage female participation in paid employment, and expansion of women's access to health care, including through the creation of a network of public, private, and NGO facilities and a cash transfer programme. It underscored the government's commitment to the provision of quality services, information and counselling, and expanding contraceptive method options in order to enable people to make voluntary and informed choices.

National AIDS Prevention and Control Policy 2002 The overall goal of the National AIDS Prevention and Control Policy 2002 was the effective containment of the infection levels of HIV/AIDS in the general population in order to achieve zero-level of new infections by 2007 (National AIDS Control Organisation 2002). To meet these objectives, the policy delineated various strategies including raising awareness, controlling STIs, ensuring the safety of blood and blood products, improving services for the care and support of people living with HIV/AIDS, and creating an enabling socio-economic environment. The policy emphasized the importance of inter-sectoral coordination, forging partnerships with multiple stakeholders including NGOs and community-based organizations, decentralized planning and implementation, and integration of services. Recognizing the special vulnerability of the youth, the policy underscored the need to promote a better understanding of HIV infection and safe sex practices among the youth. A variety of measures have been suggested to prevent risky behaviour among young people, including awareness building, condom promotion, creation of an enabling environment, and reinforcing traditional Indian moral values. It also advocated the provision of HIV/AIDS education in schools and colleges through curricular and co-curricular activities, as well as through youth organizations for those outside of educational institutions.

National Health Policy 2002 The National Health Policy 2002 provided the overarching framework for improvements in access to and standards of health services in India, ensuring more equitable access to health services, and addressing the needs of the most underserved. It called upon the Central Government to play a key role in augmenting public health investments, and specifically, to increase, by 2010, health sector expenditure to six percent of GDP, with two percent contributed as public health investment. In order to address inequities, the Policy argued for greater investment (55 per cent of total public health investment) in the primary health sector. Infrastructure and human resources were particular areas of focus; provision of essential drugs at primary health care level, the need for more frequent in-service training, expanding the pool of medical practitioners in under-served areas to include practitioners trained in Indian Systems of Medicine and nurses trained in allopathic medicine, and greater decentralization of the implementation of programmes to local self-government institutions. The Policy also envisaged Information, Education and Communication (IEC) strategies that would focus on interpersonal communication and other information dissemination activities; it recognized, in particular, the need to raise awareness among school and college students about health-promoting behaviour. The Policy made few specific recommendations with regard to sexual and reproductive health services, noting that the focus on primary health sector infrastructure would facilitate increased access of women to basic health care, and committing 'the highest priority of the Central Government to the funding of programmes relating to women's health' (Ministry of Health and Family Welfare 2002).

National Youth Policy 2003 and 2012 (draft) The National Youth Policy 2003, and the more recent draft National Youth Policy 2012, have underscored the multiple needs of the youth, and the need for holistic and multipronged action. The National Youth Policy 2003 addresses the needs of those aged 13–35 but recognizes adolescents (aged 13–19) as a special group requiring different strategies from those appropriate for young adults (aged 20–35) (Ministry of Youth Affairs and Sports 2003). With regard to health issues, it recognizes the vulnerability of the youth in the sexual and reproductive health arena, and advocates the provision of free state-sponsored counselling services for the youth, the establishment of 'adolescent clinics' to provide appropriate counselling and treatment, and the establishment of Youth Health Associations at the grassroots level to provide family welfare and counselling services. In the area of nutrition, it calls for efforts to redress gender imbalances in the nutritional status of young people. It also articulated the importance of life skills building programmes for the youth, as well as a commitment to enable the youth to attain high levels of education, access employment opportunities, and to address gender disparity in schooling and economic opportunities.

The draft National Youth Policy 2012, reiterates many of these commitments (Ministry of Youth Affairs and Sports 2012). It has redefined the age range of the population to which it refers; 16–30 instead of 13–35. It argues for programming for three groups of this population: those aged 16–21, 21–25, and 26–30, recognizing that each group is at a different stage of development and has different needs. It argues for an integrated and collaborative approach to youth development programmes, and for the mainstreaming of youth needs and concerns in overall national development policies. A key objective of the policy is to improve young people's health status. In order to do so, it seeks to facilitate access to services, notably in the areas of basic nutrition, reproductive and sexual health, mental health, as well as to information on sexual and reproductive health matters. It also seeks to promote a healthy lifestyle free of substance abuse and other unhealthy addictions, and calls for measures to dissuade youth from engaging in harmful sexual practices. Policy interventions proposed focus on developing education and training materials that integrate information and skill-based approaches that are expected to enable young people to adopt appropriate changes in their behaviours and actions, establishing linkages with agencies dealing with health issues, building the capacity of community-based organizations to create awareness about HIV-related matters, developing programmes addressing the health needs of differentlyabled youth, and conducting annual health checkups. The policy also contains a number of recommendations for promoting gender justice and equality–engaging youth clubs and youth volunteers to undertake educational programmes on such issues as female foeticide, domestic violence, girls' education, and early childbearing, for example. The policy also argues for the need to enhance educational and economic opportunities for the youth. Its recommendations include creating educational opportunities for disadvantaged youth groups, paying special attention towards making higher education vocation-oriented, and setting up networks of training institutions providing technical and/or entrepreneurship training, financial institutions, voluntary organizations and the corporate sector to promote entrepreneurship among young women and men.

National Policy for the Empowerment of Women 2001 The National Policy for the Empowerment of Women (2001) squarely acknowledges the widespread prevalence of gender disparity and discrimination against girls and women (Ministry of Women and Child Development 2001). Its goals are wide-ranging and include creating social and economic opportunities that enable women to realize their full potential, enabling women to enjoy human rights and fundamental freedoms on an equal basis with men, ensuring equal access to participation and decision-making for women in social, economic and political spheres, ensuring equal access to health care, quality education, career guidance, employment and so on, strengthening legal systems to eliminate discrimination against women, changing societal attitudes, and eliminating violence against women and girls. Specific policy prescriptions include efforts to enact or change existing laws, including in the area of ownership of property and inheritance and, more directly, to empower women economically and socially, through poverty eradication efforts, strengthening micro credit opportunities, affirmative action to ensure women's participation in decision-making, and ensuring equal access to education. A number of policy prescriptions directly address women's sexual and reproductive health: access to comprehensive, affordable, and quality health care, and recognition of their right to make informed choices, notably with regard to sexual and reproductive health matters including HIV and STIs. Mention is also made about the need to prioritize birth, death, and marriage registration as a means of tracking infant and maternal mortality, and efforts to delay marriage and address malnutrition among women and girls, including pregnant and lactating women. The elimination of all forms of violence against women is a key policy prescription, encompassing such concerns as the need to eliminate sexual harassment in the workplace and the persistence of dowry and dowry related harassment. It argues strongly for the protection of the rights of girls, including the elimination of prenatal sex selection, female foeticide and infanticide, child marriage, child abuse, and child prostitution. It also identifies adolescent girls as a vulnerable group and highlights the need to pay attention to their education and nutrition.

XIth Five-Year Plan 2007–12 and XIIth Five-Year Plan (draft) The XIth Plan reiterated the commitments articulated in policies described above. The objective of the XIth Plan is to achieve good health for people, especially the poor and the underprivileged. It has set a number of time-bound goals, including reducing maternal mortality ratio to 1 per 1,000 live births, infant mortality rate (IMR) to 28 per 1,000 live births, total fertility rate (TFR) to 2.1, malnutrition among children aged 3 years and below to half its present level and anaemia among women and girls by 50 per cent

(Planning Commission 2008a, 2008b). The Plan highlighted the role of the NRHM established in 2005 and the proposed National Urban Health Mission (not yet established), described in detail in sections later on, as the major programmes through which to achieve these goals. The XIth Plan underscored that the NRHM would represent a shift away from previous vertical health and family welfare programmes to a focus on inclusive health development in which integration of health concerns and programmes were to be emphasized. Among the key strategies outlined in the XIth Plan for implementation by the NRHM were (a) training and capacity building of Panchayati Raj Institutions (PRIs) to supervise and manage public health services and encouraging the development of Health Plans for each village through Village Health Committees of the Panchayat; (b) strengthening the role of the female health activist (Accredited Social Health Activist (ASHA)) to promote access to improved health care at household level; (c) strengthening sub-centres, PHCs and Community Health Centre (CHC); (d) regulation of the private sector, including informal rural practitioners; (e) promotion of public private partnerships to ensure quality services and the achievement of public health goals; and (f) effective and viable risk-pooling and social health insurance to provide health security to the poor. The Plan placed considerable emphasis on upgrading facilities: all sub-centres, for example, were to be made functional by 2010, with two Auxiliary Nurse Midwives (ANMs) each; all PHCs were to contain three staff nurses and provide round-the-clock services by 2010; and 6,500 CHCs were to be strengthened by 2012 with seven specialists and nine staff nurses. The Plan also makes special note of the need to enhance access to appropriate services, through improvements in infrastructure, including physical access to facilities, availability of essential drugs, supplies and equipment, and special efforts to reach the most remote and underserved, notably the tribal population. It also underscores the need to provide gender responsive health care, establish measures at state and district levels to halt declining sex ratios, improve the coverage, content, and quality of antenatal, delivery services and postpartum care services, make First Referral Unit (FRU) operational for providing emergency and essential obstetric care; decentralize power for the approval of sites authorized to provide abortion and thereby enlarge the network of safe abortion providers, provision for early detection and management of common RTIs and expansion of services for RTIs/STIs at sub-district level, and encourage home based neonatal care and other measures to address newborn health.

The Plan also recognized young people as a group with special and distinct needs, and underscored the importance of investing in them. In the area of health, it aims to give special attention to the health of adolescent girls and proposes multifaceted areas of focus, including: (a) nutrition and health education for adolescents; (b) optimum health and nutrition interventions during pregnancy; (c) orientation and training of health service delivery personnel to build awareness of and provide youth-friendly services to young people seeking reproductive and sexual health services; (d) development of materials for communication and behavioural change; (e) provision of adolescent/youth friendly services at all PHCs and CHCs, including the establishment of a special window to serve their needs; and (f) the appointment of counsellors in all schools and the provision of helplines equipped to reach out to youth in need of mental health services. The Plan stresses advocacy efforts to delay age at marriage, as well as special attention to strengthening enforcement mechanisms for the implementation of the Prohibition of Child Marriage Act. It also emphasizes the importance of compulsory registration of marriages. It introduced the Integrated Child Protection Scheme and the Scheme for Relief and Rehabilitation of Victims of Sexual Assault. The Plan similarly emphasizes the provision of life skills, youth empowerment, and greater female participation in youth development programmes. It also advocates a strengthening and expansion of the youth club movement, including a larger female membership. It also highlights the nutritional needs of adolescents, especially girls, and aims to reduce anaemia among women and girls by 50 per cent by the end of the XIth Plan. It recommends that adolescents (ages 11–18) and school aged children (ages 6–10) should be served under the National Nutritional Anaemia Prophylaxis Programme (NNAP), and that iron and folic acid supplementation be provided to adolescent girls weekly. The XIth Plan also prioritizes the need to attain an educated youth population. It aims to raise the minimum level of education to class X and universalize access to secondary education. Indeed, it proposes to increase the gross enrolment ratio (GER) in secondary education from 52 per cent in 2004–05 to 75 per cent by 2011–12, and to provide a secondary school within 5 km of every habitation. In addition, the Plan focuses on improving quality, both of curriculum content and teacher skills. For example, ICT infrastructure is to be established at government and government aided secondary and senior-secondary schools (about 80,000) during the Plan period. It recognizes adolescent girls as particularly disadvantaged and proposes measures to enhance their school enrolment and continuation.

The XIth Plan has also recognized the pervasiveness of violence against women and girls, and argued for the strengthening of the justice delivery mechanism, the legislative environment, and the health system to better address the needs of women. In order to increase women's political participation at the grass roots level, the XIth Plan proposed to accelerate the process of women's participation in PRIs by recommending that the arbitrary use of the no-confidence clause be discontinued, laws in some states preventing women with more than two children from holding office are repealed, and resources are allocated for capacity building of PRIs including women. The XIth Plan devotes a full chapter to women's agency and child rights (Planning Commission 2008a). It recognizes that interventions must be multipronged and must ensure women's basic entitlements, prioritize economic empowerment for women, ensure that they are free from all forms of violence and are adequately represented in political and policy making spheres, and that institutional mechanisms are in place for gender mainstreaming. It set specific targets for women and children, including (a) an increase in the child (0–6) sex ratio from 927 in 2001 to 935 by 2011–12; (b) a minimum of 33 per cent of direct and indirect beneficiaries of government schemes to be women and girls; (c) a reduction in infant mortality from 57 to 28 and the maternal mortality ratio from 301 to 100 per 100,000 births; (d) a reduction by half in child (0–3) malnutrition and in anaemia among women and girls by 2011–12; and (e) a 10 per cent reduction in primary and secondary school discontinuation among both girls and boys.

The Approach Paper for the XIIth Plan maintains that health, education and skill development will continue to be focus areas (Planning Commission 2011). In the area of health, it notes that the NRHM needs to expand to a more comprehensive vision of health care than the current focus on antenatal and delivery care and to bring forth convergence among all existing national health programmes. It calls for paying special attention to reducing gender-based inequities in health outcomes of girls and women, meeting special requirements of different sub-groups including adolescents and elderly, improving the skills of health care providers and encouraging public-private partnership. Of relevance to adolescents and young people, the approach paper advocates making secondary education nearly universal, providing vertical mobility options for students of vocational courses to pursue graduate and post-graduate courses and improving the quality of teachers' training programmes. The approach paper also highlights the need for ending gender-based inequities, discrimination and violence faced by girls and women.

Other Policies, Particularly of Relevance to Adolescents and Young People Several other policies also acknowledge the need to pay special attention to the sexual and reproductive health and development of young people. The National Policy on Education (as modified in 1992) stresses the need to reduce gender imbalances in school attendance and completion (Ministry of Human Resource Development 1998). It highlights the importance of universal school enrolment and completion, and stresses the need to reduce gender imbalance in school attendance and completion. It also emphasizes that educational programmes should actively motivate and inform the youth about family planning and responsible parenthood. Also of special importance to young people is the proposed National Skill Development Policy. The policy calls for establishing a National Skills Development Initiative that aims to empower individuals through improved skills, knowledge, and qualifications to gain access to employment in an increasingly competitive global market (Ministry of Labour 2009). The policy aims to meet, by 2022, the skill needs of 500 million individuals, with special attention to women, the youth, and school drop-outs. The policy seeks to motivate the youth to participate in training programmes through activities conducted by village or block skills development centres, as well as in incentive mechanisms. It also proposes to strengthen the capacity of schools to lay a solid foundation that enables young people to acquire employable skills and to engage in continuous skill upgradation throughout their working life, use school education as a tool to increase awareness of vocational skill building options among young people, and to give alternative education in combination with skill development opportunities to out of school youth (Ministry of Labour 2009). The National Plan of Action for Children (2005), similarly, called for greater attention to young people's education and development opportunities (Ministry of Women and Child Development 2005). It also recognized the special needs of adolescents up to age 18, and argued for actions to enable them to have access to physical and mental health services, to build awareness of sexual and reproductive matters, and called for greater attention to protecting young people from violence and abuse (Ministry of Women and Child Development 2005).

Summary of Targets Set in the Area of Population and Reproductive Health A number of measurable goals and targets have been set by policies and international agreements that affirm India's commitment to improving population and reproductive health. Key goals are listed in Table 1.1. They highlight two important points, one promising and the other disturbing. First, the goals and targets are clearly ambitious, and underscore India's commitment to accelerating the pace of change in improving population and reproductive health. In the area of literacy and education, they call for universal literacy among youth, the elimination of gender disparities in primary and secondary education, and the containment of school discontinuation rates. In the areas of fertility and mortality, ambitious targets were set, including with regard to the TFR, the maternal mortality ratio, the IMR, a reversal of the adverse child sex ratio, universal child immunization, access to family planning information and services, significant reductions in malnutrition and child marriage, and stemming the spread of HIV/AIDS.

Second, as Table 1.1 suggests, in several instances, notably infant and maternal mortality, virtually identical targets have been set that are to be achieved by progressively later dates. For example, the target of achieving infant mortality rates below 30 per 1,000, and maternal mortality ratios of around 100 per 100,000 live births were set to be achieved by 2010, 2012, and 2015. Moving the goalposts in this way raises questions about the rationale underlying the setting of targets on the one hand, and the seriousness with which the achievement of targets are expected to be realized, on the other.

Table 1.1 Goals and Targets Set and Commitments Made in the Areas of Population and Reproductive Health

	NPP 2000 goals to be achieved by 2010*	XIth Plan goals (to be achieved by 2012)	MDG goals and targets to be achieved by 2015**
Literacy and education			
Literacy rate (15–24 year olds)			100
Schools enrolment	Make school education free and compulsory for those aged up to 14 years	Universal enrolment of 6–14 year-olds; increase gross enrolment ratio in secondary education to 75% by 2011–12	
Ratio of girls to boys in primary/ secondary education		Gender gaps in enrolment to be eliminated by 2011–12	1
Drop out at primary and secondary school	<20%		
Fertility			
Total fertility rate (TFR)	2.1	2.1	
Family size	Promote small family norm		
Infant and child mortality, health, and nutrition			
Infant mortality rate (IMR)	<30/1,000 births	28	27
U5MR (under 5 mortality rate)			41
Child immunization	100%		
Malnutrition among 0–3 year olds		By 1/2	

(Continued)

Table 1.1 *(Continued)*

	NPP 2000 goals to be achieved by 2010*	XIth Plan goals (to be achieved by 2012)	MDG goals and targets to be achieved by 2015**
Undernourished children			27.4
Child sex ratio		935	
Underweight children aged <3			26
Maternal mortality and reproductive health			
Maternal mortality ratio	<100/100,000 births	100	109
Institutional delivery	80%		
Trained attendance at delivery	100%		
Malnourishment (% of total population)			31.1
Anaemia among females 15–49/ malnutrition		By half	
Child marriage	Promote delayed marriage for girls to age 18		
FP counselling and services	100%		
Registration of vital events	100%		
HIV/AIDS	Contain the spread, promote integration with STI/RTI services		

Note: *Goals relating to addressing unmet needs in basic RCH services, supplies and infrastructure, communicable diseases, sectoral linkages not included; **Goals relating to MDG 2–6 only; poverty, sanitation, malaria, and TB not included.

Key laws

There are a number of laws in India that have relevance, directly or indirectly, for sexual and reproductive health, young people's health and development needs, and women's empowerment. We focus here on notable laws that have been enacted in the last decade.

Prohibition of Child Marriage Act 2006 The Child Marriage Restraint Act of 1929 and the Child Marriage Restraint Act of 1978 prohibit the marriage of a girl before she reaches age 18 and of a boy before he reaches age 21. The more recent Prohibition of Child Marriage Act 2006 has considerably strengthened legislation in the case of child marriage (age 18 and 21 for girls and boys, respectively, as before). It imposes the following: (a) the district court can order both parties to the marriage and their parents to return all money, valuables and gifts received; (b) the family of the groom may be asked to pay maintenance to the bride-to-be until her remarriage; (c) the groom, if over age 18, is liable for two years imprisonment and/or a fine of up to Rs. 1 lakh; (d) anyone who 'performs, conducts, directs or abets' a child marriage will be punishable with rigorous imprisonment for up to two years and a fine of Rs. 1 lakh; (e) anyone who does anything to promote the marriage or permits it to be solemnized or fails to prevent it from being solemnized is also punishable with the same quantum; and (f) each state will appoint a Child Marriage Prohibition Officer whose task is to prevent such marriages from taking place, sensitize communities about early marriage and collect evidence for effective prosecution of those contravening the provisions of the Act (Ministry of Law and Justice 2007a).

Medical Termination of Pregnancy Act (MTP) 1971 and Amendment of 2002 The Medical Termination of Pregnancy (MTP) Act of 1971 and the 2002 amendments to the Act have ensured women's right to terminate an unwanted pregnancy safely and confidentially (Government of India 1971, 2003). It allows women to seek pregnancy termination in a wide range of circumstances, such as, when the mother's life is at risk or when her physical or mental health is compromised, in case of rape, if the pregnancy is likely to result in the birth of a child with physical or mental abnormalities; and if the pregnancy is the result of contraceptive failure. Pregnancies of up to 20 weeks may be terminated legally. However, the concurrence of at least two physicians is required for pregnancies of more than 12 weeks' gestation. However, legally, abortion services can be provided only in registered facilities and by certified providers (Government of India 1971). In 2002, medical abortion (the mifepristone-misoprostol combination) was approved for use for the termination of early pregnancies by the Drugs Controller of India, further facilitating women's access to abortion. While the Act makes no distinction between the rights of the married and the unmarried, it does require that women under 18 must have parental consent: 'No pregnancy of a woman who has not attained the age of 18 years... shall be terminated except with the consent in writing of her guardian.'

Pre-Natal Diagnostic Techniques (Regulation and Prevention of Misuse) Act 1994 and the Pre-Natal Diagnostic Techniques (Regulation and Prevention of Misuse) Amendment Act 2002 In order to curb the incidence of sex selective abortion, the Pre-Natal Diagnostic Techniques (Regulation and Prevention of Misuse) Act of 1994 (PNDT Act), and the 2002 amendments to the Act (PCPNDT), provide for the regulation of the use of prenatal diagnostic techniques and the prevention of misuse of such techniques for the purpose of prenatal sex determination leading to the selective termination of pregnancies carrying a female foetus (Ministry of Health and Family Welfare 1994, 2003). Several restrictions have been imposed: for example, all genetic counselling centres must be registered under the Act, the sale of ultrasound or imaging machines may only be made to facilities registered under the Act, all those conducting ultrasonography must declare that he or she has not disclosed the sex of the foetus to anyone; all those undergoing any such testing must declare that she does not wish to know the sex of the foetus; all facilities are expected to prominently declare in writing that disclosure of the sex of the foetus is prohibited under the law. All facilities may be inspected for violations from time to time, and the authorized officer is empowered to seize equipment and seal facilities that violate the Act. While the PCPNDT Act (Minister of Health and Family Welfare 2003) is aimed at curbing sex selection through the misuse of technology, it must be emphasized that the Act in no way deters from women's right to terminate a pregnancy in a host of conditions, as reflected in the Medical Termination of Pregnancy (MTP) Act of 1971 (Government of India 1971).

Protection of Women from Domestic Violence Act 2005 The Protection of Women from Domestic Violence Act 2005, passed in 2006, goes a long way in strengthening women's (including young women's) options and protection (Ministry of Law and Justice, 2007b). For one, it adopts a broad definition of domestic violence, including both actual abuse and the threat of abuse. Abuse covers physical (beating, pushing), sexual (including being forced into sex or into watching pornography), verbal, emotional, and economic (not providing for wife and children) violence, and it also covers dowry-related harassment. Also of relevance to young women is that it includes being forced not to attend an educational institution, and being prevented from taking a job or leaving the home. It also includes being forced to marry someone against their will or being prevented from marrying someone they wish to marry. The Act offers women considerable protection, including the right to reside in the matrimonial or shared household and the imposition of restraining orders on the perpetrator. In addition, under the Act, NGOs may register with the state as service providers, to support women's needs by way of legal aid, health care, economic support, and so on.

The Immoral Traffic (Prevention) Amendment Bill 2006 The Immoral Traffic (Prevention) Amendment Bill 2006 amended the Immoral Traffic (Prevention) Act 1956, to combat trafficking and sexual exploitation for commercial purposes (Ministry of Women and Child Development 2006). The Bill specifically covers trafficking for the purposes of prostitution, as well as punishment to those involved in trafficking of persons—usually girls—for this purpose. Key provisions include the deletion of the clause that penalized sex workers for soliciting clients, and more stringent punishment for those committing trafficking as well as the clients of trafficked victims. Additionally, it strengthens the role of authorities at central and state levels to address trafficking.

The Protection of Children from Sexual Offences Act 2012 The Protection of Children from Sexual Offences Act 2012 seeks to protect children, defined as those aged below 18 years, from sexual assault, sexual harassment and pornography, and provides for the establishment of special courts for the trial of such offences (Press

Information Bureau 2012). It seeks to prevent the inducement or coercion of a child to engage in any sexual activity, the use of children in prostitution or other sexual practices, and the use of children in pornographic performances and materials. The Act treats sexual assault as an aggravated offence when a person in authority or position of trust commits the offence. It also contains guidelines for the media to sensitively and discreetly report cases of sexual offence.

The Protection of Women against Sexual Harassment at Workplace Bill 2010 The proposed Bill for the Protection of Women from Sexual Harassment in the Workplace 2010 seeks to ensure a safe environment for women at work places, both in public and private sectors, whether organized or unorganized (Press Information Bureau 2010). The Bill proposes a definition of sexual harassment, which is as laid down in the Vishaka judgment by the Supreme Court (any unwelcome sexually determined behaviour, including physical contacts and advances, a demand or request for sexual favours, sexually coloured remarks, showing pornography and any other unwelcome physical, verbal or non-verbal conduct of sexual nature). Additionally, it recognizes the promise or threat to a woman's employment prospects or creation of hostile work environment as 'sexual harassment' at workplace. The Bill provides protection not only to women who are employed but also to any woman who enters the workplace as a client, customer, apprentice, and daily wageworker, or in ad-hoc capacity.

The Women's Reservation Bill (The Constitution 108th Amendment Bill) 2008 Amendments to the constitution have focused more on ensuring greater participation of women in political processes. The 73rd and 74th Constitutional Amendments, passed in 1993, reserve one-third of all seats in panchayats and municipal bodies for women. More recently, in 2010, the Women's Reservation Bill was passed, by way of the 108th Amendment to the Indian constitution, by the Rajya Sabha, but is still to be passed in the Lok Sabha. This amendment reserves one-third of all seats in the parliament and in state legislative bodies for women. The Bill is to be effective for 15 years once passed and aims to reduce gender disparities in representation at state and national levels (Rajya Sabha 2010).

The Right of Children to Free and Compulsory Education Act 2009 The Right of Children to Free and Compulsory Education Act 2009 places responsibility on the state to ensure free and compulsory enrolment, as well as regular attendance and completion of elementary school, particularly among children from disadvantaged groups. The availability of a neighbourhood school, infrastructure, teaching staff and learning equipment, good quality education, appropriate training of teachers, and the integration of children from socially excluded groups into the school system (Ministry of Human Resource Development 2011). The Act also places responsibility on parents for ensuring that their children are enrolled in an appropriate elementary school and remain in school until they have completed Class VIII. Additionally, the Act stipulates conditions that may well enhance continuation and regular attendance: that schools must ensure that no child will be held back, subjected to physical punishment or mental harassment, and that regular meetings are held with parents to apprise them of their children's progress.

Population and Reproductive Health Scenario

India's population reached 1.21 billion in 2011, and is characterized by a sex ratio that continues to be unfavourable to females, a large rural population, heavy reliance on agriculture and widespread poverty with significant proportions living below the poverty line. Some current demographic and reproductive health indicators, drawn from the 2011 Census of India, and various national and sub-national studies carried out over the decade of the 2000s, are reflected in Table 1.2. Findings highlight that while progress has been made, the situation continues to be disturbing, and a comparison of Tables 1.1 and 1.2 shows that there is a considerable disconnect between commitments made and the reality in several indicators. For example:

- Although literacy rates have increased and gender disparities have narrowed over time, literacy rates are far from universal and the female disadvantage in literacy persists. A significant proportion of the population remains illiterate, and wide geographic and gender disparities in enrolment, particularly middle and secondary school enrolment, persist.

- The infant mortality rate is currently 47/1,000 live births; not only has India failed to achieve the national socio-demographic goal of an infant mortality rate of below 30 per 1,000 live births by the year 2010, but achieving the XIth Plan goal of 28/1000 live births by 2012 remains a challenging task.
- The maternal mortality ratio of 212/100,000 live births remains far in excess of the Population Policy and XIth Plan goals of less than 100/100,000, and suggests that without considerable acceleration in the pace of decline in maternal mortality, the MDG goal of 109/100,000 by 2015 will be difficult to achieve.
- Institutional delivery and trained attendance at delivery reach about three-quarters of recently delivered women today, a considerable increase since the beginning of this century; however, comprehensive ante-natal care and, in particular, access to postpartum care, are limited.
- Marriage continues to take place in childhood for almost half of all young women, and while the prevalence of child marriage has declined, the pace of decline is unacceptably slow.
- Contraceptive use has increased, and just 13 per cent of women report an unmet need for contraception; yet unmet need remains much higher for married young couples, and the method mix remains highly skewed towards tubal ligation.
- Large proportions of women suffer gender based violence; while violence in marriage is widespread, other crimes against women, ranging from assault and molestation to rape, kidnapping, and murder, are also evident.

The single most disturbing finding of the 2011 Census of India has been the plummeting sex ratio of the child population. Indeed, the child sex ratio (for the population aged 0–6) fell from 927 girls to 1,000 boys in 2001 to 919 girls to 1000 boys by 2011. It is estimated that approximately 4.5 million girls are missing, as a result of the practice of prenatal sex selection in the period 2001 to 2008 (UNFPA 2010). As is well-known, the adverse child sex ratio reflects the confluence of many socio-cultural factors: wide gender disparities, continuing strong son-preference, and the combination of declining family size preferences and unchanging demand for sons, the easy availability, in practice, of technology that enables foetal sex

Table 1.2 Selected Demographic and Reproductive Health Indicators

Population size, 2011[1]	1,210,569,573
Urban population (%), 2011	31.2
Literacy rate, female[1]	64.6
Literacy rate, male[1]	80.9
Sex ratio, 2011 (females/1,000 males)[1]	943
Child sex ratio, 2011 (0–6 years)[1]	919
Infant mortality rate (2010)[2]	47
Total fertility rate (2010)[2]	2.5
Young Women	
Women aged 20–24 married by 18 years, 2005–06 (%)[3]	47.4
Estimates of premarital sexual activity among females 15–24 years (%)[4]	4
Estimates of premarital sexual activity among males 15–24 years (%)[4]	15
Married adolescents 15–24 years using contraceptives (%)[4]	27.5
Contraceptive Use Dynamics[4]	
Contraceptive prevalence rate, all methods	56.3
Contraceptive prevalence rate, modern methods	48.5
Currently married women with an unmet need (%)	12.8
Sterilized women as a proportion of all couples using modern methods (%)	76.9
Currently married couples using male methods (vasectomy or condoms) (%)	12.8
Maternal Health and Care	
Maternal mortality ratio (per 100,000 live births)[5]	212
Neonatal mortality rate[3]	39.0
Institutional delivery (%)[6]	72.9
Skilled attendance at delivery (%)[6]	76.2
Women receiving all recommended antenatal services (%)[6]	26.5
Postpartum care within two months of delivery (women delivering in the five years preceding the survey(%)[4]	41
Induced Abortion	
Estimated number of total abortions (million)[7]	6.7

(Continued)

Table 1.2 *(Continued)*

Abortion ratio (abortions per 100 live births) community-based studies[8]	5–11
Maternal deaths resulting from unsafe abortion, 1998 (%)[9]	8
Estimated number of abortions at approved centres (million, 2010–11)[10]	0.62
Infertility	
Couples experiencing primary or secondary infertility (%)[11]	8–10
Women aged 40–49 years currently married estimated to be childless (%)[3]	2
Sexually Transmitted Infections (STIs) and HIV/AIDS	
STI prevalence (adult population)[12]	5
STI/RTI prevalence (adult population, range)[12]	14–18
Estimated number of PLHA (2008) (million)[13]	2.3
HIV prevalence (%)[13]	0.29
HIV prevalence range among antenatal women[13]	0.6
HIV prevalence range among STD clinic patients[13]	3.7
Domestic Violence	
Ever married women beaten by husbands (%)[3]	39

Source: [1]Office of the Registrar General and Census Commissioner India (2013); [2]Registrar General, India (2012); [3]International Institute for Population Sciences and Macro International (2007); [4]International Institute for Population Sciences and Population Council (2010); [5]Office of The Registrar General, India (2011) [6]UNICEF (2010); [7]Chhabra and Nuna (1994); [8]Elul et al. (2004); Malhotra et al. (2003); Ganatra et al. (2008); Jejeebhoy, Zavier, and Kalyanwala (2011a; 2011b); [9]Registrar General of India (2006); [10]Ministry of Health and Family Welfare (2011); [11]Ministry of Health and Family Welfare (2010a); [12]National AIDS Control Organization (2006); [13]National AIDS Control Organization (2010).

determination, and the apparent difficulty in enforcing available laws prohibiting the revelation of foetal sex.

Wide regional and socioeconomic disparities characterize almost all of the health and development indicators described in Table 1.2, and as subsequent chapters will reveal in more depth. For example, the north-south divide continues to be observed, with population and reproductive health indicators revealing greater well-being in southern states than in central and eastern states, and the poorly educated, the poor and the socially excluded far more likely to experience ill-health, and higher mortality and fertility than others. At the same time, we note that the adverse child sex ratio is more likely to be observed in economically better developed states, and among economically better off and educated households, than others.

What This Volume Covers and What It Does Not

We start with a few words to guide the reader. In conducting this synthesis, we focused on India's population and sexual and reproductive health situation, and the policies, laws, and programmes—and those aspects of policies, laws, and programmes—that relate to this situation. The synthesis does not encompass more general health system issues, such as infrastructure, human resources for health, efficiency, health sector financing, or health insurance. Where these issues are addressed, they are discussed in a limited way, that is, in relation to population and sexual and reproductive health matters. Among thematic areas, while we present evidence on the HIV situation, education, access to livelihood skills, and international support for India's programmes, we acknowledge that these have not been addressed comprehensively, but rather, with a singular focus on their intersections with the population and sexual and reproductive health scenario.

What we know about India's population situation underscores considerable socioeconomic and region- or state-wise inequities in levels and patterns of various outcome indicators, in access to services and in socio-cultural, gender and health system determinants. Each chapter highlights these inequities. For key indicators, additional state-wise information is provided in appendix tables.

Key aspects of the population situation encompass many thematic areas. Certain cross-cutting issues, like gender double standards and power imbalances, exercise of informed choice, male involvement, quality of care and services, are central to more than one broad topic and have been addressed within the discussion of each subject. For example, the sex ratio of the child population is addressed in the discussion of population structure and composition, abortion practices, and gender inequity. Adolescent concerns are addressed as a separate theme, but aspects of young people's health and development also fall into discussions of population and development, reproductive health, and gender disparities. Key challenges are described in most chapters. A certain amount of overlap is thus inevitable and we argue that this should be retained in order that each topic is addressed as thoroughly as possible.

Structure of the Report

This report is divided into a total of seven chapters, including this first introductory one that has laid out the objectives and the design of the review. Chapter 2 addresses the population and development scenario, and identifies challenges and broad areas for future attention. Chapter 3 reviews the sexual and reproductive health situation in India and outlines challenges and future needs. Chapter 4 focuses on the situation and the needs of adolescents and the youth, and the challenges and opportunities in meeting their needs. Chapter 5 explores progress in and obstacles to achieving gender equality, equity, and the empowerment of women. Chapter 6 summarizes the role of partners, notably development agencies, and highlights the type of support these partners provide, as well as the role of civil society and types of support offered by civil society organizations in programme implementation. Chapter 7 highlights key broad, overarching recommendations for the way ahead, as it assimilates from previous chapters the outstanding gaps and needs, and the opportunities, options, and priorities, for future programme emphasis.

References

Chandrashekhar, C. P., J. Ghosh, and A. Roychowdhury. 2006. 'The Demographic Dividend and Young India's Economic Future', *Economic and Political Weekly*, 41(49): 5055–63.

Chhabra, R. and S. C. Nuna. 1994. *Abortion in India: An Overview*. New Delhi: Ford Foundation.

Elul, B., S. Barge, S. Verma, R. Ved, R. Singhi, and K. Lockwood. 2004. *Unwanted Pregnancy and Induced Abortion: Data from Men and Women in Rajasthan, India*. New Delhi: Population Council.

Ganatra, B., S. Hirve, S. Karvande, L. Garda, and V. N. Rao. 2008. 'Induced Abortions in Rural Western Maharashtra: Prevalence and Patterns', in M. Koenig, S. J. Jejeebhoy, J. Cleland, and B. Ganatra (eds), *Reproductive Health in India: New Evidence*. New Delhi: Rawat Publications.

Government of India (GOI). 1971. *The Medical Termination of Pregnancy Act (Act. No. 34)*. New Delhi: Government of India.

———. 2003. *The Medical Termination of Pregnancy Rules (Amendment)*. New Delhi: Government of India.

International Institute for Population Sciences (IIPS) and Macro International. 2007. *National Family Health Survey (NFHS-3), India, 2005–06*. Mumbai: IIPS.

International Institute for Population Sciences (IIPS) and Population Council. 2010. *Youth in India: Situation and Needs 2006–2007*. Mumbai: IIPS.

Jejeebhoy, S. J., A. J. Francis Zavier, R. Acharya, et al. 2011a. *Increasing Access to Safe Abortion in Rural Maharashtra: Outcomes of a Comprehensive Abortion Care Model*. New Delhi: Population Council.

———. 2011b. *Increasing Access to Safe Abortion in Rural Rajasthan: Outcomes of a Comprehensive Abortion Care Model*. New Delhi: Population Council.

Malhotra, A., L. Nyblade, S. Parasuraman, K. Mac Quarrie, N. Kashyap, and S. Walia. 2003. *Realizing Reproductive Choice and Rights: Abortion and Contraception in India, Report*. Washington DC: International Council for Research on Women.

Ministry of Health and Family Welfare (MOHFW). 1994. *The Pre-conception and Pre-natal Diagnostic Techniques (Prohibition of Sex Selection) Act, 1994*. New Delhi: MOHFW, Government of India.

———. 2000. *National Population Policy 2000*. New Delhi: Department of Family Welfare, MOHFW, Government of India.

———. 2002. *National Health Policy*. New Delhi: MOHFW, Government of India.

———. 2003. *The Pre-natal Diagnostic Techniques (Regulation and Prevention of Misuse) Amendment Act, 2002 (No. 14 of 2003)*. New Delhi: MOHFW, Government of India. Available at http://pndt.gov.in/writereaddata/mainlinkFile/File50.pdf [Accessed 25 March 2012].

———. 2010a. *National Rural Health Mission, State–wise Progress as on 30.09.2010*. New Delhi: Department of Family Welfare, MOHFW, Government of India.

———. 2010b. *Comprehensive Abortion Care: Training and Service Delivery Guidelines*. New Delhi: MOHFW, Government of India.

———. 2011. *Family Welfare Statistics in India, 2011*. New Delhi: MOHFW, Statistics Division, Government of India.

Ministry of Human Resource Development (MOHRD) 1998. *National Policy on Education 1986 (as modified in 1992) with National Policy on Education, 1968*. New Delhi: MOHRD, Government of India.

———. 2011. *The Right of Children to Free and Compulsory Education Act, 2009. The Gazette of India: Extraordinary, published on March 24, 2011*. New Delhi: Government of India.

Ministry of Law and Justice. 2007a. *The Prohibition of Child Marriage Act, 2006. No. 6 of 2007 Gazette of India*. New Delhi: Ministry of Law and Justice, Government of India. Available at http://www.wcd.nic.in/cma2006.pdf (Accessed 1 June 2011).

———. 2007b. *Protection of Women from Domestic Violence Act, 2005(43 of 2005). The Gazette of India: Extraordinary, Part II Section1*. New Delhi: Government of India.

Ministry of Labour. 2009. *National Policy on Skill Development*. New Delhi: Ministry of Labour, Government of India. Available at http://www.labour.nic.in/policy/NationalSkillDevelopmentPolicyMar09.pdf (Accessed 4 July 2001).

Ministry of Women and Child Development (MOWCD). 2001. *National Policy for Empowerment of Women*. New Delhi: MOWCD, Government of India.

———. 2005. *National Plan of Action for Children 2005*. New Delhi: MOWCD, Government of India.

———. 2006. *The Immoral Traffic (Prevention) Amendment Bill, 2006, Bill No. 47 of 2006*. New Delhi: Government of India.

Ministry of Youth Affairs and Sports (MOYAS). 2003. *National Youth Policy 2003*. New Delhi: MOYAS, Government of India. Available at: http://www.youth-policy.com/Policies/IndiaNATIONALYOUTHPOLICY2003.pdf (Accessed 6 June 2011).

———. 2012. *Exposure Draft National Youth Policy 2012 (NYP 2012)*. New Delhi: MOYAS, Government of India.

National AIDS Control Organisation (NACO). 2002. *National AIDS Prevention and Control Policy*. New Delhi: NACO.

———. 2006. *HIV/AIDS Epidemiological Surveillance and Estimation Report for the Year 2005*. New Delhi: MOHFW, Government of India.

———. 2010. *National AIDS Control Programme, Response to the HIV Epidemic in India*. New Delhi: NACO.

Office of the Registrar General and Census Commissioner India, 2011. *Special Bulletin on Maternal Mortality in India 2007–09, Sample Registration System*. New Delhi: Office of the Registrar General.

——— 2013. *Census of India 2011: Primary Census Abstract: Data Highlights, India, Series 1*. New Delhi: Office of the Registrar General.

Planning Commission. 2008a. *Eleventh Five Year Plan 2007–2012: Inclusive Growth. Vol. 1*. New Delhi: Government of India.

———. 2008b. *Eleventh Five Year Plan 2007–2012, Volume II, Social Sector*. New Delhi: Government of India.

———. 2011. *Report of the Working Group on National Rural Health Mission (NRHM) for the 12th Five Year Plan*. New Delhi: Planning Commission.

Press Information Bureau. 2010. *Protection of Women against Sexual Harassment at Workplace Bill, 2010*. New Delhi: Press Information Bureau, Government of India. Available at http://pib.nic.in/newsite/erelease.aspx?relid=66781 [Accessed 25 March 2012].

———. 2012. *The Protection of Children from Sexual Offences Act, 2012*. New Delhi: Press Information Bureau, Government of India. Available at http://pib.nic.in/newsite/erelease.aspx?relid=84409 [Accessed 25 March 2012].

Rajya Sabha. 2010. *Thirty Sixth Report on The Constitution (One Hundred and Eighth Amendment Bill, 2008)*. New Delhi: Rajya Sabha Secretariat, Parliament of India.

Registrar General of India. 2006. *Maternal Mortality in India: 1997–2003 Trends, Causes and Risk Factors*. New Delhi: Office of Registrar General.

———. 2011. *Sample Registration System Bulletin, Volume 45 No. 1*. New Delhi: Office of the Registrar General.

———. 2012. *Sample Registration System Statistical Report 2010, Report No. 2 of 2012*. New Delhi: Office of the Registrar General.

United Nations Population Fund, India (UNFPA). 2010. *Trends in Sex Ratio at Birth and Estimates of Girls Missing at Birth in India*. UNFPA: New Delhi.

United Nations Children Fund (UNICEF). 2010. *Coverage Evaluation Survey 2009*. New Delhi: UNICEF.

United Nations Development Programme (UNDP). 2012. *Human Development Report 2011, Sustainability and Equity: A Better Future for All*. New York: UNDP.

2

The Population and Development Scenario in India

P.M. Kulkarni

The twentieth century has witnessed remarkable changes in India's demographic situation. First, the population more than quadrupled through the century, from about 238 million at the beginning of the century to over one billion at the end of it; in contrast, the population size had remained nearly stagnant for many centuries in the past and barely doubled in the nineteenth century. The rapid growth resulted from a steep fall in mortality, especially through the middle of the twentieth century, which was not matched by fertility decline for some time. The rate of growth of population was low initially, but accelerated after the 1950s, rising to two per cent per annum. India's rapid population growth became a matter of national and international concern and fears of population explosion were loudly voiced. A decline in the pace of population growth—small but clear—was not seen until just before the turn of the twenty-first century. By 2001, India had reached a stage of moderately low mortality; while still higher than levels reached in the developed world, mortality levels were much lower than those experienced in the early 1900s. At the same time, moderately low fertility was also observed, with some parts of the country reaching replacement levels. As of 2011, at the national level, the most recent census of 2011 has confirmed that while population continues to grow, the rate of growth has declined substantially. Alarmist voices are now muted and the attainment of a zero growth stage during this century is taken for granted, although its timing cannot be predicted. It is clear that India has been passing through a classical demographic transition, a process experienced by many populations of the world in different times and at varying paces.

Side by side with these changes in population growth rates, there have been changes in the Indian society and in its economy. The close linkage between population and development is well recognized in debates on development. In one direction, population size, growth, and structure impact socioeconomic development. In the opposite direction, socioeconomic development influences the processes of fertility, mortality, migration, and urbanization. Thus, any discussion on population cannot be restricted to purely demographic factors but must take into account socioeconomic changes as well.

This chapter first examines population size, growth, and age-sex structure followed by fertility, mortality, age at marriage, contraceptive practice, migration, and urbanization. In most cases, recent trends are presented and discussed. For some factors, changes over a longer period are also noted. This is followed by a brief review of India's socioeconomic development. Given India's diversity, the timing and pace of its demographic transition have varied spatially, and demographic behaviour and conditions have also differed by socioeconomic indicators. Hence, spatial and socioeconomic differentials in key demographic indicators are also discussed. Finally, issues emerging in the context of the changing population situation are noted.

Population Growth

India has long had a tradition of decennial population censuses and this enables us to examine population trends quite clearly. The latest census revealed that India's population was 1,211 million

(1,210,569,573) on March 1, 2011 (Office of the Registrar General and Census Commissioner, India 2013). It also showed a notable drop in the rate of growth. India's population had increased from 238 million in 1,901 to 1,029 million by 2001, most of the growth having taken place in the second half of the century (Table 2.1). The pace was slow up to 1921, with some decline during the 1911–21 decade on account of a major influenza epidemic; it picked up after 1921 and was accelerated after 1951, with the decadal increase rising to 20 per cent in the first decade after independence. Indeed, in the period 1961–91, the growth rate exceeded two per cent per annum. Some slowing down in the pace of increase was noticed after the 2001 census, with the annual rate falling marginally below the two per cent mark. The latest census has shown a clear fall, to a decadal growth of 17.7 per cent and an annual growth rate of 1.63 per cent (Figure 2.1). In fact, not just that the growth rate has slowed down but the absolute increase of the population has also shown some decline though very marginal, from 182.3 million during 1991–2001 to 181.8 million during 2001–11. What is clear is that India's trajectory of growth has turned downward, although the population trajectory, that is, the size of the population, continues to grow.

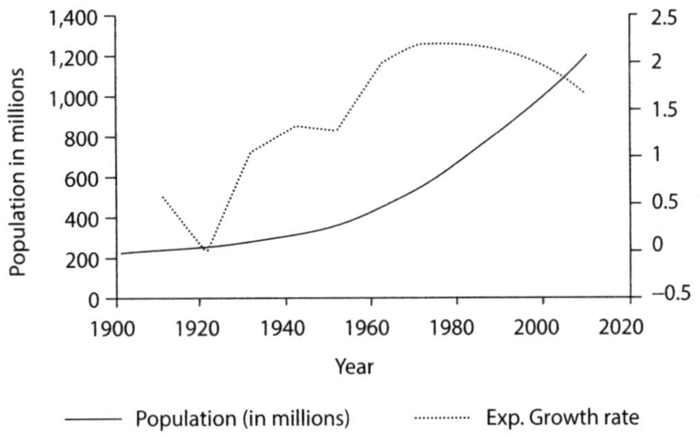

Figure 2.1 Trends in Population Size (in Thousands) and Annual Exponential Growth Rate (in Per cent), India, 1901–2011

Note: The scale for population is shown on the left and for growth rate on the right.

Source: Registrar General (2006b); Office of the Registrar General and Census Commissioner, India (2013).

Table 2.1 Population Trends in India, 1901–2011

Year	Population (in thousands)	Inter-censal increase			Density (Persons per sq. km.)
		Number of persons (in thousands)	Per cent	Annual exponential growth rate (per cent)	
1901	238,396				75
1911	252,093	13,697	5.75	0.56	80
1921	251,321	–772	–0.31	–0.03	79
1931	278,977	27,656	11.00	1.04	88
1941	318,661	39,683	14.22	1.33	101
1951	361,088	42,428	13.31	1.25	114
1961	439,235	78,147	21.64	1.96	139
1971	548,160	108,925	24.80	2.20	173
1981	683,329	135,169	24.66	2.22	216
1991	846,421	163,092	23.87	2.14	267
2001	1,028,737	182,316	21.54	1.95	325
2011	1,210,570	181,832	17.68	1.63	382

Source: Registrar General (2006b); Office of the Registrar General and Census Commissioner, India (2013).

As will be seen in later sections, the acceleration of the growth rate during the middle to late twentieth century was on account of mortality declines, whereas the recent slowing down has resulted from a substantial fall in fertility. The population is yet to reach replacement level, and, in addition, there is the momentum effect, namely, the continued growth of a population for some time after reaching replacement level. As a result of these forces, population growth continues to take place, albeit at a slower pace.

India has 29 states and six union territories (UTs). Uttar Pradesh in the largest state in population size, with the 2011 population just under 200 million (199,812,341), followed by Maharashtra and Bihar, with populations exceeding 100 million (Table A2.1). The UT of Lakshadweep is the smallest, with a population below 100,000 (64,473); the UTs of Daman and Diu, Dadra and Nagar Haveli, Puducherry, and the state of Sikkim have populations below one million. Over the twentieth century, growth occurred in all parts of the country, that is, all the states and UTs showed large increases. However, this growth has not been uniform. Delhi and Chandigarh, essentially city states, have, as expected, experienced larger rates of population increase than others. On the other hand, Goa, Himachal Pradesh, Punjab, and Tamil Nadu have grown at a relatively slower pace. Moreover, the timing of growth patterns has also varied. Kerala led in experiencing both rapid growth and a slowing down of the pace of growth. The latest decade, 2001–11, exhibits vast differences in the rate of growth; among large states, it has varied between a mere 0.48 per cent in Kerala to 2.27 per cent in Bihar (Table A2.1). Growth rates in some smaller states and UTs were either very high (over 4 per cent in Dadra and Nagar Haveli, Daman and Diu) or very low (negative in Nagaland, and below 1 per cent in Lakshadweep, Andaman and Nicobar Islands and Goa). A consequence of the inter-state variation in growth rates is that the share of states in India's population has changed. While for many states, the change is not much, Uttar Pradesh and Tamil Nadu have lost 2–3 percentage points and Assam, Gujarat, and Maharashtra have gained more than one point.

An obvious consequence of population growth is a corresponding rise in population density. The population density rose from just 75 persons per sq. km. in 1901 to 382 persons per sq. km. in 2011. There are large variations in density across the country (Table A2.1). Density is very high, over 2000, in Delhi, Chandigarh, Puducherry, Daman and Diu, and Lakshadweep. It is also high, over 1000, in the large states of Bihar and West Bengal, with Kerala and Uttar Pradesh not far behind. At the other end, Arunachal Pradesh, Andaman and Nicobar Islands, Mizoram, and Sikkim have densities below 100.

What are India's population prospects in the near future? A technical group, constituted by the National Commission on Population, has provided projections for India, its large states and groups of small states up to the year 2026 (Registrar General 2006a); these are commonly called as Registrar General of India (RGI) projections and have the status of 'official' projections. These projections assume that the total fertility rate (TFR) will fall to 2.1 by 2021 and the life expectancies for males and females rise to 69.8 and 72.3 respectively by 2021–25. Besides, the United Nations Population Division routinely makes projections for all countries including India, and these are updated regularly; the 2010 revision provides projections up to the year 2100 (United Nations 2011). The UN gives alternate projections and the 'Medium' variant used here assumes that the TFR will fall to 2.1 by 2020–25 and further to 1.85 by 2045–50. The Population Foundation of India (PFI), in collaboration with the Population Reference Bureau (PRB), has also made projections for India and its states, up to 2101 (Population Foundation of India and Population Reference Bureau 2007). Of the two scenarios presented, 'Scenario B' assumes that the TFR will fall to 2.1 by 2041–46 and to 1.9 by 2061–70 (Scenario A assumes a slower fall in fertility, to 2.1 by 2061–66, and is not used here). In addition, individual demographers have made projections of India's population. For example, Dyson (2004) has made projections for large states up to 2026 and at the all-India level up to 2051. In the 'Standard' run (falling between the 'High' and Low' ones), these projections assume that the TFR will reach 2.1 by 2016–21, and, ultimately, 1.8 by 2031–36 (in the 'High' version TFR falls slowly, to 2.1 by 2026–31 and in the 'Low' version, rapidly to 2.0 by 2016–21 and further to 1.5 by 2031–36). Of these projections, the PFI/PRB has assumed the slowest fertility decline.

Summary results of these projections are shown in Figure 2.2 and Table A2.2. For 2011, all the projections are close to the provisional totals; this is to be expected, since projections typically do well for a short projection period of 10 years. In the long run, the PFI/PRB projections show higher values than others because of its assumption of a slower fertility transition than others, as noted above. All the projections show a slowing down of population growth over time. However, though fertility is assumed to reach the replacement level and fall somewhat after that in all the projections, zero growth is not seen at least up to the middle of the century. This continued growth clearly reflects the effect of population momentum, The UN projections, which are for a longer period, indicate zero growth (and subsequent small declines) after 2070 with the population reaching a level of just below 1.8 billion; the PFI/PRB projections show a decline after 2080 and a peak of just below 1.9 billion.

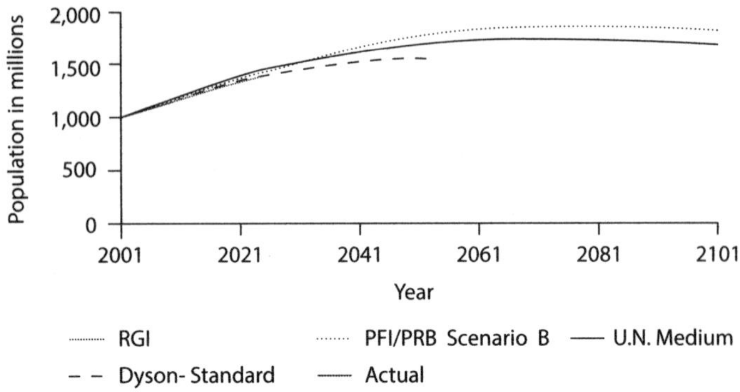

Figure 2.2 Alternate Population Projections, India, up to 2101 (population in millions)

Sources: Registrar General (2006a); Office of the Registrar General and Census Commissioner, India (2013); Population Foundation of India and Population Reference Bureau (2007); Dyson (2004); United Nations (2011).

Age Structure

The age structure of a population is the result of demographic processes and in a way tells us much about the recent demographic history of the population. Changes that occur in the course of the demographic transition from a regime of high fertility-mortality to one of low fertility-mortality, are typically accompanied by changes in the age structure of populations. Such changes are clearly evident in India's age distribution over the last few years. The population pyramid was wide at the bottom, narrowing steeply over age some time ago; this pattern is characteristic of a population with high fertility, moderate mortality, and high growth. But by 2001 (as a result of recent declines in fertility), there was a clear shrinking at young ages with the population bulge moving upwards (Figure 2.3); detailed data from the 2011 census would almost certainly show a continuing of the trend. The most conspicuous changes are seen in the shares of the youngest age groups, 0–4 and 5–9. The Indian census has been providing, over several censuses, the share of the population aged 0–6 (that is, below seven years); there has been a steady fall in the share of this age group in recent years, of about two percentage points per decade. The results of the 2011 census reveal that the share of this

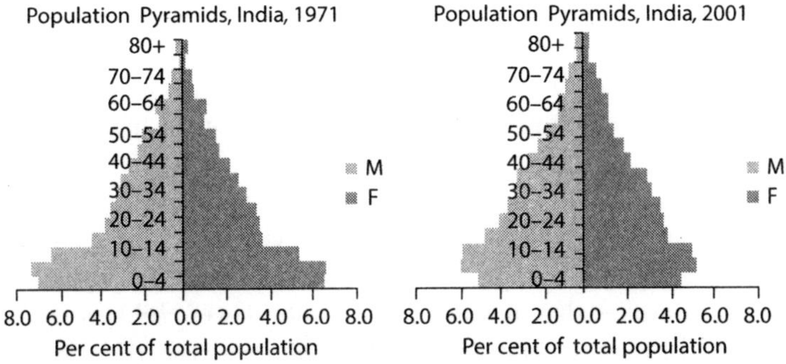

Figure 2.3 Population Pyramids, India, 1971 and 2001
Source: Based on age distributions in Registrar General (2004a).

age group fell from 15.9 per cent in 2001 to 13.6 per cent by 2011, reflecting the rapid decline in fertility that has occurred in recent years and is described in a subsequent section.

In broad terms, the population has begun to age. Corresponding to the fall in the share of the child population has been a rise in the share of adults (Table 2.2); most of the latter has accrued to the working ages. The share of the broad age group 15–59, generally labelled as working ages, has gained by over five points between 1971 and 2001, from 52.0 per cent to 57.1 per cent (for the 15–64 age group,

Table 2.2 Changes in Percentage Shares of Various Broad Age Groups and Dependency Ratios, India, 1971–2001

Age Group	1971	2001
0–14 years	42.0	35.4
15–59 years	52.0	57.1
60 years and above	6.0	7.5
Total	100.0	100.0
Dependency Ratio (per cent)		
Overall	92.3	75.2
Young age	80.8	62.1
Old age	11.5	13.1

Source: Computed from Registrar General (2004a).

the increase was from 54.6 per cent to 59.8 per cent). The older ages (60 and above) have also gained but only marginally, from 6.0 to 7.5 per cent (and from 3.3 to 4.8 per cent for those aged 65 and above). Clearly, ageing has begun to occur in India, but at the moment, only just so.

A consequence of the change in the age distribution is that the dependency ratio has fallen, from 92 per cent to 75 per cent. The decline is largely the result of a fall in the young age dependency ratio and implies that as couples are having fewer children than in the past, the requirement of supporting children has correspondingly declined.

The age structure varies across states. Focusing on the 0–6 age group data for which are available from the latest census of 2011, one can see a wide range, from 9.9 per cent in Goa to 19.2 per cent in Meghalaya (Table A2.3). All the states in the southern region and many in the western and eastern regions show small percentages in this young age group, clearly exhibiting low fertility in these states. On the other hand, the share is large in the north-central states known to have relatively high fertility. Notwithstanding these differences however, we note that, with the sole exception of Jammu and Kashmir, all states have shown a fall in the share of the population aged 0–6 between 2001 and 2011, again indicating fertility decline.

The age distribution implied by the UN Medium projections shows a drastic change in the shape of the age pyramid, with a bulge in the middle ages, shrinking of the young ages and a notable share of the elderly population aged 60+ (Figure 2.4). Clearly, by the middle of the century, India's population will be ageing. Of the broad age groups, the share of the population in young ages, 0–14 years, will fall to nearly half the level it was in 2001, and that of the old age group 60 years (or 65 years) and above will more than double. The share of the working ages will rise for some time, reaching a peak of 65 or 70 per cent for the age group 15–59 and 15–64, respectively, before beginning to decline. This bulge in the population of working ages yields the demographic dividend. India will thus enjoy a huge demographic dividend, a situation in which the working age population is well over 60 per cent and the dependency ratio is low. This demographic dividend or window of demographic opportunity will be experienced in India through the first half of the twenty-first century.

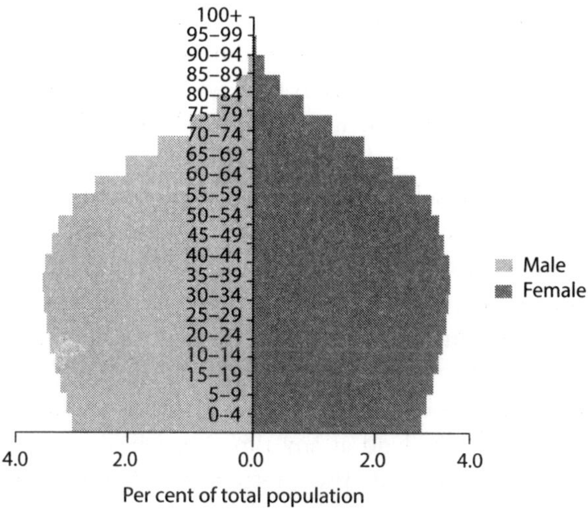

Figure 2.4 Population Pyramid: U.N. Projections, Medium Variant, India, 2050

Source: Based on age distributions in United Nations (2011a).

As noted earlier, regions of India are at different stages of demographic transition. As a result, the growth trajectories of these regions also differ. Growth in states that have already achieved replacement level fertility will result only from population momentum. Thus, as the PFI/PRB projections (these are long-term and available for all states) reveal, Kerala and Tamil Nadu will not grow much (Population Foundation of India and Population Reference Bureau 2007), barring a large rise in net in-migration. On the other hand, the populations of Bihar, Rajasthan, and Uttar Pradesh are likely to double during the first half of the century. These states and many others, such as Chhattisgarh, Jharkhand, Madhya Pradesh and some small states will grow in the near future because fertility has not yet reached replacement level, and later due to momentum. In-migration will also contribute to significant population growth in Delhi and Maharashtra. Of course, trends in net migration are quite unpredictable and could change, as happened between 1991–2001 and 2001–11.

A consequence of the staggered fertility transition suggested above is that the demographic dividend experienced in the country will also be staggered. In other words, the window of demographic opportunity will remain open in different regions during different time periods. Therefore, nationally, at any given time, some regions will be at the peak of their demographic dividend, while others will have just begun to experience a demographic dividend. For example, Kerala and Tamil Nadu have already gained their dividend but by the time other states—the north-central states for example—reap their demographic dividend, the window of opportunity will have closed in Kerala and Tamil Nadu and population ageing will have been experienced. Thus, although at individual state-level, the share of the population aged 15–64 will be high at some time, the share at national level will not be very high at any given time (Kulkarni 2010). As a result, India will not achieve a high dividend at any time but will derive a moderate dividend over a long period. This contrasts with China, which is currently reaping a huge dividend, but whose window of opportunity is much shorter than that of India.

As in the case of the demographic dividend, the share of the population in the elderly ages will also rise in some states earlier than in others. At present, less than 10 per cent of the population of most states is over 60 years of age. However, some states, notably Kerala and Tamil Nadu, have begun to show a rise in the share of the elderly population; other states will follow gradually. By the middle of the century, all states will have large populations in the older ages.

Changes in the Sex Ratio of the Population

In contrast to the global situation, India's population, like that of other south Asian countries and China, has long contained more men than women. The sex ratio of India's population actually worsened through the twentieth century, reaching a low of 930 females per thousand males (or 107.5 males per 100 females, following the international convention of defining sex ratio) in 1971 and 927 (107.9 males/100 females) in 1991 (Table 2.3). Some improvement was seen in 2001, and the 2011 census shows a further increase in the sex ratio, to 943 (106.1 males/100 females). This sex ratio is, however, still more masculine than observed globally.

While the overall sex ratio of the population has improved, that is, the female deficit has declined; the last three censuses have revealed that

Table 2.3 Trends in Population Sex Ratio, India, 1901–2011

Year	Females per 1,000 males		Males per 100 females	
	All ages	Ages 0–6	All ages	Ages 0–6
1901	972		102.9	
...				
1951	946		105.7	
1961	941		106.3	
1971	930	964	107.5	103.7
1981	934	962	107.1	104.0
1991	927	945	107.9	105.8
2001	933	927	107.2	107.9
2011	943	919	106.1	108.9

Source: Office of the Registrar General and Census Commissioner, India (2011a, 2013).

the sex ratio in the young ages has actually become more unbalanced (Figure 2.5). For the 0–6 year age group, for example, the ratio has fallen from 962 girls per 1,000 boys in 1981 to 945, 927, and 919 in the three successive censuses of 1991, 2001, and 2011, respectively. The worsening of the sex ratio in this age group is largely attributed to the growing imbalance in the Sex Ratio at Birth (SRB), for which there is independent evidence from the Sample Registration System (SRS); the child sex ratio is also affected by female disadvantage in child mortality, but the degree of disadvantage is too small to explain the observed imbalance. By using male and female child survival probabilities obtained from life tables constructed from SRS data on age-specific death rates for the period 2004 –10, and applying the procedure of reverse survival, the sex ratio of 919 at ages 0–6 yields an SRB of 923 for the cohort born during the seven-year period before the 2011 census. Assuming an SRB of 952 (equivalent to 105 male births per 100 female births) under normal conditions, of the gap of 33 points (952 –919), only 4 points (923–919) are attributable to sex differentials in child mortality, and 29 points (952–923) are attributable to deviations in the SRB from normal.

The SRB in India was somewhat unfavourable to females even in the past (Visaria 1968). While for most populations, the SRB

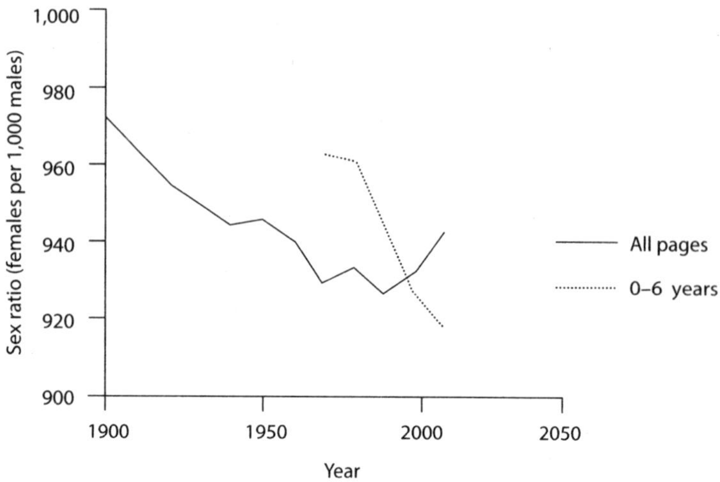

Figure 2.5 Trends in Sex Ratio, India, 1901–2011
Source: Office of the Registrar General and Census Commissioner, India (2011a, 2013).

is close to 105 males per 100 females, and generally in the range 103–107, most estimates show that in India it has been well over 106 males per 100 females (or lower than 943 females per 1,000 males). However, recent evidence from the SRS shows that the SRB has become even more adverse to females over time (Figure 2.6). Since the 1990s, it has been generally below 910 girls per 1,000. Largely the result of this adverse SRB, the observed sex ratio of the population aged 0–6 was 927 in 2001 and has fallen even further, to 919, in 2011. This adverse sex ratio of the population aged 0–6 has drawn attention to its principal cause, namely, sex-selective abortions. The practice of pre-natal sex detection via sonographic scans and subsequent sex selective abortion (of female foetuses) is prevalent in many parts of the country. Though legal steps have been taken, via the Pre-Conception and Pre-Natal Diagnostic Techniques (PCPNDT) Act, to ban this practice, sex selective abortions continue to take place as the evidence so clearly demonstrates.

The rise in the overall sex ratio but fall in the child sex ratio may appear paradoxical. For long, the relatively higher mortality

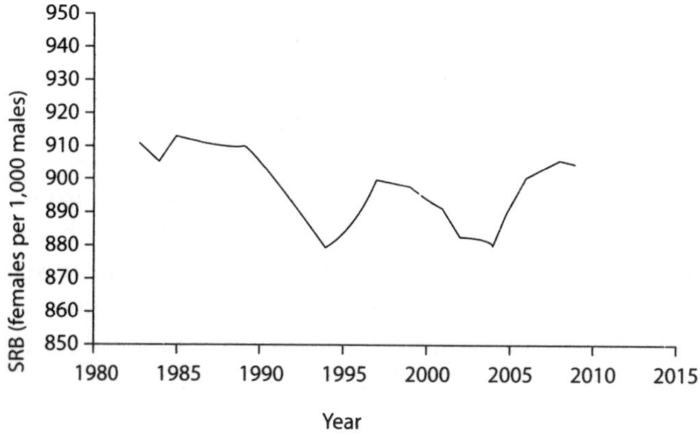

Figure 2.6 Trends in SRB, India, SRS, 1982–2010
Source: Registrar General (2001, 2002, 2003, 2004b, 2004c, 2005b, 2006c, 2006d, 2007, 2008b, 2009, 2010, 2011b, 2012a).

of women was the major factor responsible for the masculinity in India's sex composition. The recent rise in the population sex ratio could be attributed, at least partly, to the fact that female mortality is now lower than mortality overall (evidence on this is presented later in this chapter). Besides, special efforts have been made in recent censuses to ensure that women are not missed and this would have reduced the under-enumeration of females. Further, the age distribution has changed. As population ages, and the share of the older age groups rises, the overall sex ratio is influenced more by the sex ratio at older than younger ages. Since the sex ratio at older ages is higher than that at younger ages (in 2001, the sex ratio for ages below 10 was 928 whereas for ages above 60 it was 1029), it has influenced the population sex ratio positively. Thus, even with worsening of the child sex ratio, the population sex ratio has improved. A detailed analysis of census age–sex distributions can provide clearer answers.

For the population as a whole, sex selective migration has been a major factor influencing the sex ratio. In fact, the migrant receiving regions such as urban areas show greater masculinity because more males than females migrate for employment. On the other hand, for the child population, especially the population below seven years of age, migration is unlikely to be sex selective and imbalances clearly result from those in the SRB and possibly in child survival. Data show that the imbalance in the 0–6 age group is much larger for some states than others (Table A2.4). Among large states, Haryana, Punjab, Jammu & Kashmir, Delhi, Rajasthan, Gujarat, and Maharashtra, have particularly poor sex ratios that fall below 900 girls per 1,000 boys. The regional pattern is quite evident; states in the western and northern regions have very low sex ratios, whereas those in the eastern and southern regions, by and large, seem to have ratios in the range 930–970, close to what is observed in most populations globally.

The 2011 census shows that the sex ratio for the population aged 0–6 has fallen in many states, pointing out to a widening imbalance (Table A2.4). Jammu & Kashmir, Rajasthan, and Maharashtra are notable in this regard. On the other hand, Punjab has shown a marked rise in the sex ratio of its population aged 0–6, from 798 per 1,000 in 2001 to 846 in 2011. Even so, its sex ratio is much lower than normal and among the lowest in the country; its child sex ratio may best be described as revealing a change from 'extremely bad' to 'very bad'.

There is close, though not perfect, correspondence between the observed sex ratio in the population aged 0–6 years and the SRB over the last seven years in large states (Table A2.4; note that data on SRB are available only for large states and as three-year averages). Sex selection at birth has quite clearly been the leading factor underlying the imbalance in the sex ratio of the child population.

From the sex ratio of the population aged 0–6 years, as revealed by the 2011 census, it is possible to obtain a rough idea of the number of sex-selective abortions that are likely to have taken place during the period preceding the census. Computations based on the observed sex ratio and SRS estimates of fertility and sex-specific child survival, and on the assumption of a normal SRB of 952, show that in India, about 2.5 million sex-selective abortions took place during the seven-year period 2004 –10, that is, an average of about 375 thousand annually. The intensity of sex selection (as measured by the per cent of sex selective abortions to births) is the highest in Punjab and Haryana, but the volume of sex selective abortions is the highest in Uttar Pradesh (nearly 95 thousand per year), followed by Maharashtra (about 60 thousand per year) and Rajasthan (about 50 thousand per year).

Trends and differentials in fertility

Fertility, along with mortality and migration, account for population change, and levels and trends in these determine trends in population size and structure. Since the civil registration system has not effectively recorded all births in India, the estimates of birth rate (as also of death rate) for the past are indirect, obtained from censuses by census actuaries or demographers, and thus refer to inter-census periods. However, since the 1970s, the SRS has been providing annual estimates of indicators of fertility and mortality, both at the national and the state levels. Besides, a number of household surveys have also been undertaken and these give a good idea of the levels and pattern of, and differentials in fertility; the three rounds of the National Family Health Survey (NFHS) are most prominent in this regard, as these were nationwide surveys covering all states and following a common methodology.

As in all populations, fertility was high in India in the past, with the Crude Birth Rate (CBR) in the upper 40s (per thousand population) during the early part of the twentieth century (Table 2.4), and mostly unregulated, except that fertility took place primarily within marriage. Some decline was noticed in the 1940s, followed by a plateau through the 1960s, with the birth rate hovering around the 40 point mark (Figure 2.7). However, since the 1970s, a steady fall has been observed (note that while the estimates up to 1971 are indirect, based on census data, the post-1970 estimates are from the SRS, as depicted in Figure 2.8). Both the CBR and the TFR show a declining trend, with the CBR reaching 22.1 and the TFR 2.5 by 2010. There was some stalling of fertility, through the late 1970s to the mid-1980s, but since then the decline has been fairly smooth.

During the process, the age pattern of fertility has undergone a change. Age-specific Fertility Rates (ASFRs) in the age range 25–39 have fallen much more steeply than have those in other age groups, though a decline is seen at all the ages (Figure 2.9

Table 2.4 Trends in Crude Birth and Death Rates, India, 1901–2010

Period	CBR	CDR
	Census based estimates	
1901–10	49.2	42.6
1911–20	48.1	48.6
1921–30	46.4	36.3
1931–40	45.2	31.2
1941–50	39.9	27.4
1951–60	41.7	22.8
1961–70	41.1	19.0
	SRS based estimates	
1971–75	35.6	15.5
1976–80	33.4	13.8
1981–85	33.6	12.1
1986–90	31.4	10.6
1991–95	28.9	9.5
1996–2000	26.6	8.8
2001–05	24.6	7.9
2006–10	22.8	7.3

CBR: Crude Birth Rate, per 1,000 population; CDR: Crude Death Rate, per 1,000 population

Sources: Rele (1982) and Jain (1982) (for the years 1901–70); 1971 onwards averages obtained from SRS series. Registrar General (2009, 2010, 2011b, 2012a).

and Table A2.5). Fertility is now much more concentrated in the prime ages, 20–29 years, than in the past. In fact, childbearing at ages over 35 is not common in recent periods, a consequence of the practice of sterilization as a means of limiting family size. The latest SRS figures show that 72 per cent of births were of first- or second-order in 2010 in contrast to 57 per cent in 1991 (Registrar General 2010; 2012a). Fertility has also declined in the adolescent age group (15–19), though marital fertility in this group has hardly changed (Registrar General 2010). Clearly, a rise in age at marriage has made an impact on fertility in the young ages, although fertility regulation within marriage does not seem to be very common at these ages.

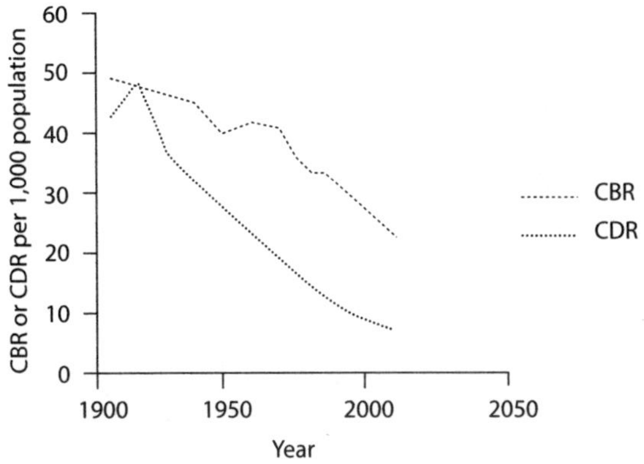

Figure 2.7 Trends in CBR and CDR, India, 1901–2010
Source: Jain (1982); Rele (1982); Registrar General (2009, 2010, 2011b, 2012a).

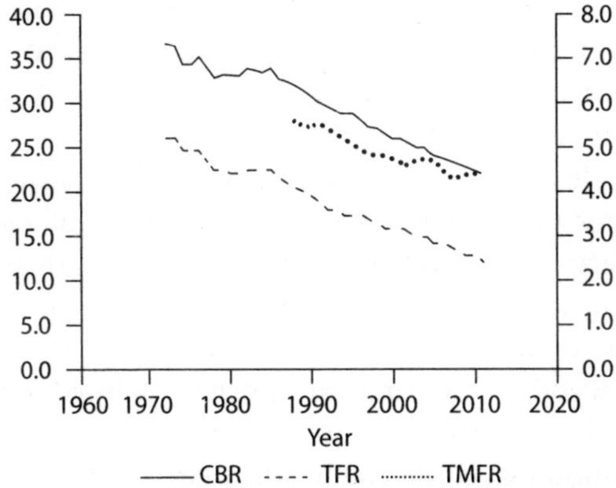

Figure 2.8 Trends in CBR, TFR, and TMFR, India, 1971–2010
Note: The scale for CBR is shown on the left and for TFR and TMFR on the right.
Source: Registrar General (2009, 2010, 2011c, 2012a).

It is well recognized that fertility levels differ by the socioeconomic background of women. The three rounds of the NFHS allow us to assess not only the differentials at a point in time, but changes in these as well, since the surveys are spread over the period 1992–93 to 2005–06, a period in which large fertility declines took place (Table 2.5). Fertility is lower in urban areas than rural, among the

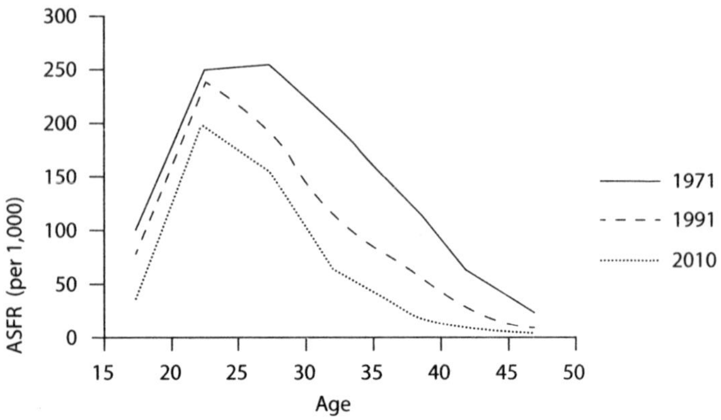

Figure 2.9 Changes in the Age Pattern of Fertility, India, 1971–2010
Source: Registrar General (2009, 2012a).

more than the less educated, among the rich and middle classes than the poor. Differentials by caste exist but are not very wide. Religion-wise differentials show that Sikhs and Christians have lower fertility than Hindus, whereas fertility among Muslims is higher than that among Hindus. Observed differentials are, of course, gross, not controlled for other factors. Obviously the effect of various socio-economic factors on fertility may be confounded by their association with other factors, and hence, ideally, net effects that eliminate the effect of confounding are needed. Many analysts have carried out such analyses and, by and large, the differentials by education persist, as do some by religion, but rural-urban, income/wealth and caste differences diminish considerably when effects of other factors are controlled.

The trends over the three rounds of the NFHS clearly reveal that India's fertility decline has been quite pervasive: decline has occurred among all sections of society, the poor and the rich, the illiterate and the educated, residents of villages and towns or cities, and in various caste and religion groups. The trends also suggest a narrowing of socioeconomic gaps in fertility, implying that the fertility transition has been occurring in all sections; some groups are, however, ahead of others and have lower fertility than average.

Fertility has declined throughout India, but the degree and timing of decline have varied. States like Tamil Nadu, Kerala, and Goa

Table 2.5 Socioeconomic Differentials in TFR, India, NFHS-1, 2, 3

Socioeconomic background	NFHS-1	NFHS-2	NFHS-3
All	3.39	2.85	2.68
Place of residence			
Rural	3.67	3.07	2.98
Urban	2.70	2.27	2.06
Education of woman			
Illiterate	4.03	3.47	3.55
<5 years	3.01	2.64	2.45
5–7 years	2.49	2.26	2.51
8–9 years			2.23
10–11 years	2.15	1.99	2.08
12+ years			1.80
Social group			
SC	3.92	3.15	2.92
ST	3.55	3.06	3.12
OBC		2.83	2.75
Other	3.30	2.66	2.35
Religion			
Hindu	3.30	2.78	2.59
Muslim	4.41	3.59	3.40
Christian	2.87	2.44	2.34
Sikh	2.43	2.26	1.95
Standard of living/Wealth class			
Poorest			3.89
Second	$	3.37*	3.17
Middle		2.85	2.58
Fourth		2.10	2.24
Highest			1.78

Note: $: Wealth/standard of living categories were not provided in NFHS-1; *: For NFHS-2, the categories are for Standard of Living: Low, Medium and High

Source: IIPS (1995), IIPS and ORC Macro (2000), IIPS and Macro International (2007).

began to experience fertility decline much earlier than other regions, so that by 1991, the TFRs in Goa, Kerala, and Delhi and in the smaller states/UTs of Puducherry, Mizoram, and Chandigarh, had fallen below 2.1, the well-recognized mark signifying replacement level fertility in a low mortality regime (Table A2.6). Tamil Nadu followed soon thereafter, and by 2010 all the southern states, the large states of Maharashtra, Punjab, Himachal Pradesh, West Bengal, Jammu & Kashmir, and Delhi and most of the small northeastern states and UTs had TFRs below the 2.1 mark. Bihar, Uttar Pradesh, Rajasthan, Madhya Pradesh, Jharkhand, and Meghalaya are the only states with TFRs 3.0 or above. A broad regional pattern is discernible: the southern, western and northern regions have low fertility, and the north-central regions have higher—but moderate—levels of fertility. The current fertility scenario emphasizes that not a single part of the country can be said to have high fertility.

Clearly, fertility transition is well underway throughout India. While fertility differentials across states were evident even in 1971 and are seen even today, there have been substantial declines in fertility in all states. In some north-central states, the TFRs have declined from 6–7 to 3–4, and in many others it has declined from 4–5 to about 2. These trends suggest that all states will reach fertility levels near or below replacement in the coming decades, though the date by which replacement will be reached cannot be predicted.

Decline in fertility has obvious advantages for women's reproductive health. Fewer pregnancies mean fewer episodes of obstetric risk for women, and correspondingly, lower levels of maternal mortality and morbidity, as also maternal depletion. Fewer pregnancies and deliveries may also have a positive impact on investments in women's health care in general and pregnancy related care in particular, both at household and at state levels.

Trends and differentials in mortality

A hundred years ago, a child born in India was expected to live for only about 20 years. Mortality at all ages was high—extremely high during infancy and early childhood but high even in adult ages. Influenza, cholera, tuberculosis, and epidemics of plague killed a large number of people. Frequent famines aggravated the situation. Improvements began to be witnessed after 1920 and the pace increased substantially after independence. Though reliable data on the registration of deaths for the early years are not available (and even now, the registration of deaths is not satisfactory), census actuaries and demographers have estimated CDR indirectly and constructed life tables for inter-census periods on the basis of age distributions; these estimates allow us to examine trends in mortality up to 1970. Since 1971, the SRS has been providing CDRs and Age-specific Death Rates (ASDRs) and has also constructed life tables by sex for India and large states. The under-five mortality rate, commonly used as a measure of early childhood mortality, can also be obtained from these life tables.

Long-term trends in CDR are shown in Table 2.4. The CDR was very high, over 40 per thousand, during the early years of the twentieth century, but fell below 40 in the 1920s, below 30 in the 1940s, and below 20 after 1960. It has been less than 10 since the 1990s. Mortality trends can be assessed more scientifically with the help of the expectation of life at birth, or life expectancy, a more refined measure of overall mortality than the CDR. Life expectancy in India increased from a low of 20 years during 1911–20 (there was a fall from 1901–10 to 1911–20, primarily on account of the widespread influenza epidemic) to over 30 during 1931–40; it crossed 40 years during 1951–60, 50 years in the mid-1970s, and 60 in the early 1990s (Figure 2.10 and Table A2.7). Broadly, there has been a rise of about 10 years in life expectancy every two decades. The most recent

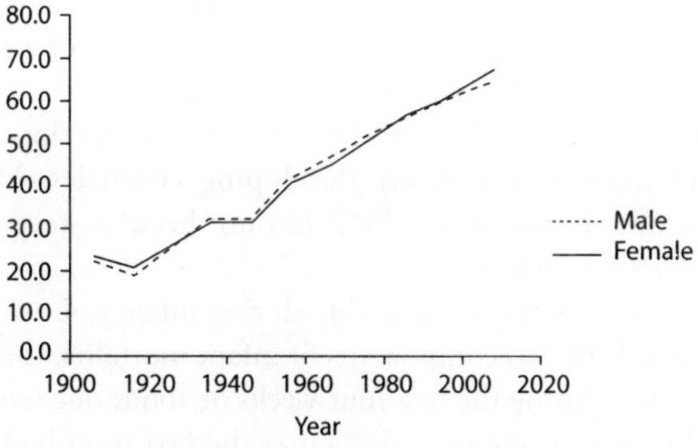

Figure 2.10 Trends in Life Expectancy, India, 1901–2010

Source: Jain (1982) (for the years 1901–1971); Registrar General, 2010 (for the years 1971–1995); and Registrar General, 2012b (for 1996 onwards).

data show a life expectancy of 66.1 years (64.6 for males and 67.7 for females) during 2006–10 (Registrar General 2012b).

On average, globally, women live longer than men by quite a margin (the reason why population sex ratios favour females). But during most of the twentieth century, female life expectancy in India was actually lower than male expectancy. This differential was reversed after 1980 with female expectancy exceeding male, although only barely so. While the gap has since widened, it is still not of the order observed in other countries with a similar level of life expectancy. Thus, although Indian women have gained more than men in terms of life expectancy over the past 30 years, and are no longer more disadvantaged than men in survival, they do not enjoy the same advantage as women in other countries do.

The age pattern of death rates in India broadly follows the standard, with high mortality during early childhood, low during late child and young adult ages, and rising with age after middle ages. Declines in mortality have occurred at all ages, but much more in the early childhood ages and relatively less in old ages.

The IMR was well over 100 per 1,000 live births through the 1970s (estimates of the IMR for periods in the past, coming mainly from civil registration, are obvious underestimates and hence not used here to assess trends) implying that over ten per cent of newborn died during infancy (Table 2.6). By 2010, the IMR had fallen below 50 (Registrar General 2012a). Similarly, the U5MR has declined from over 200 per 1,000 live births (one fifth of newborn dying before completing five years of age) to just below 60 in 2010. Though early childhood mortality has fallen, the level is still quite high, well above that in the developed world, but higher than that in many developing countries. Moreover, after 1991, the decline in the IMR has not been as steep as it was during the 1970s and 80s.

For an understanding of mortality during infancy, it is important to review trends in two components of infant mortality, that is, neonatal mortality (during the first four weeks or about one month after birth) and post-neonatal mortality (after the first month but within the first year). These reveal that the fall in post-neonatal mortality has been greater than that in neonatal mortality (Registrar General 2010). The latter is much more (though not entirely) influenced by

Table 2.6 Trends in Early Childhood Mortality, India, 1970–2010

Period	Infant Mortality Rate (IMR)* *(per 1,000 births)*			Under-five Mortality Rate (U5MR)** *(per 1,000 births)*		
	Male	Female	Combined	Male	Female	Combined
1970–75	130	135	132	196	224	210
1976–80	121	127	124	181	206	193
1981–85	104	104	104	152	169	161
1986–90	87	87	90	126	142	137
1991–95	81	79	80	108	119	113
1996–2000	71	72	71	93	104	98
2001–05	64	67	65	80	88	84
2006–10	52	53	52	64	71	67

Source: * Registrar General (2009, 2010, 2011b, 2012a, 2012b).

endogenous factors, especially conditions originating during pregnancy and at birth, than the former. There has been considerably less success in preventing deaths during the neonatal than during the post-neonatal period of infancy.

While differentials by sex are not seen in the IMR, the U5MR has consistently been higher for girls than for boys (Table 2.6) pointing towards relative neglect of girls. While the female disadvantage is especially evident in the younger ages, some disadvantage can also be observed during ages 15–24 (earlier it was for the range 15–29), likely to be a consequence of maternal mortality which has been quite high in India (this issue is addressed in Chapter 3).

Large socioeconomic differentials in mortality are commonly seen in all populations and India is no exception. Life tables constructed separately for rural and urban populations show that life expectancy for the urban populations is 6–8 years higher than that of rural populations (Registrar General 2010). As life tables are normally not constructed for various socioeconomic groups, we rely on surveys to enable assessments of early childhood mortality for different socioeconomic groups. The three rounds of the NFHS show clearly higher levels of U5MR among the children of uneducated than educated women, poorer than richer, the socially disadvantaged in terms of scheduled castes and tribes than others, and Hindus and Muslims than Sikhs and Christians (Table 2.7). Differentials by education and income/wealth persist when controlling for other factors. At the same time, mortality has declined in all sections. The narrowing of differentials over time, the inter-survey period, is also quite conspicuous.

The level of mortality also varies considerably spatially in India, although, since the 1970s, mortality decline has occurred in all states. Among the large states, Kerala has for long enjoyed higher survival levels than others. In the 1970s, while life expectancy in Kerala was 60 years, many states, especially those in the north-central belt, had life expectancies well below 50 years (Registrar General, 2010). Recent estimates, for the quinquennium 2006–10, show that life expectancy is now well over 70 years in Kerala but near 60 years in Assam, Madhya Pradesh, Odisha, and Uttar Pradesh. Under 5 Mortality Rates (U5MR) also show a similar pattern (Table A2.8). Recent estimates show a low level (below 20 per 1,000) in Kerala, moderate (20–40 per 1,000) in Maharashtra, Tamil Nadu, Delhi, and West Bengal, and high (over 60 per 1,000) in the large states of Uttar Pradesh, Bihar, Rajasthan, Madhya Pradesh, Odisha, and Assam. Although the decline in the U5MR has been very steep in several states that had experienced very high child mortality in the past, and although gaps from better performing states are narrowing, these states have a long way to go in achieving satisfactory U5MR.

Trends in age at marriage

Age at marriage, especially of women, has social, psychological as well as demographic implications. In India, child marriages have been fairly common, and social reformers, concerned about socio-psychological consequences of subjecting a young girl to married life, depriving her of childhood, education, and normal development, campaigned for specifying a minimum age for the marriage of girls, leading to the passing of the Child Marriage Restraint Act (CMRA) as early as in 1929. Currently, the Child Marriage Act (CMA) specifies the minimum ages of marriage as 18 years for women and 21 for men.

Whether due to the Act (CMA) or otherwise, age at marriage has increased in India over the years. The commonly accepted measure, the Singulate Mean Age at Marriage (SMAM), computed from

Table 2.7 Socioeconomic Differentials in U5MR, India, NFHS-1, 2, 3 (probability of dying before completing five years of age × 1,000)

Socioeconomic background	NFHS-1	NFHS-2	NFHS-3
All	118.8	101.4	74.3
Place of residence			
Rural	130.9	111.5	82.0
Urban	78.3	65.4	51.7
Education of woman			
Illiterate	140.5	122.8	94.7
< 5 years	83.9	75.8	78.8
5–7 years	64.8	58.1	60.5
8–9 years			46.9
10–11 years	43.2	37.1	40.0
12+ years			29.7
Social group			
SC	149.1	119.3	88.1
ST	135.2	126.6	95.7
OBC		103.1	72.8
Other	111.5	82.6	59.2
Religion			
Hindu	124.0	107.0	76.0
Muslim	106.3	82.7	70.0
Christian	68.4	68.0	52.8
Sikh	64.8	64.9	52.1
Wealth class/Standard of living			
Poorest			100.5
Second	$	130.0*	89.6
Middle		94.6	71.9
Fourth		51.5	51.2
Highest			33.8

Note: $: Wealth/standard of living categories were not provided in NFHS-1; *: For NFHS-2, the categories are for Standard of Living: Low, Medium and High
Source: IIPS (1995); IIPS and ORC Macro (2000); IIPS and Macro International (2007).

census data, was as low as 13 years for women and 20 for men during 1901–11 (Goyal 1988). After 1931, a clear and steady rise occurred. Figures since 1961 show a large rise especially for females (Table 2.8) with the SMAM for 2001 being 20.2. The increase for males has been modest; the initial level was not very low and increases have been slow.

A consequence of the rise in the age at marriage is that proportion of women single (never married) in the ages 15–19 has increased, from less than one third in 1961 to three fourths in 2001; increases have been observed for the 20–24 age group as well. However, in spite of the impressive rise in age at marriage, the proportion of girls marrying before the specified minimum age is large. Nonetheless, the fall in proportions married at young ages has resulted in perceptible declines in fertility.

Notable differences are seen across states in the age at marriage. The SMAM for females is high in Nagaland, Mizoram and Goa and among large states, in Jammu & Kashmir and Kerala. On the other hand, the mean is very low (below 19 years) in Rajasthan and Bihar even in 2001.

Contraceptive prevalence

In the past, fertility within marriage was unregulated in India. Contraceptive use was minimal, effective contraceptive options were not available, and even the idea of fertility regulation was not

Table 2.8 Trends in SMAM, and Proportion Never Married, India, 1961–2001

Census year	SMAM Female	Per cent of single females		SMAM Male
		Age 15–19	Age 20–24	
1961	15.9	29.2	6.0	21.9
1971	17.2	42.9	9.1	22.6
1981	18.3	55.8	14.0	23.3
1991	19.3	64.7	18.2	23.9
2001	20.2	75.1	23.0	24.8

Sources: Goyal (1988); Registrar General (1998, 2008a).

acceptable to many, notwithstanding the efforts of social reformers who campaigned for contraceptive services. After 1951, fertility regulation was promoted by the government's family planning programme and gradually modern contraceptives became available. But according to estimates provided by the government programme, only about 10 per cent of couples of reproductive ages practised any form of contraception in 1971 (Table 2.9). Thereafter, there was an increase in contraceptive practice, with a jump in 1977 reflecting the sterilization drive during the national emergency, followed by a plateau for some time due to the post-emergency backlash suffered by the programme, and a gradual increase after the mid-1980s. Programme estimates are obtained from data on acceptance and hence suffer from inflated reporting by programme administrators as well as the exclusion of contraceptive adoption from outside of the programme. Fortunately, reliable estimates from surveys are available and can be used to assess trends. The three rounds of the NFHS revealed contraceptive prevalence of 36 per cent (of couples of reproductive age) during 1992–93, rising to 42 per cent by 1998–99 and 48 per cent by 2005–06 (lower panel of Table 2.9). It is well known that contraceptive use in India is dominated by sterilization; vasectomy was the principal method up to 1976 and female sterilization took this role after the post-emergency set-back. Limiting family size through female sterilization is the most common mode of fertility regulation in India. Spacing is less popular, although recent trends do show some increase in the use of non-terminal methods.

We invoke the Bongaarts' proximate determinants model to assess the impact of increases in contraceptive use, in comparison with that of the rise in age at marriage, on fertility. Lactational amenorrhoea and induced abortion, the remaining two proximate determinants of fertility in this model are not assessed, because not much change has been seen in lactational amenorrhoea and reliable data on induced abortion are not available. Hence, the focus here is on the two proximate determinants, proportions married (Cm) and contraceptive use (Cc) in the Bongaarts model. It is seen that between 1971 and 2005, the TFR declined from 5.2 to 2.9 and the total marital fertility rate (TMFR) from 6.5 to 4.4. With the rise in contraceptive prevalence, from a level of merely 10 per cent in the early 1970s to one close to 50 per cent in the recent years, the Cc index fell sharply from 0.89

Table 2.9 Trends in Contraceptive Prevalence Rate in India, 1971–2006

Year	Per cent Couples of Reproductive Age Effectively Protected by			
	Sterilisation	IUD	Other Modern Methods	All Modern Methods
Programme estimates*				
1971	8.0	1.4	1.0	10.4
1991	30.3	6.7	7.2	44.1
NFHS Estimates**				
1992–93 NFHS-1	30.7	1.9	3.6	36.3 *(40.6)$*
1998–99 NFHS-2	36.1	1.6	5.2	42.8 *(48.2)$*
2005–06 NFHS-3	38.3	1.7	8.5	48.5 *(56.3)$*

Note: IUD: Intra-uterine device. $: Including traditional methods. Programme estimates of prevalence rate are based on acceptance obtained from the government programme and reported to the programme.
Sources: * Department of Family Welfare, 1993; ** IIPS, 1995; IIPS and ORC Macro, 2000; IIPS and Macro International, 2007.

to 0.51 (decline of 42 per cent). As noted earlier, there has been some rise in female age at marriage and this too has made an impact; the Cm index also fell from 0.80 to 0.66 (or by 18 per cent) but to a smaller degree than that the Cc index. Clearly in recent years, increased contraceptive practice has made a huge impact on fertility.

Patterns of migration and urbanization

Migration, the third component of population change, results in population redistribution over space or geographic units. While migration is a move from one geographic unit to another, whether within the district, within the state, or to another state, it is inter-state migration that attracts much attention since it leads to inter-state population redistribution. Besides, the relative sizes of streams of migration, rural to urban and urban to rural, have implications for urbanization. In India, information on migration is routinely collected in the census. According to the 2001 census (the 2011 census data on migration are not yet available), 307 million, or about 30 per cent of India's population, lived at a place other than their place of birth (Registrar General 2006e). Migration, measured in this way, was greater among women (217 million or 44 per cent of women) than men (90 million or 17 per cent of men). It is well known that the higher rates of migration observed among women result from the practice of women moving to their husband's place of residence following marriage (the virilocal system) in many parts of India. International migration rates—if not volume—have been negligible in India.

Census tabulations of migrants by place of last residence and duration of residence at the place of enumeration allow for the estimation of inter-censal migration. Of India's enumerated population of 2001, 98 million, or 9.6 per cent had migrated within the 10-year period preceding the census, 65 million of these migrants were women and 33 million were men. Most of this migration—82 per cent—took place within the state itself (Table 2.10). The rural to rural stream was far larger than other streams. The rural to urban stream was three times as large as the urban to rural stream, suggesting an overall net shift from villages to cities and towns, and urbanization. The extent of inter-state migration is small, though for men, about one fourth of the total migration was inter-state (clearly, most marriage related migration was within states).

A majority of women (65 per cent) who migrated moved on account of marriage (Registrar General 2006e). On the other hand, for men, employment was the principal reason for migration 38 per cent moved for this reason. Besides, a large proportions of both male and female (25 and 29 per cent respectively) migrants moved along with families.

Inter-state migration has generally not been large. In some states, however, it has been considerable and thus has become a political issue. For the 1991–2001 decade, Delhi, and a number of small states and UTs had high positive net migration rates (Table A2.9). Among large states, Haryana and Maharashtra showed moderate levels of net in-migration, 3–5 per 1,000 per annum. On the other hand, Uttar Pradesh and Bihar reported moderate net out-migration rates.

Table 2.10 Streams in Inter-censal Migration, India, 1991–2001

Migration stream	Persons	Males	Females
	(As percent of inter-censal migrants)		
Intra state			
Rural to Rural	49.7	30.4	59.5
Rural to Urban	14.5	19.8	11.8
Urban to Rural	5.3	6.3	4.8
Urban to Urban	10.1	13.3	8.4
Unclassified	2.6	3.2	2.2
Total intra-state	82.1	72.9	86.7
Inter-state			
Rural to Rural	4.6	5.3	4.2
Rural to Urban	6.5	11.6	3.9
Urban to Rural	1.1	1.6	0.8
Urban to Urban	4.6	6.7	3.5
Unclassified	0.4	0.7	0.3
Total inter-state	17.1	25.9	12.7
International	0.8	1.1	0.6
Total Migrants	100.0	100.0	100.0
Total inter-censal migrants as per cent of population	9.6	6.2	13.2
Number of inter-censal migrants(in millions)	98.3	32.9	65.4

Source: Computed from Migration Data Highlights, Registrar General (2006e).

While estimates for the 2001–11 decade are not available, indirect estimates, that is, the difference between the inter-censal and natural increase (as computed from average SRS birth and death rates for the inter-censal years) show high net in-migration into some small states and UTs. Among large states, Jammu & Kashmir, Delhi, Tamil Nadu, and Maharashtra experienced moderate net in-migration. On the other hand, Kerala, Uttar Pradesh, and Rajasthan were out-migrating states. We note a caveat here. Estimates for 2001–11 are indirect, based on the assumption that the SRS birth and death rates are fairly accurate. Small errors in birth and death rates can cause large relative errors in the estimates of migration rates; the estimate for Jammu & Kashmir shown in the table appears improbably high. In general, for very small states and UTs, the residual method may not give reliable results since the SRS estimates of birth and death rates for these are based on small samples. Hence, we acknowledge that, migration rates provided here must be interpreted cautiously; reliable estimates of migration will become available once migration tables from the 2011 census are published.

The level of urbanization in India is not high. As of 2011, 31.2 per cent of India's population live in urban areas (Office of the Registrar General and Census Commissioner India 2013), a level much lower than that observed in many developing countries. However, we note that criteria for classifying a place as urban are stringent in India; it must be declared as a town or a city by the government or must satisfy conditions of size, density, and structure of the male workforce. This makes comparisons with other countries difficult. However, trends in urbanization show that the tempo of urbanization has been slow. In 1901 just over 10 per cent of the population lived in urban areas, this rose to 14 per cent by 1941, increased another 17 per cent over the next decade, and after that, except for the decade 1971–81, the increments have been small (Figure 2.11 and Table 2.11). The Urban-Rural Growth Differential (URGD) has been close to or below 2 per cent since 1951. The decade of 2001–2011 shows some increase in the tempo, with urbanization rising from 27.8 per cent to 31.2 per cent, or by 3.4 percentage points, in comparison to an increase between 1991 and 2001 of only 2.1 percentage points. We note, however, that this increase does not necessarily imply that rural to urban migration has increased substantially. The number of census towns (settlements that are not declared as urban by the state but have urban characteristics as specified by the census organization) has nearly tripled, from 1,362 to 3,894 and this has also contributed to the increase in the population classified as urban. The relative contributions of the change in classification of urban areas and the increase in rural-urban migration to the decadal increase in the urban population will become clearer once more detailed census data become available.

Urbanization varies considerably across states. In Delhi and Chandigarh, which are nearly city states, and in Puducherry, Lakshadweep, and Daman and Diu, a majority of the population was

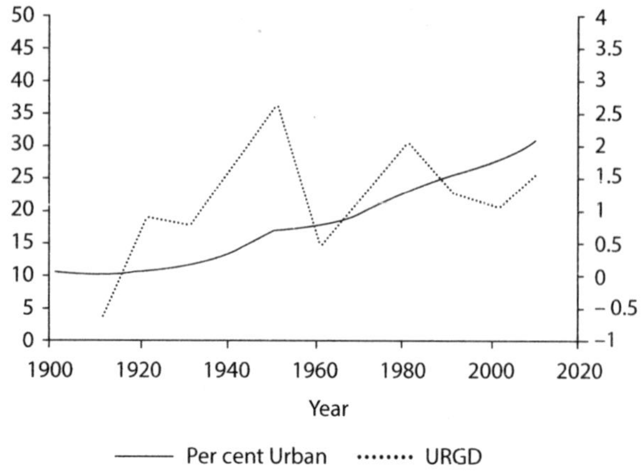

Figure 2.11 Trends in Urbanization and URGD, India, 1901–2011

Note: The scale for per cent urban is shown on the left hand and for URGD on the right hand.

Source: Computed from Office of the Registrar General and Census Commissioner, India (2006b, 2013).

urban in 2011 (Office of the Registrar General and Census 2013). Goa, Mizoram, Tamil Nadu, Kerala, Maharashtra, and Gujarat are also highly urbanized with over 40 per cent living in urban areas. There has been a large increase in urbanization in Kerala; however, this appears to be largely due to reclassification of many villages as census towns in the 2011 census. At the other end, in Himachal Pradesh, Bihar, and Odisha among the large states and Sikkim, Arunachal Pradesh, Tripura, Nagaland, and Meghalaya among the north-eastern states, less than one fifth population lived in urban areas. Uttar Pradesh, the largest state, is also predominantly rural.

While the level of urbanization has been low, crowding in metropolitan areas remains a major concern. In particular, a large section of the population in large cities resides in slums. The enumeration of slum population in cities and towns of population over 50,000 in the 2001 census yielded a figure of 42.6 million (Registrar General 2005a). Mumbai itself had 6.5 million slum dwellers, constituting a majority of the city's population. Delhi, Kolkata, Chennai, Nagpur, Surat, and Pune also had large slum populations.

Table 2.11 Trends in Urbanization in India, 1901–2011

Year	Population (in thousands) All	Urban	Percent Urban	Growth Rate All	Urban	Inter-censal Increase in % Urban	URGD
1901	238,396	25,855	10.85				
1911	252,093	25,948	10.29	0.56	0.04	–0.56	–0.58
1921	251,321	28,091	11.18	–0.03	0.79	0.89	0.92
1931	278,977	33,463	11.99	1.04	1.75	0.81	0.80
1941	318,661	44,162	13.86	1.33	2.77	1.87	1.66
1951	361,088	62,444	17.29	1.25	3.46	3.43	2.62
1961	439,235	78,937	17.97	1.96	2.34	0.68	0.47
1971	548,160	1,09,114	19.91	2.20	3.21	1.94	1.25
1981	683,329	1,59,463	23.34	2.22	3.83	3.43	2.04
1991	846,421	2,17,611	25.71	2.14	3.11	2.37	1.28
2001	1,028,737	2,86,120	27.81	1.95	2.74	2.10	1.07
2011	1,210,570	3,77,106	31.15	1.63	2.76	3.35	1.61

Source: Office of the Registrar General and Census Commissioner, India (2006b; 2013).

Economy

India has long been categorized as a low income country but incomes have been rising impressively in the recent years. Trends based on the national income data provided by the Central Statistical Organisation (CSO), which releases various indicators over time at both current and constant prices thereby allowing a meaningful assessment, show that at constant prices (base: 2004–05) India's Gross National Product (GNP) rose from Rs. 2,78,677 crores in 1950–51 to Rs. 48,33,178 crores in 2010–11 (Ministry of Finance, 2012). Thus, the GNP in 2010–11 was over 16 times as large as the GNP in 1950–51 (Table 2.12).

There have been huge changes over time in the relative contributions of the three major sectors: Primary (agriculture, fishery, forestry, mining, and allied), Secondary (manufacturing, construction,

Table 2.12 Trends in Gross National Product, Per Capita Income, and Shares of Sectors

Year	GNP (in Rs. Crores at constant prices: base 2004–05)	Ratio to 1950–51 GNP	Per capita income (2004–2005 prices)	Ratio to 1950–51 PCI	Percentage shares of various sectors in GDP		
					Primary	Secondary	Tertiary
1950–51	278677	1.00	7114	1.00	55.0	14.7	30.3
1960–61	408739	1.51	8889	1.25	50.9	18.3	30.8
1970–71	585672	2.12	10016	1.41	44.5	21.7	33.8
1980–81	798504	2.85	10712	1.51	38.7	23.3	38.1
1990–91	1331040	4.71	14330	2.01	33.1	24.2	42.7
2000–01	2318974	8.12	20362	2.86	25.3	24.3	50.4
2010–11 Q	4833178	16.71	35993	5.06	16.0	25.0	59.0

Source: Computed from CSO estimates: Ministry of Finance (2012); Q: Quick Estimate.

electricity, etc.), and Tertiary (trade, transport, finance, and administrative services). The primary sector dominated in the 1950s, but its share has fallen continuously, and, in recent years, steeply, so that by 2010–11, this sector contributed only 16 per cent to the GDP (Table 2.12). On the other hand, the tertiary sector, comprising trade, transport and various services has become dominant, contributing to over half of the GDP. The share of the secondary sector (manufacturing, construction, electricity, water supply etc.) has also increased to one fourth of the total GDP. This amounts to a major structural transformation of the Indian economy.

Of special interest is the Per Capita Income (PCI). At constant (2004–05) prices, PCI increased from Rs. 7,114 in 1950–51 to Rs. 35,993 in 2010–11. This shows that in real terms the PCI quintupled over the period. The rate of growth was slow up to 1992, and in some years, the real PCI actually declined, but it has been higher since then, especially after 2002–03. Trends since 1950 show a larger rise in the Net National Product (NNP) than in population size; thus, though India's population has more than doubled since 1951, the NNP (in constant prices) has increased even more than that, with the result that real has also raised over the period (Figure 2.12).

Per capita income varies spatially. In 2009–10 (the year for which data on most states are available), Goa, Delhi, and Chandigarh had relatively high incomes (more than Rs. 100,000, in current prices), followed by Puducherry, Haryana, Maharashtra, Andaman and Nicobar Islands, Sikkim, Gujarat, Tamil Nadu, and Punjab (Rs. 60,000–100,000). Lowest incomes were seen in Bihar, below Rs. 20,000. Most of the states in the north-central region also have low incomes. Even if small states and city states are not taken into account (because of their special circumstances), state-level incomes vary from a low of Rs. 17 thousand in Bihar to Rs. 78 thousand in Haryana. Inter-state variations are, quite clearly, very large.

In all populations, incomes vary across households. For a low income country like India, this also means that many are poor. For long, India's Planning Commission has been estimating the level of poverty in the country and in states by specifying a 'poverty line,' such that those living below the line are considered to be 'poor'. The percentage of persons living below this line is a measure of poverty, the headcount ratio measure. While more sophisticated measures have

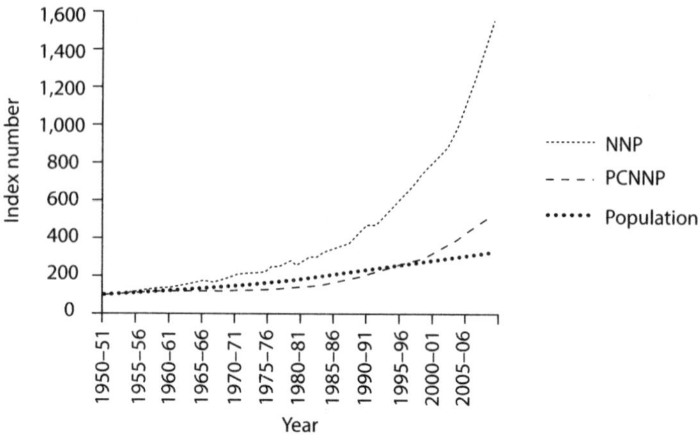

Figure 2.12 Index Numbers of Population (NNP) at constant prices and Per Capita NNP (PCNNP) at constant prices, India, 1950–51 to 2010–11; Base: 1950-51

Source: Computed from CSO estimates: Ministry of Finance (2012); the population figures are from census with interpolation for intermediate years.

been suggested in the literature, the headcount ratio is very commonly used as a simple measure of the extent of poverty. Data on household consumption expenditure from the National Sample Survey (NSS) are used to obtain estimates of the poverty ratio. The measurement of poverty has long been a contentious issue in India and questions have been raised about criteria employed to specify the poverty line, and the fact that the poverty line used by the Planning Commission does not match some of the international lines (such as one dollar a day or two dollars a day); there is also the problem of making adjustments for purchasing power parity to facilitate international comparisons.

Instead of getting into the debate, only the Planning Commission estimates based on the recent methodology recommended by the Tendulkar Committee (2009) are presented here (Table 2.13). These show that poverty levels are high, but show a declining trend. This declining trend is observed in both rural and urban areas. While in the early 1990s nearly half the rural population was categorized as poor, in 2009–10 only about a third of rural population and a fifth of urban population was classified as poor. Regardless of the methodology adopted, one can conclude that there is considerable poverty in

Table 2.13 Poverty Ratios in India *(percent below poverty line, headcount ratios)*

Year	Rural	Urban	Combined
1993–94	50.1	31.8	45.3
2004–05	41.8	25.7	37.2
2009–10	33.8	20.9	29.8

Note: These are based on the new methodology by the Tendulkar Committee (2009).

Source: Planning Commission (2012).

India and though there has been some decline, a large proportion of the population is quite poor.

The level of poverty also varies across states. In 2009–10, poverty was relatively high (over 40 per cent) in Bihar, Chhattisgarh and Manipur and moderately high (30–40 per cent) in Assam, Jharkhand, Odisha, Madhya Pradesh, Uttar Pradesh, Uttarakhand, Dadra and Nagar Haveli, and Daman and Diu. The level was low (below 10 per cent) in Goa, Himachal Pradesh, Jammu & Kashmir, Puducherry, Lakshadweep, Andaman and Nicobar Islands, and Chandigarh (Planning Commission 2012).

Work Participation and Unemployment

Individuals play a dual role in the economy, as consumers and producers. While all are consumers, only some are producers in economic terms, and are called workers and the numbers of workers and the level of participation are important indicators for any economy. Data on work participation are available both from decennial censuses and special surveys, such as the NSS, which collects data on employment in its various rounds. As the NSS collects data on work participation in more detail than the census does, these are considered more dependable than census data to assess trends (Visaria 1996). Trends in work participation rates from various rounds of the NSS that had covered employment and had large samples are provided in Table 2.14, assessed on the basis of the 'usual activity status' of individuals. The level of work participation is higher among males than females; this is a common pattern globally, although in some populations, female participation rates are close to those of males, and in others, very low

Table 2.14 Work Participation Rates, India, NSSO, 1983 to 2009–10 *(usual activity status, principal, and subsidiary status)*

NSS round	Year	Rural		Urban	
		Male	Female	Male	Female
		Work participation rate (per cent of population)			
38	1983	54.7	34.0	51.2	15.1
43	1987–88	53.9	32.3	50.6	15.2
50	1993–94	55.3	32.8	52.1	15.5
55	1999–2000	53.1	29.9	51.8	13.9
61	2004–05	54.6	32.7	54.9	16.6
66	2009–10	54.7	26.1	54.3	13.8

Source: NSSO (2009, 2011).

rates of female work participation are observed. Since 1983, the work participation level has been fairly steady in India, with a small decline in work participation rates of rural females, and an increase in the work participation rates of urban males.

It is essential to look at work participation by age, as changes in age structure are expected in India. Participation is nearly universal for males aged 30–59 years in both rural and urban areas; these are the prime working ages (Table 2.15). On the other hand, in childhood ages, 5–14, participation is quite low yet non-negligible, pointing towards some continuation of child labour. In the older ages, 60 years and above, participation is high among rural males and substantial among urban males as well. Apparently, a large section of the work force, being outside the organized sector, does not retire as such.

A majority of workers are engaged in the primary sector (agriculture, fisheries, forestry, mining, etc.). Though there has been some decline in the share of this sector since 1961 (Alagh 2004), even in 2009–10, over half of all workers (53.2 per cent) were engaged in primary activities, compared to only 21.5 per cent in secondary activities, and 25.4 per cent in tertiary activities (NSSO 2011). Thus, although the share of the primary sector in the gross domestic product has fallen to less than one fifth, the share of workers in this sector is disproportionately high, resulting in relative impoverishment of those in agriculture. Moreover, while the size of the population has increased, land under

Table 2.15 Work Participation Rates by Age and Sex, India, 2009–10 (usual activity status, principal, and subsidiary status) *(per cent of population)*

Age group	Rural		Urban	
	Male	Female	Male	Female
5–14 years	1.4	2.0	1.5	0.7
15–29 years	62.6	28.8	56.4	14.4
30–59 years	97.9	47.1	96.4	24.0
60 years and higher	63.6	22.6	34.2	7.0
15–59 years	82.2	39.2	78.5	19.8

Source: Computed from NSSO (2011).

cultivation has not, nor has there been a large shift of workers out of agriculture. As a result, there has been a fall in the average size of the agricultural holdings of rural households. Earlier, most Indian farmers were in the category of small and marginal holders, having less than two hectares of land. Now, a majority of holdings are marginal; the share of holdings of marginal size (less than one hectare) increased from 39 per cent in 1960–61 to 63 per cent in 2002–03 (Bhalla 2007). Population pressure on land is clearly felt.

Unemployment in India is not very high. The unemployment rate (per cent of labour force unemployed) is quite low, about 2 per cent, in rural areas, among both males and females but non-negligible in urban areas, 3 per cent for males and 7 per cent for females (NSSO 2011). The low level of unemployment in rural areas should not be taken as full employment, since a large part of the rural work force is engaged in agriculture where employment is seasonal.

Literacy and Education

One key indicator of social development is the level of education. Results from India's censuses show that literacy was low in the past. In 1951, less than one fifth of the population (aged above 5) was literate (Table 2.16). Even at this low level of literacy, gender disparities were quite clear, as less than one tenth of women were literate. There has been a steady rise in literacy so that by 1991, a majority of the population (aged 7 years and above) was literate; relatively small proportions of females were literate, however. By 2001, the literacy rate for females also crossed the halfway mark. The most recent data show that about three fourths of persons (age 7+) are literate. Though gender disparities persist, the gap seems to be narrowing. Evidently, some catching up has been accomplished, with female literacy rates showing more rapid progress than male literacy.

The level of literacy varies across states. Literacy is now almost universal (over 90 per cent) in Kerala, Lakshadweep, and Mizoram; it is high (80–90 per cent) in Goa, Tripura, Daman & Diu, Andaman & Nicobar Islands, Delhi, Chandigarh, Puducherry, Himachal Pradesh, Maharashtra, Sikkim, and Tamil Nadu, but low (below 70 per cent) in Bihar, Arunachal Pradesh, Rajasthan, Jharkhand, Andhra Pradesh, Jammu & Kashmir, and Uttar Pradesh. As of 2011, the gender gap remains wide in Rajasthan, Jharkhand, Chhattisgarh, Dadra & Nagar Haveli, Madhya Pradesh, Jammu & Kashmir, and Bihar. We note here that, by and large, states with low levels of male literacy show narrow gender gaps; as male literacy rates rise, gender gaps become more evident, and the gap narrows as both male and female literacy become near universal; the Indian states seem to follow this pattern. The gender gap, thus, indicates the stage of development in literacy.

As expected, literacy is lower among the older than the younger population. Tabulations from the 2001 census reveal that less than

Table 2.16 Trends in Literacy, India, 1951–2011 *(per cent literate: for ages 5 and over for 1951–71 and 7 and over for 1981–2011)*

Year	Persons	Males	Females	Gender Gap (M–F)
1951	18.3	27.2	8.9	18.3
1961	28.3	40.4	15.4	25.1
1971	34.5	46.0	22.0	24.0
1981	43.6	56.4	29.8	26.6
1991	52.2	64.1	39.3	24.8
2001	64.8	75.3	53.7	21.6
2011	73.0	80.9	64.6	16.3

Source: Office of the Registrar General and Census Commissioner, India (2011a; 2013).

half of those over 60 years of age were literate (Table 2.17). Moreover, gender gaps are wider among this group than among younger groups, again reflecting the stage of development. It must be noted here that while literacy is generally accepted as the best single indicator of education at the macro level, from a human capital perspective, it is desirable to see whether educational achievement goes beyond mere literacy. School enrolment is near universal among young children now and this is reflected in the high literacy rates observed among the young. However, dropout rates are also high and many children do not continue beyond primary school. In order to obtain a more meaningful indicator of educational achievement, percentages of persons who have completed at least high school education by age and sex are presented (Table 2.17). While a majority of India's population is now literate, only a minority of men and women has completed high school. The percentages for women are particularly low and, as expected, high school completion is higher among younger persons

Table 2.17 Literacy and Completion of High School by Age and Sex, India

Age Group	Per cent Literate, 2001[1]			Per cent with at least High School education, 2005–06[2]		
	Persons	Males	Females	Persons	Males	Females
7–9	71.0	74.1	67.7	–	–	–
10–14	81.7	86.0	77.0	–	–	–
15–19	79.3	85.0	72.7	–	–	–
20–24	73.2	83.3	62.5	36.4	42.6	30.7
25–29	67.0	79.1	55.1	31.4	38.9	24.9
30–34	61.7	74.8	48.4	28.7	38.5	19.8
35–59	54.3	68.7	38.7	22.0	30.7	13.3
60+	36.3	52.8	20.3	10.0	16.3	3.6
7+	64.9	75.3	53.7			
20+	–	–	–	24.6	32.2	17.2

Note: Percentages for high school completion are shown only for those over 20 years of age.

Source: [1]Computed from Table C9 from the 2001 Census (Office of the Registrar General and Census Commissioner, CD 2013); [2]computed from household data file from NFHS-3 (2005–06).

than older. Thus, while improvements in literacy have been impressive, educational achievement, in terms of completion of high school, has remained quite low; completion of a college (university) degree is even rarer.

Even more worrying is the quality of education of those reportedly enrolled in schools. Recent studies on actual scholastic abilities of children showed that many school children have very poor reading and arithmetical skills. The latest survey (carried out in 2011) in the ASER series by Pratham showed that of the fifth grade children in rural areas, less than half (48.2 per cent) could read the second standard text book and only 27.6 per cent could perform a division (Pratham 2012). Even among the seventh grade students, less than half could do a division. Clearly, while the rise seen in literacy and school enrolment is good news, the impact in terms of human resource development is not very high.

Food Security

The very basic requirement of any population is food, and the availability of food for populations growing in size was the central issue of the Malthusian thesis. The question of whether the rapidly growing populations in the developed world will have adequate food or suffer massive starvation was raised often during neo-Malthusian debates. In fact, in the 1960s and 70s, some had predicted that a few countries including India would face severe food shortages resulting in starvation deaths on a large scale. It is, therefore, necessary to look at trends in the food situation in India.

The evidence shows that overall the production of food grains has increased in India, from 51 million tons in 1950–51 to 234 million tons in 2008–09, quadrupling since the early 1950s. The land under crops has increased to some extent; from 97 million hectares in 1950–51 to 123 million in 2008–09 (Ministry of Agriculture 2009). But there has been significant increase in the percentage of land under irrigation: from 18 per cent in 1950–51 to 46 per cent in 2007–08. Most of the increase in agricultural production has come from improved yields, expansion in irrigation and new technologies, broadly the green revolution. Food grain yields have increased from 522 kg/hectare in 1950–51 to almost 1,900 kg/hectare in 2008–09.

A comparative view of trends in population, food grain production and per capita food grain availability can be seen in Figure 2.13 (as index numbers). Trends reveal that while population size has increased, so has the production of food grains and the long-run growth in the production of food grains is slightly greater than that of population. The per capita availability of food grains (in grams per day) has fluctuated in a narrow range, mostly 400–500 gm/day, and shows only a marginal increasing trend (of 0.6 gm/day per year); this contrasts with the clear increasing trend in per capita real income noted earlier. Further, given that much of Indian agriculture is dependent on the monsoons, there is always uncertainty about agricultural production and India has had to face food shortages in some years as a result. Sharp falls in the production of food grains were seen in 1958, later in two consecutive years, 1966 and 1967, and again in 1973, 1980, and 2003. During the last 60 years, per capita food grain availability crossed the level of 500 gm. in only two years, 1991 and 1997. Besides, any shortages raise prices of food items and this affects the poorer sections of society much more than others, since the latter can divert some of their income from non-food expenditure to food while the poor have no such flexibility. Thus, though mass

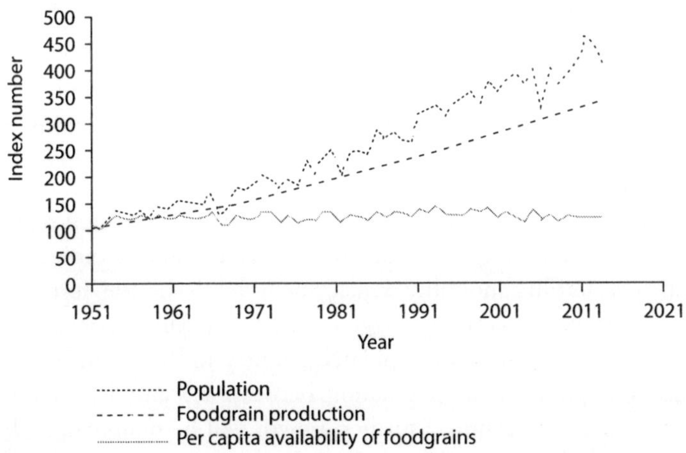

Figure 2.13 Trends in Index numbers of population, food grain production, and per capita food grain availability, India, 1951–2009: Base 1951
Source: Obtained from the data on agricultural production in Ministry of Agriculture (2009) and census population figures with interpolation.

starvation has been avoided in India, with improved productivity, public distribution schemes, and imports in some years, the food situation remains a matter of concern. Recent surveys have shown that the level of malnutrition is high among children and women. According to the NFHS-3, in 2005–06, 48 per cent of children less than five years of age were stunted (24 per cent were severely stunted) and 43 per cent were undernourished (IIPS and Macro International 2007). Similarly, 36 per cent of women in childbearing ages were undernourished (had a Body Mass Index lower than the normal range).

Challenges and the Way Forward

This overview of the demographic and development situation in India points to a number of challenges that India must address. In this section, these challenges and broad areas for future attention are outlined.

Population growth

India's population grew rapidly for quite some time. At one time, there were apprehensions of population explosion that would compromise the quality of life in India in a disastrous way. However, recent changes show that these fears were unfounded. Although population continues to grow, and will grow for some more time, the long-term perspective is that the growth will not be large. India's demographic transition is now in the phase of falling fertility, resulting in reduced natural growth; many states have already reached or crossed replacement levels of fertility, and the country as a whole is projected to reach low fertility-mortality replacement levels in the foreseeable future. Various projections suggest that India will overtake China and will become the most populated country in the world by 2030. Projections place India's population between 1.5 and 1.8 billion at the middle of the century; further growth will be marginal, and, in fact, some decline is anticipated. Thus, while uncontrolled population growth is no longer an issue, the size of the population will be much larger than at present, and policies and programmes must be designed with this in mind.

Fertility decline

The fall in fertility has been a welcome change, with implications not just in terms of meeting population stabilization goals, but also in terms of meeting reproductive rights, addressing women's autonomy, and affecting the health and development of women and children (Bhat 2002). The fall in fertility may be attributed to declining family size preferences and the adoption of fertility regulation by all sections of society. Parental aspirations about children, especially on education of children, sons as well as daughters, have risen; these involve costs, and there is quality-quantity trade-off resulting in desires for small families. This is true across income and education classes, the rich and the poor, the educated and the illiterate parents, though some differentials remain. Thus, couples can now spend more time and money on the children they have. Moreover, women are freed from the burden of frequent childbearing, allowing them to participate more fully in other activities, market, or otherwise. Fertility declines have not, however, been uniform across the country. In some parts of the country, especially in the north-central region, there is considerable unmet need for fertility regulation. There is a need for attention to this region; efforts to meet this need will have a positive impact on the life of women and children, and, at the same time, have implications for reducing fertility in ways that are respectful of reproductive rights.

Infant mortality

Mortality has no doubt fallen and life expectancy has risen impressively; the process began long before fertility began to decline. Yet, mortality in India continues to be higher than that in many developing countries; for example, India's life expectancy is 6–8 years lower than that of China. Much of the sluggish pace of decline in mortality may be attributed to show declines in infant mortality since 1991; while infant mortality has indeed declined, current levels of about 50 per 1,000 live births, remain unacceptably high. Of particular concern is neonatal mortality, which remains high and is declining far too slowly; this is attributable to the poor health and nutritional status in pregnancy. Inequities by region and socioeconomic factors are particularly evident in infant mortality and concerted efforts are needed to combat these high rates of neonatal and infant mortality in worse-off sections of society and in affected regions of the country.

Sex selection

The unbalanced sex ratio of the child population has drawn the attention of civil society in the recent years. No doubt discrimination against girls in matters of health care and nutrition has long been recognized, and was manifested in gender disparities in early childhood mortality. But during the last three decades the availability of prenatal sex detection combined with continued strong son preference has resulted in selective terminations of pregnancies carrying a female foetus, and has created a huge sex imbalance in the country. This practice is quite common in some regions of the country, especially the northern-western states, but appears to be spreading to other regions as well. Legal measures have not been adequate to prevent the misuse of this technology. Efforts are needed that stem this spread, that implement regulatory measures indicated in the law, and address the continuing strong preference for sons in the country.

Urbanization

India is not highly urbanized and the evidence suggests that the tempo of urbanization had slowed down after 1981. The results of the 2011 census show some increase in the pace of urbanization but as the details are not yet available, it is not clear whether this implies that rural to urban migration has increased substantially. We note, however, that while at the national level the degree of urbanization is not high, some urban areas, especially metropolitan cities, have long experienced overcrowding, and poor housing, sanitation, and hygiene conditions. In many cities, very large sections of the urban population live in slums, and if the tempo of urbanization increases, especially with rapid growth in the tertiary and secondary sectors, this segment of the population may increase. Accommodating the needs of the populations residing in slums calls for major investments in infrastructure—housing, water supply, sanitation, and other amenities—for the urban poor, without which quality of life for this large urban population will be severely and adversely affected.

Persistent regional and social inequalities

This chapter has emphasized the persistence of both inter-state variations and differences by socioeconomic indicators in India's demographic situation. While the demographic transition is in progress or has been completed in all regions, its timing has varied. For example, some regions—especially the north-central states—have experienced a far more gradual demographic transition than other states, and are likely to double their populations during the first fifty years of the twenty-first century, raising concerns about population density, distress out-migration, and the potential for related social and political tensions. At the same time, wide socioeconomic disparities persist in India, notably in terms of poverty levels, educational attainment and social status; these inequalities are evident both at national level, and in individual states. As far as demographic outcomes are concerned, the implications of these disparities are stark with regard to mortality; for example, the risk of child mortality is much higher among those belonging to scheduled castes and scheduled tribes, the poorly educated, the poor and those from lesser developed states than others. Notwithstanding improvements in overall conditions, these persistent disparities must be addressed.

Demographic dividend

As India moves through its demographic transition, significant changes are taking place in its age structure, such that the share of the child population will decline, and that of the population in the working ages will increase, resulting in lowering the dependency ratio, and thereby yielding the demographic dividend. Work by Bloom et al. (2003) has emphasised the extent to which this dividend will benefit national economies. Indeed, the demographic dividend is the most talked about benefit of the demographic changes—in particular, the sharp fertility decline—that the nation has recently undergone. This dividend provides India with a window—available only for a few more decades—of demographic opportunity. The extent to which India can capitalize on this depends however on how skilled and healthy its population is, and how well its workers can be employed. Issues relating to the quality of India's labour force and the capacity of its economy to harvest the potential dividend have been highlighted (James 2008). While some dividend will accrue naturally because of changes in the age structure and the dependency burden, the full impact of reaping the demographic dividend will not accrue unless India's labour force is efficiently utilized. The quality of school education, that has been found to be quite poor, must be raised if the dividend is to be gained. Health status of population is also an important factor in utilizing the dividend.

Employment

Population growth brings in the possibility of unemployment and raises questions about the economy's ability to absorb an increasing number of workers. In India, open unemployment has not been large but underemployment is widespread and a serious concern. Given the seasonal nature of Indian agriculture, and the domination of the agriculture sector in the workforce, many are not engaged in work for large parts of the year. On the other hand, many elderly persons are employed (again because they are not in the organized sector) although their participation is likely to fall. Female work participation, low at present, is expected to rise. For all of these reasons, India's labour force is likely to grow considerably in the foreseeable future, and concerted efforts towards employment generation are urgently required.

Food availability

Over the past decades, India has managed to raise levels of food production substantially and food grain production has, by and large, kept pace with population growth. However, per capita food availability has not really improved and overall nutritional conditions remain poor. At the same time, even with declines in fertility, further population growth in inevitable. The need to increase per capita food grain availability is imperative and calls for further improvements in agricultural production.

Ageing

Over time, the large bulge of population will move from the working ages to old ages, giving rise to increased old age dependency. This inevitable ageing of the population suggests changes at both the macro-level and also at the micro or household level. At household level, at present, supporting elderly parents has been the responsibility of working adult children; low fertility means smaller numbers of children and elderly parents may have fewer grown up children on whom they can depend than in the past. In such circumstances, as in other countries, the state will need to intervene to ensure the wellbeing of the elderly. At macro-level, this possibility raises the need to develop mechanisms to provide old age support. Such mechanisms need to be put into place very soon in some states, that is, those leading the demographic transition, and later, in the rest of the country as well. The need for programmes for the elderly has been recognized and a National Policy for Older Persons (NPOP) and several schemes to support the elderly have been introduced. But these have not received much attention in the public sphere. The present low share of the elderly in India is perhaps the reason for this matter not getting adequate attention. But this is one consequence of the demographic transition that is inescapable and therefore the state and the society need to take steps for addressing it well in advance.

This chapter has shown that fertility decline has been achieved and that India will reach replacement level fertility in the coming decades. Key issues now facing the nation are to ensure the timely completion of the demographic transition in regions whose demographic change has been lagging, and to take steps to ensure the quality of life and well-being of India's population. The principal population issues are well-identified, and the focus now must be on anticipating and planning efficiently for the future.

Appendix

Table A2.1 Population Growth in States and UTs, India, 2001–2011

India/state	Population (in thousands)		Annual growth rate* (%)	Density (persons per sq. km.)
	2001	2011		
India	1,028,737	12,10,570	1.63	382
Jammu & Kashmir	10,144	12,541	2.12	124
Himachal Pradesh	6,078	6,865	1.22	123

(*Continued*)

Table A2.1 *(Continued)*

India/state	Population (in thousands)		Annual growth rate* (%)	Density (persons per sq. km.)
	2001	2011		
Punjab	24,359	27,743	1.30	551
Chandigarh	901	1,055	1.59	9,258
Uttaranchal	8,489	10,086	1.72	189
Haryana	21,145	25,351	1.81	573
Delhi	13,851	16,788	1.92	11,320
Rajasthan	56,507	68,548	1.93	200
Uttar Pradesh	166,198	199,812	1.84	829
Bihar	82,999	104,099	2.27	1,106
Sikkim	541	611	1.21	86
Arunachal Pradesh	1,098	1,384	2.31	17
Nagaland	1,990	1,979	–0.06	119
Manipur	2,294	2,570	1.71	115
Mizoram	889	1,097	2.11	52
Tripura	3,199	3,674	1.38	350
Meghalaya	2,319	2,967	2.46	132
Assam	26,656	31,206	1.58	398
West Bengal	80,176	91,276	1.30	1,028
Jharkhand	26,946	32,988	2.02	414
Odisha	36,805	41,974	1.31	270
Chhattisgarh	20,834	25,545	2.04	189
Madhya Pradesh	60,348	72,627	1.85	236
Gujarat	50,671	60,440	1.76	308
Daman & Diu	158	243	4.30	2,191
Dadra & Nagar Haveli	220	344	4.44	700
Maharashtra	96,879	112,374	1.48	365
Andhra Pradesh	76,210	84,581	1.04	308
Karnataka	52,851	61,095	1.45	319
Goa	1,348	1,459	0.79	394
Lakshadweep	61	64	0.61	2,149
Kerala	31,841	33,406	0.48	860
Tamil Nadu	62,406	72,147	1.45	555

India/state	Population (in thousands)		Annual growth rate* (%)	Density (persons per sq. km.)
	2001	2011		
Puducherry	974	1248	2.47	2547
Andaman & Nicobar Islands	356	381	0.66	46

*: The growth rate is annual exponential rate computed from the population figures; for Manipur this is computed from the per cent increase as reported in Office of the Registrar General and Census Commissioner (2013).
Source: Office of the Registrar General and Census Commissioner, India (2013).

Table A2.2 Population Projections for India, 2011–2101
(Population in millions)

Year	Projection and variant				
	RGI	PFI/PRB Scenario B	U.N. Medium	Dyson-Standard	Actual
2011	1193	1201	1250	1204	1211
2016	1269	1283	1335	1290	
2021	1340	1371	1415	1362	
2026	1400	1445	1488	1419	
2031		1523	1555	1465	
2036		1585	1616	1508	
2041		1651	1667	1543	
2046		1700	1709	1566	
2051		1751	1742	1579	
2061		1822	1783		
2071		1864	1792		
2081		1881	1771		
2091		1876	1728		
2101		1853	1675		

Sources: Office of the Registrar General and Census Commissioner (2006a, 2013); PFI and PRB, 2007, United Nations (2011); Dyson (2004).

Table A2.3 Per cent Population in Ages 0–6, States, India, 2001, 2011

State	2001	2011	Decline
India	15.93	13.59	2.34
Jammu & Kashmir	14.65	16.10	–1.45
Himachal Pradesh	13.05	11.33	1.72
Punjab	13.02	11.09	1.93
Chandigarh	12.84	11.32	1.52
Uttaranchal	16.02	13.44	2.58
Haryana	15.77	13.34	2.43
Delhi	14.56	11.99	2.57
Rajasthan	18.85	15.54	3.31
Uttar Pradesh	19.03	15.41	3.62
Bihar	20.25	18.38	1.87
Sikkim	14.46	10.50	3.96
Arunachal Pradesh	18.75	15.33	3.42
Nagaland	14.56	14.71	–0.15
Manipur	14.23	13.16	1.07
Mizoram	16.18	15.36	0.82
Tripura	13.64	12.47	1.17
Meghalaya	20.18	19.16	1.02
Assam	16.87	14.86	2.01
West Bengal	14.24	11.59	2.65
Jharkhand	18.40	16.34	2.06
Odisha	14.56	12.56	2.00
Chhattisgarh	17.06	14.33	2.73
Madhya Pradesh	17.87	14.88	2.99
Gujarat	14.87	12.87	2.00
Daman & Diu	13.01	11.07	1.94
Dadra & Nagar Haveli	18.23	14.81	3.42
Maharashtra	14.11	11.86	2.25
Andhra Pradesh	13.35	10.81	2.54
Karnataka	13.59	11.72	1.87
Goa	10.83	9.91	0.92
Lakshadweep	14.99	11.25	3.74
Kerala	11.91	10.40	1.51
Tamil Nadu	11.59	10.29	1.30
Puducherry	12.02	10.65	1.37
Andaman & Nicobar Islands	12.57	10.74	1.83

Source: Office of the Registrar General and Census Commissioner, India (2013).

Table A2.4 Sex Ratio in Population (females per 1,000 males), Large States, India, 1991–2011

State	All ages				Children ages 0–6 years				SRB
	1991	2001	2011	Change 2011–2001	1991	2001	2011	Change 2011–2001	2006–08
India	927	933	943	10	945	927	919	–8	904
Jammu & Kashmir		892	889	–3		941	862	–79	862
Himachal Pradesh	976	968	972	4	951	896	909	13	938
Punjab	882	876	895	19	875	798	846	48	836
Haryana	865	861	879	18	879	819	834	15	847
Delhi	827	821	868	47	915	868	871	3	877
Rajasthan	910	921	928	7	916	909	888	–21	870
Uttar Pradesh	876	898	912	14	928	916	902	–14	877
Bihar	907	919	918	–1	959	942	935	–7	914
Assam	923	935	958	23	975	965	962	–3	933
West Bengal	917	934	950	16	967	960	956	–4	941
Jharkhand	922	941	949	8	979	965	948	–17	922
Odisha	971	972	979	7	967	953	941	–12	937
Chhattisgarh	985	980	991	2	984	974	969	–5	975
Madhya Pradesh	912	919	931	12	952	932	918	–14	919
Gujarat	934	920	919	–1	928	883	890	7	898
Maharashtra	934	922	929	7	946	913	894	–34	884

(*Continued*)

Table A2.4 *(Continued)*

State	All ages				Children ages 0–6 years				SRB
	1991	2001	2011	Change 2011–2001	1991	2001	2011	Change 2011–2001	2006–08
Andhra Pradesh	972	978	993	15	974	961	939	–22	917
Karnataka	960	965	973	8	960	946	948	2	935
Kerala	1036	1059	1084	25	958	960	964	4	964
Tamil Nadu	974	987	996	9	974	942	943	1	936

SRB: SRB (females per 1,000 males) from the SRS.

Source: Office of the Registrar General and Census Commissioner, India (2001, 2013); Registrar General (2009).

Table A2.5 Trends in Age-Specific Fertility Rates (ASFR), India, 1971–2010

(ASFR)					
Age group	Year			1971 to 2010	
	1971	1991	2010	Absolute Decline	Per cent Decline
15–19	100.8	76.1	37.2	63.6	63
20–24	250.8	234.0	198.6	52.2	21
25–29	254.8	191.3	156.8	98.0	38
30–34	202.2	117.0	66.0	136.2	67
35–39	137.8	66.8	29.7	108.1	78
40–44	62.2	30.6	9.3	52.9	85
45–49	24.4	12.1	3.9	20.5	84
TFR	5.2	3.6	2.5	2.7	51

Source: SRS: Registrar General (2010; 2012a).

Table A2.6 TFR in States and UTs, India, 1971–2010

State	TFR		
	1971*	1991#	2010
INDIA	5.2	4.5	2.5
Jammu & Kashmir		2.6	2.0
Himachal Pradesh		3.0	1.8
Punjab	5.2	3.1	1.8
Chandigarh		1.5	*2.1a*
Uttarakhand			
Haryana	6.7	4.0	2.3
Delhi		1.8	1.9
Rajasthan	6.3	4.6	3.1
Uttar Pradesh	6.6	5.1	3.5
Bihar	5.7	4.4	3.7
Sikkim		3.0	*2.0a*
Arunachal Pradesh		4.1	*2.7a*
Nagaland		2.3	*2.0a*
Manipur		2.5	*1.6a*
Mizoram		1.7	*2.0a*

(*Continued*)

Table A2.6 *(Continued)*

State	TFR		
	1971*	1991#	2010
Tripura		2.7	*1.7a*
Meghalaya		4.1	*3.1a*
Assam	5.7	3.5	2.5
West Bengal	4.2	3.2	1.8
Jharkhand			3.0
Odisha	4.7	3.3	2.3
Chhattisgarh			2.8
Madhya Pradesh	5.6	4.6	3.2
Gujarat	5.6	3.1	2.5
Daman & Diu		3.7	*1.9a*
Dadra & Nagar Haveli		5.0	*3.3a*
Maharashtra	4.6	3.0	1.9
Andhra Pradesh	4.6	3.0	1.8
Karnataka	4.4	3.1	2.0
Goa		1.6	*1.6a*
Lakshadweep		3.9	*2.1a*
Kerala	4.1	1.8	1.8
Tamil Nadu	3.9	2.2	1.7
Puducherry		1.8	*1.6a*
Andaman & Nicobar Islands		2.5	*1.8a*

Note: * for Bihar and West Bengal the values refers to 1981; # For Jammu & Kashmir to 2000; for Mizoram to 1997; for Dadra & Nagar Haveli to: 1994; [a]For small states and UTs the values refer to average for 2005–07.
Source: Registrar General (2010; 2012a).

Table A2.7 Trends in Expectation of Life at Birth, India, 1901–2010

Period	Expectation of Life at Birth		
	Males	Females	Persons
1901–10	22.6	23.3	22.9
1911–20	19.4	20.9	20.0
1921–30	26.9	26.6	26.8
1931–40	32.1	31.4	31.8

Period	Expectation of Life at Birth		
	Males	Females	Persons
1941–50	32.4	31.7	32.1
1951–60	41.9	40.6	41.3
1961–70	46.4	44.7	45.6
1970–75	50.5	49.0	49.7
1976–80	52.5	52.1	52.3
1981–85	55.4	55.7	55.4
1986–90	57.7	58.1	57.7
1991–95	60.3	59.7	60.9
1996–2000	61.2	62.7	61.9
2001–05	63.1	65.6	64.3
2006–10	64.6	67.7	66.1

Sources: Jain (1982) (Census based estimates for the years 1901–70); Registrar General (2010) (SRS Life Tables for the years 1971–95); Registrar General (2012b) (SRS Life Tables for the years 1996–2010).

Table A2.8 U5MRs, Large States, India, 1970–75 to 2010

State	Male		Female	
	1970–75*	2010	1970–75	2010
INDIA	196	55	224	64
Jammu & Kashmir	119	46	122	50
Himachal Pradesh	153	43	184	57
Punjab	143	38	182	48
Haryana	138	51	180	59
Delhi		33		35
Rajasthan	221	60	266	79
Uttar Pradesh	271	71	344	87
Bihar	163	60	187	68
Assam	213	79	207	87
West Bengal	131	37	131	38
Jharkhand		52		66
Odisha	219	76	227	79
Chhattisgarh		52		70

(*Continued*)

Table A2.8 *(Continued)*

State	Male		Female	
	1970–75*	2010	1970–75	2010
Madhya Pradesh	237	79	264	85
Gujarat	222	52	248	60
Maharashtra	167	31	174	35
Andhra Pradesh	195	46	194	51
Karnataka	151	43	157	47
Kerala	94	14	99	16
Tamil Nadu	197	26	193	28

Note: *For Jammu & Kashmir and Rajasthan the figures refer to 1972–75; for Karnataka and Kerala to 1971–75 and for Bihar and West Bengal to 1981–85.
Source: For 1970–75, based on life tables, Registrar General (2010) (For the years 1970–75); Registrar General (2012a) (For the year 2010).

Table A2.9 Net Inter-censal Inter-state Migration in India, 1991–2001 and 2001–11

State	Net Migration Rate (per 1,000 per annum)	
	1991–2001	2001–11 (Indirect)
Jammu & Kashmir	–0.4	8.0
Himachal Pradesh	1.0	0.3
Punjab	1.7	1.3
Chandigarh	21.4	3.9
Uttaranchal	0.4	4.5
Haryana	4.1	0.5
Delhi	18.7	5.8
Rajasthan	–0.6	–2.3
Uttar Pradesh	–2.0	–2.9
Bihar	–2.7	0.5
Sikkim	5.9	–2.3
Arunachal Pradesh	7.2	6.9
Nagaland	–1.4	–8.8
Manipur	–1.4	–1.1
Mizoram	–0.1	8.5
Tripura	1.0	3.9

State	Net Migration Rate (per 1,000 per annum)	
	1991–2001	2001–11 (Indirect)
Meghalaya	0.8	7.2
Assam	–0.7	–0.4
West Bengal	0.4	0.7
Jharkhand	–0.5	1.7
Odisha	–0.7	0.4
Chhattisgarh	–0.6	2.4
Madhya Pradesh	0.0	–1.6
Gujarat	1.7	1.3
Daman & Diu	44.1	29.0
Dadra & Nagar Haveli	32.6	21.3
Maharashtra	3.0	2.8
Andhra Pradesh	–0.3	–1.2
Karnataka	0.3	1.1
Goa	8.0	1.1
Lakshadweep	6.4	–5.7
Kerala	–0.6	–4.1
Tamil Nadu	–0.7	5.0
Puducherry	8.8	15.2
Andaman & Nicobar Islands.	7.9	–5.1

Source: 1991–2001: Office of the Registrar General and Census Commissioner, India (2006e): 2001–2011: Indirect estimates computed by residual method using SRS natural increase and inter-censal growth.

References

Alagh, Y.K. 2004. *An Overview: State of the Indian Farmer—A Millennium Study Vol. 1*. New Delhi: Academic Foundation.

Bhalla, G.S. 2007. *Indian Agriculture since Independence*. New Delhi: National Book Trust.

Bhat, P.N. 2002. 'Returning a Favor: Reciprocity Between Female Education and Fertility in India', *World Development,* 30(10): 1791–1803.

Bloom, David, D. Canning, and J. Sevilla. 2003. *The Demographic Dividend: A New Perspective on Economic Consequences of Population Change*. Santa Monica CA: The Rand Corporation.

Department of Family Welfare. 1993. *Family Welfare Programme in India, Yearbook, 1989–90*. New Delhi: Ministry of Health and Family Welfare.

Dyson, Tim. 2004. 'India's Population—The Future', in Tim Dyson, Robert Cassen, and Leela Visaria (eds.), *Twenty-first Century India: Population, Economy, Human Development, and the Environment*. New York: Oxford University Press. pp. 74–107.

Goyal, R.P. 1988. *Marriage Age in India*. New Delhi: B.R. Publishing.

International Institute for Population Studies (IIPS). 1995. *National Family Health Survey (NFHS), India, 1992–93*. Mumbai: IIPS.

International Institute for Population Sciences (IIPS) and ORC Macro. 2000. *National Family Health Survey (NFHS-2), India, 1998–99*. Mumbai: IIPS.

International Institute for Population Sciences (IIPS) and Macro International. 2007. *National Family Health Survey (NFHS-3), India, 2005–06*. Mumbai: IIPS.

Jain, S.P. 1982. 'Mortality Trends and Differentials', in *Population of India, Country Monograph Series No.10, ST/ESCAP/220*. New York: ESCAP. U.N. pp. 135–157.

James, K.S. 2008. 'Glorifying Malthus: Current Debate on "Demographic Dividend" in India', *Economic and Political Weekly*, 38: 63–69.

Kulkarni, P.M. 2010. 'Demographic Changes, Opportunities and Challenges in India', in Moneeer Alam and Armando Barrientos (eds.), *Demographics, Employment and Old Age Security and Challenges in South Asia*. New Delhi: Macmillan. pp. 25–36.

Ministry of Agriculture. 2009. *Agricultural Statistics at a Glance 2009*. New Delhi: Directorate of Economics and Statistics, Ministry of Agriculture.

Ministry of Finance. 2012. *Economic Survey, 2011–12*. New Delhi: Ministry of Finance.

National Sample Survey Organisation (NSSO). 2009. *Employment and Unemployment Situation in India 2007–08, NSS 64th Round*. New Delhi: NSSO.

———. 2011. *Key Indicators of Employment and Unemployment in India 2009–10, NSS 66th Round*. New Delhi: NSSO.

Office of the Registrar General and Census Commissioner, India. 2011. Provisional Population Totals, Paper 1 of 2011: Census of India 2011, Series 1-India. New Delhi: Controller of Publications.

Office of the Registrar General and Census Commissioner 2013. *Census of India 2011: Primary Census Abstract: Data Highlights, India, Series 1*. New Delhi: Controller of Publications.

Office of the Registrar General and Census Commissioner 2013. CD. Social and Cultural Tables, Table C–9, Census of India. New Delhi: Office of Registrar General and Census Commissioner.

Planning Commission. 2012. *Press Note on Poverty Estimates 2009–10*. New Delhi: Press Information Bureau, Govt. of India. Available at www.pib.nic.in (accessed 10 March, 2012).

Population Foundation of India and Population Reference Bureau. 2007. *The Future Population of India—A Long-Range Demographic View*. New Delhi: Population Foundation of India.

Pratham. 2012. *Annual Status of Education Report (Rural) 2011—ASER 2011 (Provisional)*. Mumbai: Pratham.

Registrar General. 1998. *State Profile 1991—India Census of India*. New Delhi: Controller of Publications.

———. 2001. *Provisional Population Totals, Paper 1 of 2001: Census of India 2001, Series 1—India*. New Delhi: Controller of Publications.

———. 2002. *Sample Registration System Statistical Report, 1999*. New Delhi: Controller of Publications.

———. 2003. *Sample Registration System Statistical Report, 2000. Report No.5 of 2003*. New Delhi: Controller of Publications.

———. 2004a. *Report and Tables on Age, C-14, C-14SC, C–14ST, Series 1—India*. New Delhi: Controller of Publications.

———. 2004b. *Sample Registration System Statistical Report, 2001. Report No.1 of 2004*. New Delhi: Controller of Publications.

———. 2004c. *Sample Registration System Statistical Report, 2002. Report No.3 of 2004*. New Delhi: Controller of Publications.

———. 2005a. *Slum Population. Vol. I Census of India 2001, Series 1—India*. New Delhi: Controller of Publications.

———. 2005b. *Sample Registration System Statistical Report, 2003. Report No.2 of 2005*. New Delhi: Controller of Publications.

———. 2006a. *Population Projections for India and States 2001–2026, Report of the Technical Group on Population Projections*. New Delhi: Controller of Publications.

———. 2006b. *General Population Tables, India, States and Union territories (Tables A–1 to A–3) Part I: Census of India 2001, Series 1—India*. New Delhi: Controller of Publications.

———. 2006c. *Sample Registration System Statistical Report, 2004. Report No.1 of 2006*. New Delhi: Controller of Publications.

———. 2006d. *Sample Registration System Statistical Report, 2005. Report No. 2 of 2006*. New Delhi: Controller of Publications.

———. 2006e. *Migration Data Highlights: Migration Tables D1, D2 D3: Census of India 2001*. New Delhi: Controller of Publications.

———. 2007. *Sample Registration System Statistical Report, 2006. Paper No.4 of 2007*. New Delhi: Controller of Publications.

———. 2008a. *Marital Status and Age at Marriage- An Analysis of 2001 Census data: Census of India 2001, Series 1—India*. New Delhi: Controller of Publications.

———. 2008b. *Sample Registration System Statistical Report, 2007. Paper No. 2 of 2008*. New Delhi: Controller of Publications.

Registrar General 2009. *Sample Registration System Statistical Report, 2008. Paper No. 1 of 2009*. New Delhi: Controller of Publications.

———. 2010. *Compendium of India's Fertility and Mortality Indicators 1971–2007: Based on the Sample Registration System (SRS)*. New Delhi: Office of the Registrar General.

———. 2011a. *Provisional Population Totals, Paper 1 of 2011: Census of India 2011, Series 1—India*. New Delhi: Controller of Publications.

———. 2011b. *Sample Registration System Statistical Report, 2009. Report No. 1 of 2011*. New Delhi: Controller of Publications.

———. 2012a. *Sample Registration System Statistical Report, 2010. Report No. 1 of 2012*. New Delhi: Controller of Publications.

———. 2012b. *Sample Registration System Based Abridged Life Tables*. Available at www.censusindia.gov.in.

Rele, J.R., 1982. 'Trends and Differentials in Fertility', in *Population of India, Country Monograph Series No.10, ST/ESCAP/220 pp 91–108*. New York: ESCAP, U.N.

Tendulkar Committee. 2009. Report of the Expert Group to Review the Methodology for Estimation of Poverty. New Delhi: Planning Commission, Government of India.

United Nations. 2011. *World Population Prospects: the 2010 Revision*. New York: U.N., Dept. of Economic and Social Affairs, Population Division. Available at www.esa.un.org/unpd.wpp (accessed 10 March, 2012).

Visaria, P. 1968. *Sex Ratio of India's Population, 1961 Census Monograph*. Delhi: Controller of Publications.

———. 1996. 'Structure of the Indian Work Force, 1961–1994', *Indian Journal of Labour Economics*, 39(4): 725–740.

3

Sexual and Reproductive Health

Current Status and Future Needs

Shireen J. Jejeebhoy

K.G. Santhya

India's sexual, reproductive, and newborn health situation has improved considerably in recent decades. The maternal mortality ratio and the Infant Mortality Rate (IMR) have, for example, declined, contraceptive prevalence and skilled attendance at delivery have increased, and HIV prevalence estimates suggest that the situation is not as dire as assumed earlier. However, while levels of these indicators have undeniably improved, the pace of change remains slow and on many indicators it is unlikely that India will meet the milestones set by its National Population Policy, the IXth Five Year Plan, or the Millennium Development Goals (MDGs).

There have been, however, a number of initiatives intended to accelerate the pace of improvements in the reproductive health situation. Political commitment has been articulated in a number of programmes, including the National Rural Health Mission(NRHM), the introduction of the *Janani Suraksha Yojana* (JSY), the Accredited Social

Health Activist (ASHA) scheme, and the Adolescent Reproductive and Sexual Health Strategy (ARSH), all of which are intended to address the needs of the most vulnerable.

Policies and laws affecting sexual and reproductive health have been outlined in Chapter 1. This chapter reviews key programmes and describes what is known about India's sexual and reproductive health situation, and highlights remaining challenges, at individual, programme, and policy levels, that must be overcome to accelerate the pace of improvement in this situation.

Key Programmes Addressing Sexual and Reproductive Health

As is well known, programmes in the area of sexual and reproductive health underwent significant changes since the 1990s, notably with regard to addressing the needs of the underserved, addressing previously neglected issues and strengthening a focus on informed choice and reproductive rights. A number of programmes have been implemented, including the Reproductive and Child Health Programme, the NRHM (2005–12), the JSY (launched in 2005), and the National AIDS Prevention and Control Programme (NACP-III, 2007–12). Below we describe the key elements of key programmes.

Key Programmes: The NRHM

NRHM was launched in 2005 with the intention of providing accessible, affordable, and accountable quality health services to all, including the poorest and those residing in the most remote rural areas of the country. It marks a clear commitment to improving maternal, newborn, and child health. Indeed, its goals, similar to those of the National Population Policy, are to reduce the maternal mortality ratio to 100 per 100,000 births and infant mortality to 30 per 1,000 live births, to attain universal access to women's health services and achieve population stabilization Total Fertility Rate (TFR) of 2.1, gender and demographic balance (Ministry of Health and Family Welfare 2005a). The main focus of the NRHM has been on improving the public health infrastructure including the construction or upgrading of facilities; improving the availability of critical health care providers including the provision of an additional Auxiliary Nurse Midwive (ANM) at each sub-centre, three staff nurses at Primary Health Centre (PHC) level in 24×7 PHCs, and additional specialists and paramedical staff at Community Health Centres (CHCs), contractual appointments of medical and paramedical staff as necessary and empowering PRIs and Rogi Kalyan Samitis to ensure the presence of providers at health facilities; and the establishment of a network of some 4 lakh community health workers or ASHAs, to act as a link between communities and the health system (Ministry of Health and Family Welfare 2005a). A broad range of services are provided through the network of facilities, including delivery, safe abortion, treatment of reproductive tract infections(RTIs) and family planning services. The need to train a wide cadre of providers; provide multi-skill training to medical officers, ANMs, and paramedics; and address behaviour change communication needs as well as adolescent health needs are clearly recognized.

The NRHM proposed several measures to enhance access to services and has taken bold steps in this direction. It proposed task shifting and task sharing by encouraging the placement of AYUSH physicians in PHCs and empowering them to provide AYUSH and allopathic treatment. It has initiated the upgrading of skills enabling general physicians to provide emergency obstetric care including caesarean-section deliveries and trained ANMs to manage basic obstetric emergencies when doctors are not available (for example the provision of injectable antibiotics to treat postpartum infection, the provision of anti-hypertensive medication in cases of pre-eclampsia or uterine evacuations in cases of incomplete abortion) and involved nurses-midwives in specialized obstetric and contraceptive tasks.

Efforts to serve the urban poor have also been undertaken, although the proposed National Urban Health Mission, designed for this purpose in a total of 430 cities with populations of 100,000 and above has not yet been launched (Ministry of Health and Family Welfare 2008; 2010a). Under the RCH-2 programme's urban health programme, the focus is on providing quality integrated primary health care services in poor urban communities, strengthening the existing urban health infrastructure by upgrading existing facilities or providing new facilities in urban slums not covered, supporting the development of a referral system for institutional deliveries, emergency obstetric care and sterilization services, involving the NGO or private sector in the provision of health care or referral system for the urban poor, and ensuring that services become integrated with the existing health infrastructure. In large cities, the focus is on improving the quality of services. Activities focus on 395 cities with populations of 1 to 10 lakhs (as per the 2001 census), through a two tier model. Tier 1 comprises urban health centres, managed by a medical officer, one or more ANMs, and community link volunteers to act as a link between the community and the health system; facilities provide only out-patient services. Tier 2 comprises the referral facility, providing a range of services including delivery, emergency obstetric care and sterilization. Public-private partnerships and links with private hospitals are also proposed to enhance access to services among the urban poor. For both tiers, the RCH-2 programme envisages ensuring infrastructure and equipment, need based drugs and supplies, and support for services to be provided by NGOs (Ministry of Health and Family Welfare 2005b).

Key Programmes: Improving Maternal and Newborn Health

Several existing schemes have been revamped and new schemes have been launched to improve maternal and newborn health under the NRHM as well as through other sources. A major initiative under the NRHM is the JSY, the largest conditional cash transfer programme in the world in terms of the number of beneficiaries, currently implemented in all states and UTs with a special focus on low performing states (Ministry of Health and Family Welfare 2006). Under the scheme, in low performing states, all pregnant women—irrespective of age, parity, and economic status—who undergo institutional delivery in a government health facility or accredited private facility in rural areas are given Rs. 1,400, and in urban areas, Rs. 1,000. Additionally, ASHAs who assist pregnant women in accessing maternal health services are provided an incentive amount of Rs. 600 and Rs. 200 in rural and urban areas, respectively. In high performing states in contrast, the scheme is restricted to women bearing up to two live births, women aged 19 and older and those belonging to families registered as Below the Poverty Line. In both low and high performing states poor pregnant women, aged 19 years and above, who prefer to deliver at home are entitled to cash assistance of Rs. 500/- per delivery for up to two live births (Ministry of Health and Family Welfare 2006).

Another innovation of the NRHM, with huge potential for improving maternal and newborn care, is the implementation of the ASHA scheme. This scheme aims for each village or large habitat to be served by an ASHA who is selected by the panchayat and acts as the interface between the community and the public health system. The ASHA is expected to have at least eight years of education and reside in the village. She is compensated on the basis of her performance in the promotion of universal immunization, referral and escorting women for RCH services, and raising awareness of health promoting practices. She is also expected to act as a depot holder for essential provisions including ORS, IFA, disposable delivery kits, oral pills and condoms, and is entrusted with such responsibilities as (i) identifying pregnant women and facilitating their registration for ANC; (ii) ensuring that pregnant women receive at least three antenatal check-ups including TT injections and IFA tablets; (iii) identifying a functional government health facility or an accredited private health facility for referral and delivery; (iv) counselling pregnant women to undergo an institutional delivery; (v) arranging transport for pregnant women to reach the health centre for delivery or treatment of complications; (vi) escorting pregnant women to a pre-determined health facility and staying with them till they are discharged; (vii) counselling women about breastfeeding the newborn within one-hour of delivery and its continuation till 3–6 months; (viii) arranging immunization of the newborn till age of 14 weeks; (ix) making a postpartum visit within 7 days of delivery to track the mother's health after delivery and facilitate obtaining care; and (x) promoting family planning services (Ministry of Health and Family Welfare 2006).

The NRHM also places emphasis on the upgrading and strengthening of facilities and infrastructure. All PHCs are to provide basic emergency obstetric care, and half of all PHCs are to be upgraded into round the clock facilities. Also, 3,222 CHCs are to be upgraded into 24 hour First Referral Unit (FRU) with an anaesthetist posted at each such FRU; these would include facilities for caesarean sections, and blood transfusion. Transport facilities are to be readily available. In-service courses in emergency obstetric care for general medical officers have been instituted with the aim of deploying them in district hospitals and CHCs.

Supplementing the schemes implemented by the NRHM is the recently introduced Indira Gandhi Matritva Sahyog Yojana (IGMSY) that supplements JSY entitlements among women in 52 districts of the country, and is implemented by the (Ministry of Women and Child Development 2010). The cash incentive is larger than that provided in the JSY: Rs 4,000. Moreover, not all women are eligible: for example, the scheme is applicable only for women aged 19 and above for their first two live births and on condition that they fulfil a range of conditions. Cash transfers are made at three points: Rs 1,500 is provided at the end of the second trimester to women who had registered their pregnancy within four months, had at least one antenatal check-up, had taken IFA and TT, and had attended at least one counselling session. A second instalment of Rs 1,500 is provided three months following delivery to women who have registered the birth of their child, have immunized the infant and who attend growth monitoring and counselling sessions. The third instalment of Rs 1,000 is provided six months following delivery to those women who have breastfed exclusively for six months and provided complementary feeling thereafter, whose infant has received all immunization and who have attended growth monitoring and counselling sessions as above. While the scheme has been initiated very recently, it is not clear how payments will be made or the achievement of conditions verified.

In the area of newborn health, emphasis has been placed on implementing the integrated management of neonatal and childhood illness (IMNCI) package. The IMNCI package targets care of the newborns and young infants aged less than 2 months and care of infants aged between 2 months and 5 years. Interventions for newborns and infants aged less than 2 months focus on keeping the newborn warm, initiation of breastfeeding immediately, cord, skin and eye care, recognition and management of illness in newborn and immunization. Home visits are an integral part of these interventions. Interventions for infants aged between 2 months and 5 years emphasize the management of infant and childhood illness such as diarrhoea, acute respiratory infections, malaria, and so on; prevention and management of iron and Vitamin A deficiency; counselling on feeding and immunization (Ministry of Health and Family Welfare n.d.). In 2009, a new training programme was launched on Basic Newborn Care and Resuscitation that addresses important interventions for newborns, such as, the prevention of hypothermia and infection, early initiation of breastfeeding and basic newborn resuscitation (Ministry of Health and Family Welfare 2010b).

Key Programmes: Reducing Unmet Need for Contraception

To increase access to contraceptive services and reduce the unmet need for contraception, several strategies have been initiated under the RCH Programme 2 of the NRHM. A major focus has been on increasing the pool of public sector providers, for example, by ensuring that at least one medical officer trained in providing sterilization method is available in each CHC or PHC that has an operation theatre facility, and by providing skill-based clinical training for Lady Health Visitors (LHVs) and ANMs in the area of Intrauterine Contraceptive Devices (IUCD) insertion and removal, counselling on the lactational amenorrhea method (LAM), the standard days method (SDM) and the provision of emergency contraception. Likewise, accredited private facilities and empanelled private health care providers have been covered under the revised compensation scheme and the National Family Planning Insurance Scheme to promote public-private partnerships in family planning services. To address demand-side barriers, compensation payments were increased in all states in 2007, the National Family Planning Insurance Scheme was introduced in 2005 to compensate acceptors of sterilization or his/her nominee in the event of failures, complications or death following sterilization, and satisfied users have been roped in to serve as promoters of various services (for example, the Prerna Strategy promoted under the JSKY. Efforts have also focused on expanding the choice and operational research studies to assess the feasibility of immediate postpartum insertion of IUCD and introduction of multi load copper 375 IUCD are underway. (Ministry of Health and Family Welfare 2010b).

Key Programmes: Preventing Unsafe Abortion

Over the last forty years, following the enactment of the Medical Termination of Pregnancy (MTP) Act of 1971, women in India have been entitled to legal abortion services in registered facilities and by certified providers (Government of India 1971). In 2002, medical abortion (the mifepristone-misoprostol combination) was approved for use for the termination of early pregnancies by the Drugs Controller of India, further facilitating women's access to abortion. Women have the right to access abortions across a range of situations: when the mother's life is at risk or when her physical or mental health is compromised; in case of rape; if the pregnancy is likely to result in the birth of a child with physical or mental abnormalities; and if the pregnancy is the result of contraceptive failure. Besides, abortions may be performed up to 20 weeks of gestation and the consent of the husband or guardian is not required for adult women (aged 18 and above). To curb the incidence of sex selective abortion, the PNDT Act, passed in 1994, and the PCPNDT Act amended in 2002, have banned pre-conception, pre-implantation, and prenatal procedures for sex determination in the country (Ministry of Health and Family Welfare 1994).

Concerted efforts have been made to increase access to safe abortions. The National Population Policy recommended expanding the provision of abortion to the primary health centre level. Certification procedures have been rationalized, training of medical officers in manual vacuum aspiration has been expanding, medical abortion was legalized, and rules and regulations amended so that abortions can now be undertaken by certified providers in unregistered facilities as long as they have access to a registered facility for back-up (Government of India 2003). The NRHM operational guidelines indicate that all 24×7 PHCs and CHCs should provide manual vaccum aspiration (MVA) up to 8 weeks of pregnancy and medical abortion up to 7 weeks of pregnancy; CHCs functioning as FRUs must provide, in addition, second trimester abortions as per the MTP Act and services for the management of all post-abortion complications (Ministry of Health and Family Welfare 2010c). Even so, there is a recognition that bold steps are needed to ensure access to safe abortion services;

an expert group has been formed that has made recommendations for the amendments to the MTP Act in this regard.

Key Programmes: Management of Reproductive Tract and Sexually Transmitted Infections (STIs)

Expanding access to services for prevention, screening and management of RTIs/STIs has been a thrust area under the Reproductive Child Health Programme 2 and the NACP-III. Under the RCH-2 programme, RTI/STI services are to be made available at PHCs, CHCs, FRUs, and district hospitals (Ministry of Health and Family Welfare 2005b). The NACP-III contains a number of strategies to expand the provision of RTI/STI services and emphasis has been on the Enhanced Syndrome Case Management approach with minimal laboratory tests. The Strategy and Implementation Plan (2006–2011) makes a strong argument for expanding access to the package of STI management services both in general population groups and among groups exhibiting high risk behaviours. It seeks to strengthen STI/RTI service provision at all public health facilities at district level and above. The Strategy and Implementation Plan also acknowledges that expanding access to services will entail engaging the private sector in the provision of services; for example, the preferred private provider scheme was launched in 2009 under which high risk group populations receive free STI/RTI treatment and providers receive a token fee of Rs 50 for each consultation (National AIDS Control Organisation 2010a).

In order to systematize diagnostic criteria and strengthen the convergence of activities conducted under the RCH-2 and NACP programmes, national guidelines are available that focus on the prevention, management, and control of RTIs/STIs, and serve as a resource for programme managers and service providers in both the RCH-2 and NACP-III programmes. Guidelines enable RCH service providers to organize effective case management services through the public health system, especially though the network of 24×7 PHCs and CHCs. At the same time, the guidelines offer direction to NACP-III programme managers regarding the upscaling of targeted interventions particularly for sex workers, and the provision of quality of STI management services (Ministry of Health and Family Welfare 2007).

Key Programmes: HIV/AIDS

The AIDS Control programme is now in its third phase (NACP-III, 2007–2012), with a five-fold increase in funding (from \$0.5 billion to \$2.5 billion). The primary goal of NACP-III is to halt and reverse the epidemic by integrating programmes for prevention, care, support, and treatment, notably, prevention of new infections in high risk groups and the general population, provision of care, support and treatment to people living with HIV/AIDS, as well as by strengthening infrastructure and information management systems (National AIDS Control Organisation 2006a). More than 70 per cent of its resources go towards the scaling up of prevention efforts, notably among groups at highest risk. Prevention activities are diverse: they include targeted interventions for high risk groups; interventions for bridge populations such as truckers, prison inmates, and migrants, maintaining integrated counselling and Testing Centres, initiating blood safety measures, as well as awareness building and social mobilization and condom promotion. Indeed, the goal is to increase condom usage to 3.5 billion pieces by 2012, ensure easy access to condoms, through increasing the number of condom outlets to 3 million, with a special focus on 294 high priority districts. Behaviour change communication is stressed and campaigns are envisaged that normalize condom use and position condoms as a new age norm (National AIDS Control Organisation 2010b; 2010c).

Care and support activities are also stressed. For example, ARV therapy is to be available to all those in need. Other activities include strengthening of PLHA networks including support to 350 community care centres and mainstreaming HIV issues into government schemes and activities as well as into the corporate and civil society sectors (National AIDS Control Organisation 2010a).

The Sexual and Reproductive Health Situation

Maternal and Newborn Health

Maternal mortality

The maternal mortality ratio has declined over the course of this century, from 301 per 100,000 births in 2001–03 to 254 per 100,000 births in 2004–06 and further to 212 in 2007–09 (Office of Registrar

General, India 2009; 2011), that is, an average decline of about 15 deaths per 100,000 births per year. Even so, the level remains high: about 67,000 maternal deaths take place are estimated to take place each year (Ministry of Health and Family Welfare 2009a; Rajan, Machanda, and Nagarajan 2010). Most recent estimates, made by the WHO, suggest that the maternal mortality ratio has fallen further to 200 per 100,000 births in 2010 and that almost one fifth (19 per cent) of maternal deaths globally take place in India (World Health Organisation 2012).

The National Population Policy's goal of reducing the maternal mortality ratio to 100 per 100,000 live births by 2010 was not reached; nor will the NRHM's goal of reaching this ratio by 2012. Indeed, a recent assessment concludes that if maternal mortality continues to decline at the pace observed in the period 1990 to 2004–06, the ratio will reach 153 by the year 2015 (Paul et al., 2011). State-wise disparities in maternal mortality are wide (Table A3.1). For example, as of 2007–09, the maternal mortality ratio ranged from 81 per 100,000 births in Kerala to 359 in Uttar Pradesh/Uttarakhand and 390 in Assam. Indeed, the maternal mortality ratio in such states as Assam, Bihar/Jharkhand, Madhya Pradesh/Chhattisgarh, Odisha, Rajasthan and Uttar Pradesh/Uttarakhand is about 2.4 times as high as it is in the four southern states (308 and 127, respectively).

Common causes of maternal death are those seen in most developing country settings and are largely preventable (Table 3.1). Estimates derived from data on maternal deaths, collected through the Sample Registration System (SRS) using post-death verbal autopsies, provide a useful picture of the causes of death in the period 2001–03 (Registrar General of India 2006). Haemorrhage was the leading cause of maternal death, accounting for 38 per cent of all maternal deaths. Other identifiable causes of death during pregnancy, childbirth and the postpartum period were sepsis (11 per cent), unsafe abortions (8 per cent), obstructed labour (5 per cent) and hypertensive disorders (5 per cent).

Neonatal mortality

India did not achieve the goal set by the National Population Policy to reach an INR of 30 per 1,000 live births by 2010, nor

Table 3.1 Causes of Maternal Death, 1998 and 2001–03

Cause	1998 %	2001–03 %
Direct causes		
Haemorrhage	30	38
Puerperal sepsis	16	11
Obstructed labour	10	5
Abortion	9	8
Toxaemia	8	5
Other	25	34

Source: Registrar General of India (2000; 2006).

is it likely to achieve the NRHM goal of reaching an IMR of 28 per 1,000 live births by 2012. Indeed, the neonatal mortality rate itself stood at 39.0 per 1,000 live births for the five years preceding NFHS-3 (International Institute for Population Sciences and Macro International 2007); corresponding rates were 43.4 and 48.6 in the five years preceding NFHS-2 and NFHS-1, respectively. Declines have been modest, not exceeding 1 point per year in the period 1992–3 to 2005–06. Perinatal mortality (the sum of the number of stillbirths and early neonatal deaths divided by the number of pregnancies of seven or more months duration) was 48.5 per 1,000 pregnancies. Indeed, it has been estimated that about one quarter of all neonatal deaths globally occur in India (Baqui et al. 2006). Within India, neonatal mortality accounts for two-thirds of all infant deaths (International Institute for Population Sciences and Macro International 2007; Lahariya and Paul 2010). Half of all deaths occur by day three suggesting that greater coverage of antenatal, delivery and early postpartum interventions is critical to reduce neonatal deaths (Baqui et al. 2006; Lahariya and Paul 2010).

The neonatal mortality varies considerably by state as well (Table A3.1). While Goa and Kerala reported a neonatal mortality rate (for the five-year period preceding NFHS-3) of 8.8 and 11.5, respectively, some six states reported neonatal mortality rates of 45 or more per 1,000 births (Chhattisgarh 51, Madhya Pradesh 45, Jharkhand 49, Odisha 45, Assam 46, Uttar Pradesh 48). Differences were equally wide in the case of perinatal mortality: Goa and Kerala reported rates of 11–12 per 1,000 pregnancies, compared with rates above 55 in six states (Chhattisgarh 64, Uttar Pradesh 60, Bihar 59, Jharkhand 58, Odisha 56, Assam 63) (International Institute for Population Sciences and Macro International 2007).

Socio-demographic disparities were also wide as evident from Figure 3.1. Neonatal mortality rates were considerably higher among adolescents (54/1,000) than among those aged 20–49 (34–43/1,000); disparities in perinatal mortality rates were also wide (67/1,000 among adolescents and 43–51/1,000 among older women). Differences by education, wealth status, rural-urban residence, antenatal care and perceived small size at birth were also pronounced (see also Paul et al. 2011).

Both neonatal and perinatal mortality are largely the result of inadequate or inappropriate care during pregnancy, childbirth or the first critical hours after birth. Major identifiable causes of neonatal mortality include neonatal infections (pneumonia, tetanus, sepsis, and diarrhoea), prematurity and birth asphyxia, accounting for 35 per cent, 24 per cent, and 18 per cent of all deaths nationally (Paul et al. 2011; Baqui et al., 2006). Roughly one third of all infants (7.8 million) are born with birth weights less than 2,500 gm; low birth weight is closely linked with being underweight, stunting, and wasting in the first five years of life (Paul et al. 2011). Evidence suggests that within two to three years of the JSY programme, a reduction of about four perinatal and two neonatal deaths per 1,000 births could be attributed to the programme, suggesting the potential for steeper declines in infant mortality in the upcoming years (Lim et al. 2010).

Maternal and neonatal morbidity

Self-reported data of problems during pregnancy and complications following delivery are available for women who gave birth during the five years preceding the NFHS survey (International Institute for Population Sciences and Macro International 2007) and in the 12 months preceding the 2009 Coverage Evaluation Survey (CES) (United Nations Children's Fund 2010). Findings must be interpreted cautiously as self-reported morbidity experiences may be influenced by recall problems (as they were collected retrospectively) or by women's tendency to consider many conditions as normal events in a woman's life.

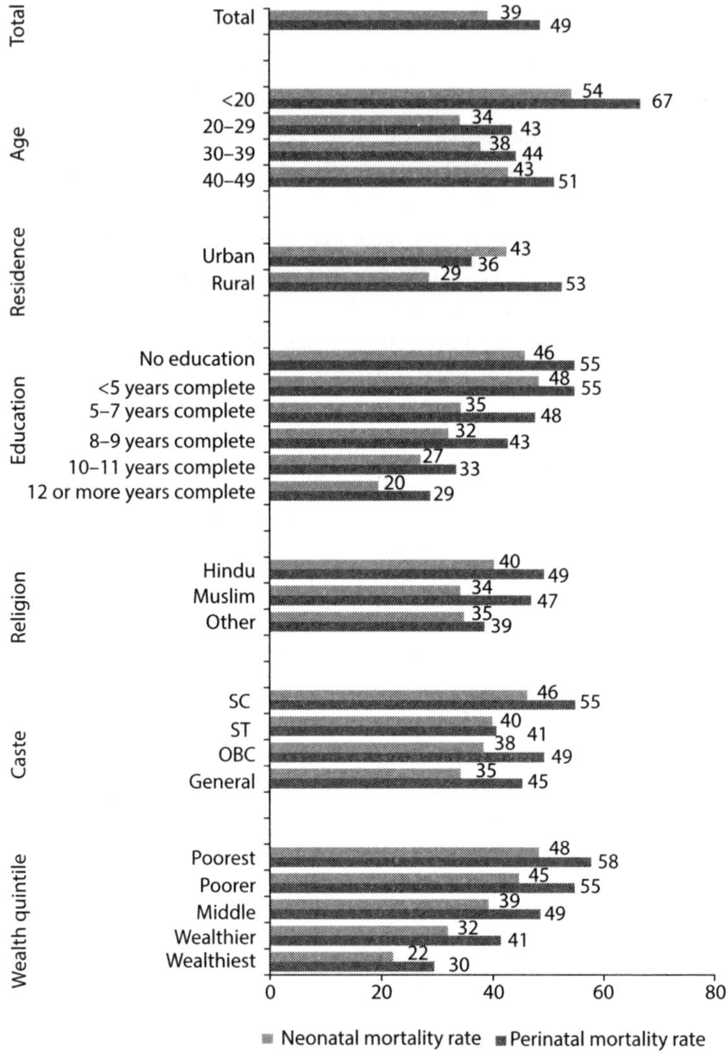

Figure 3.1 Neonatal and Perinatal Mortality Rates by Selected Background Characteristics, India, 2005–06

Source: International Institute for Population Sciences and Macro International (2007).

At the national level, findings suggest that half of all ever-married women were anaemic (56 per cent, compared to 48 per cent at the time of NFHS-2) and some 17 per cent suffered from moderate or severe anaemia (no change since NFHS-2). Considerable state-wise variation is evident in percentages with moderate to severe anaemia, ranging from 7 per cent in Kerala to 15–25 per cent in several northern, central, eastern, and north-eastern states. There has been little improvement, moreover, in percentages experiencing serious morbidity. Health problems during pregnancy, clearly exacerbated by already compromised levels of anaemia, include excessive fatigue (reported by 48 per cent of women who had a birth in the five years preceding NFHS-3), swelling of the legs, body or face (25 per cent), and convulsions (10 percent).

A comparison of findings from NFHS-2, NFHS-3 and the 2009 CES suggests that there has been little change in the percentage of women reporting the experience of haemorrhage, for example over the period 1998–99 to 2009: massive vaginal bleeding in the two months following delivery was reported by 10 per cent of women who gave birth in the 12 months preceding the (United Nations Children's Fund 2010), compared to 11–12 per cent of women who gave birth in the five years preceding NFHS-3 and the three years preceding the NFHS-2 (International Institute for Population Sciences and Macro International 2007; International Institute for Population Sciences and ORC Macro 2000). Likewise, little improvement has been observed in the experience of sepsis: the percentage of women experiencing very high fever in the two months following delivery was reported by 13–14 per cent of women who gave birth in the five years preceding NFHS-3 and the three years preceding the NFHS-2. While not recorded in large surveys, a small prospective study of pregnant women in Goa followed up to six months postpartum noted depressive disorders among 23 per cent at 6–8 weeks, and for about 12 percent at six months postpartum (Patel, Rodrigues, and DeSouza 2002).

Neonatal morbidity studies, particularly community-based ones, are relatively rare in India. Studies conducted in Gadchiroli (Bang et al. 2001; 2005) have noted a 48 per cent incidence of high-risk morbidities and a 72 per cent incidence of low-risk morbidities (those associated with a >10 per cent and <10 per cent case fatality, respectively). Leading high risk morbidities, that is, neonatal sepsis, hypothermia, and failure to suckle, were experienced by 16–17 per cent of all neonates. Leading low risk morbidities, that is, low birth weight, upper respiratory symptoms, and umbilical infection, were experienced by 20–32 per cent of all neonates. A large number of morbidities were experienced in the first week of life, however a number of infections appeared to have been acquired postpartum and attributable to environmental factors, and seasonal variation was evident in a number of morbidities.

Maternal and newborn health care utilization

We explore the extent to which maternal and newborn health care practices have changed over time, using data from NFHS (1992–93, 1998–99, and 2005–06, International Institute for Population Sciences and Macro International 2007) and the 2009 CES (United Nations Children's Fund 2010). We note that while findings from NFHS refer to women with a live birth in the 3–5 years preceding the survey drawn from a sample of women aged 15–49, CES data were collected from women who had delivered in the 12 months preceding the interview to assess maternal health care utilization patterns, and those with an infant aged 12–23 months to assess newborn care practices; we therefore advise caution in interpreting changes in indicators. Table 3.2 presents the percentages of women who received care during pregnancy, delivery and the postpartum period during 1992–93 to 2009, and highlights that while health care utilization has been increasing over the last two decades, maternal and newborn health care utilisation is, for the most part, far from adequate.

Care during the antenatal period As evident from Table 3.2, remarkable increases have been observed in the extent of care during pregnancy over the period 1992–93 to 2009, much of this increase occurred in the period following the introduction of the JSY. Even so, the achievement—even by 2009—falls far short of the goals set in the Xth Plan and to have been achieved by 2007. For example, the percentage of pregnant women who had availed of three or more antenatal check-ups increased from 52 in 2005–06 to 69 by 2009, compared to a goal of 90 by 2007; and those receiving two or more doses of tetanus toxoid increased from 76 to 87 in the same period, as against a goal of 100 (International Institute for Population Sciences and Macro International 2007; United Nations Children's

Table 3.2 Pregnancy-Related Care: The Situation 1992–93 to 2009

	1992–93[1]	1998–99[2]	2005–06[3]	2009[4]
Antenatal Care				
Women receiving any antenatal check-ups	64.6	65.8	76.9	89.6
Pregnant women receiving at least three antenatal check-ups	43.9	44.2	52.0	68.7
Pregnant women receiving ante-natal check-up in the first trimester	24.0	33.0	43.9	59.2
Pregnant women receiving two or more doses of tetanus-toxoid	53.8	66.8	76.3	86.9
Women who received all recommended components of antenatal care[5]	NA	20.0	15.0	26.5[6]
Intrapartum Care				
Women who delivered in a health facility/institution	26.1	33.6	38.7	72.9
Women whose delivery was attended by trained health personnel	35.1	42.4	46.6	76.2
Postpartum Care				
Women who received a postpartum check-up within 42 days of delivery	NA	NA	41.2	NA
Women who received a postpartum check-up within 2 days of delivery	NA	NA	37.3	NA
Women who received a postpartum check-up within 10 days of delivery	NA	NA	NA	74.4
Women who received a postpartum check-up within 3–7 days of delivery	NA	NA	NA	69.1

Source: [1]International Institute for Population Sciences (1995); [2]International Institute for Population Sciences and ORC Macro (2000); [3]International Institute for Population Sciences and Macro International (2007); [4]United Nations Children's Fund (2010); [5]3 or more antenatal check-ups, with the first check-up in the first trimester of pregnancy, two or more tetanus toxoid injections, iron and folic acid for 3 or more months; [6]3 or more antenatal check-ups, one or more tetanus toxoid injections, iron and folic acid for 3 or more months.

NA = not applicable.

Fund 2010). Indeed, as of 2009, just 27 per cent of women who had delivered in the 12 months preceding the survey had received all recommended components of antenatal care.

Wide state-wise variation is consistently evident (International Institute for Population Sciences and Macro International 2007; United Nations Children's Fund 2010). The 2009 Coverage Evaluation Survey shows, for example, that in such states as Arunachal Pradesh, Nagaland, Uttar Pradesh and Uttarakhand, more than 25 per cent had not received a single ANC service, and just 29–55 per cent had made three or more visits. In contrast, in states such as Andhra Pradesh, Goa, Karnataka, Kerala, and Tamil Nadu, over 90 per cent had made three or more visits (Table A3.2). As evident from Figure 3.2, moreover, urban and educated women, and those from general castes and economically better off households were significantly more likely, than their respective counterparts, to have made three or more visits and obtained full antenatal care.

While reasons for not obtaining any antenatal care were largely related to knowledge and attitudes, such system based factors as cost, access, and quality of care also play a role. For example, among women who had not obtained any antenatal care, most cited that care was unnecessary (56 per cent), that they were unaware of the need (15 per cent) and that a family member had objected (12 per cent); however, a considerable proportion did also cite high costs (18 per cent) and lack of access (9 per cent) and poor quality of care (5 per cent) (United Nations Children's Fund 2010).

Services provided in the course of antenatal visits also varied. Just 74–79 per cent of women who had obtained antenatal care for the birth in the year preceding the 2009 CES reported that they had been weighed, their blood pressure, urine, or blood had been tested, or that their abdomen had been examined; far fewer had been informed about danger signals (20–30 per cent), and just 58 per cent had been told where to go in case of complications. While these percentages represent an impressive increase from the situation reported among women who had delivered in the five years preceding the NFHS-3 and had received antenatal care (58–72, 15–20, and 41, respectively, had essential tests, were informed about danger

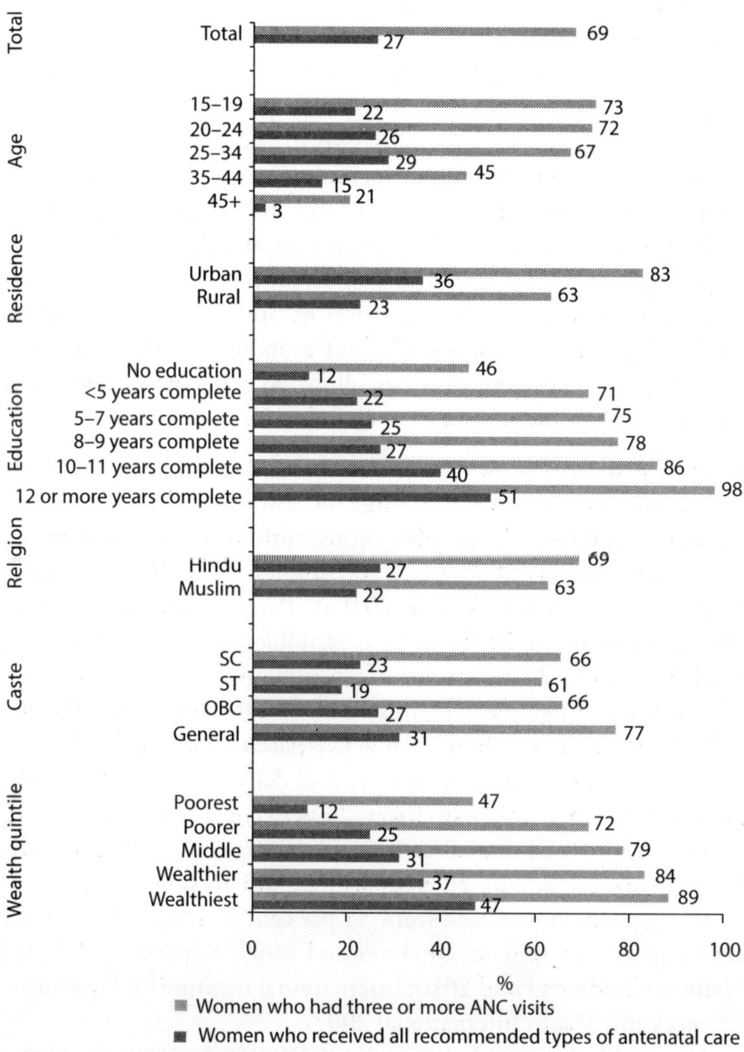

Figure 3.2 Percentage of Women Who Received Antenatal Care by Selected Background Characteristics, India, 2009
Source: United Nations Children's Fund (2010).

signals and told where to go in case of complications), receipt of basic services remains far from universal.

Small-scale studies with health care providers also confirm that service provision during antenatal visits is skewed; not much attention has been paid towards providing comprehensive information related to pregnancy care or comprehensive pregnancy-related care. For example, a study of ASHAs and ANMs in two districts in Rajasthan reports that just one-third and one-quarter had typically discussed danger signs during pregnancy and birth preparedness, respectively, with pregnant women (Santhya, Jejeebhoy, and Zavier 2011a). Not surprisingly, birth preparedness and readiness to seek care in case of complications are far from satisfactory among pregnant women, particularly among those socially and economically disadvantaged, including those residing in urban slums, as observed in a study of slum dwellers in Indore (Agarwal et al. 2010).

Delivery practices Following the introduction of the JSY, effectively late 2006, there has been a surge in institutional deliveries; for example, nationally, the number of institutional deliveries increased from 10.8 million in 2005–06 to 16.2 million by 2009–10 (Ministry of Health and Family Welfare 2010a). JSY beneficiaries increased from 0.7 million in 2005–06 to 10.2 million women in 2009–10; as of September 2010, a total of 35 million women had benefitted from the programme (Ministry of Health and Family Welfare 2010a). As Table 3.2 shows, while the pace of increase in the percentage of women reporting institutional delivery was modest in the period 1992–93 to 2005–06 (from 26 per cent to 39 per cent or 13 points), it increased dramatically to 73 per cent, or by 34 points by 2009. A similar picture emerges with regard to skilled attendance at delivery, which increased from 35 per cent in 1992–93 to 47 per cent and 76 per cent in 2005–06 and 2009, respectively (United Nations Children's Fund 2010; International Institute for Population Sciences and Macro International 2007).

Along with the spurt in institutional delivery, there has also been a significant shift from private to public sector deliveries following the introduction of the JSY programme. Indeed, much of the increase observed in institutional deliveries over the periods covered by NFHS-1, NFHS-2, and NFHS-3 was the result of increases in deliveries conducted in private sector facilities. For example, while about half of all institutional deliveries had taken place in the private sector in 2005–06, the situation had reversed by 2009, at which time almost two-thirds (64 per cent) of institutional deliveries were conducted in the *public* sector (International Institute for Population Sciences and Macro International 2007; United Nations Children's Fund, 2010). Deliveries conducted by traditional birth attendants (TBAs) also declined, from 37 per cent in 2005–06 to 19 per cent in 2009.

Wide differentials in institutional delivery and trained attendance at delivery continue to be observed by age, rural–urban residence, education, caste and wealth status; however, these differentials have narrowed considerably since the introduction of the JSY programme, as clear from Figure 3.3. For example, 54 per cent of uneducated women compared to 93 per cent of those with 12 or more years of education reported an institutional delivery in 2009, that is, a 39 point difference. In 2005–06, corresponding percentages were 18 and 86, that is, a 68 point spread (not shown in figure). In 2009, likewise, 57 per cent of women from scheduled tribes compared to 76 per cent of those from general castes reported an institutional delivery, compared to 25 per cent and 53 per cent, respectively, in 2005–06 (not shown in figure). State-wise differences also persist. As shown in Table A3.2, fewer than half of all deliveries were conducted institutionally in such states as Bihar, Chhattisgarh, Jharkhand and Nagaland in 2009, compared to almost all—98–100 per cent—in Goa, Kerala and Tamil Nadu. Similarly, 44–56 per cent of deliveries in Bihar, Chhattisgarh, Himachal Pradesh, Jharkhand, and Nagaland were assisted by a trained professional compared to more than 95 per cent in Goa, Kerala, and Tamil Nadu.

Harmful delivery practices Of serious concern is the unmonitored intrapartum oxytocin use in home and hospital deliveries, administered by untrained rural medical practitioners and perceived as a means of speeding up delivery or *dard badana* (Jeffery et al. 2007; Barnes; 2007; Iyengar et al 2009a; 2009b; Sharan, Strobino, and Ahmed 2005; Santhya et al 2011b). Studies in Rajasthan (Iyengar et al 2009a; 2009b) note that the application of forceful fundal pressure was widely practised both in home and facility deliveries.

While rates of caesarean section are not high overall (9 per cent), considerable variation in C-section rates by rural-urban status, education and wealth status is evident and suggests a trend towards unnecessary C-sections. For example, 6 per cent of rural women

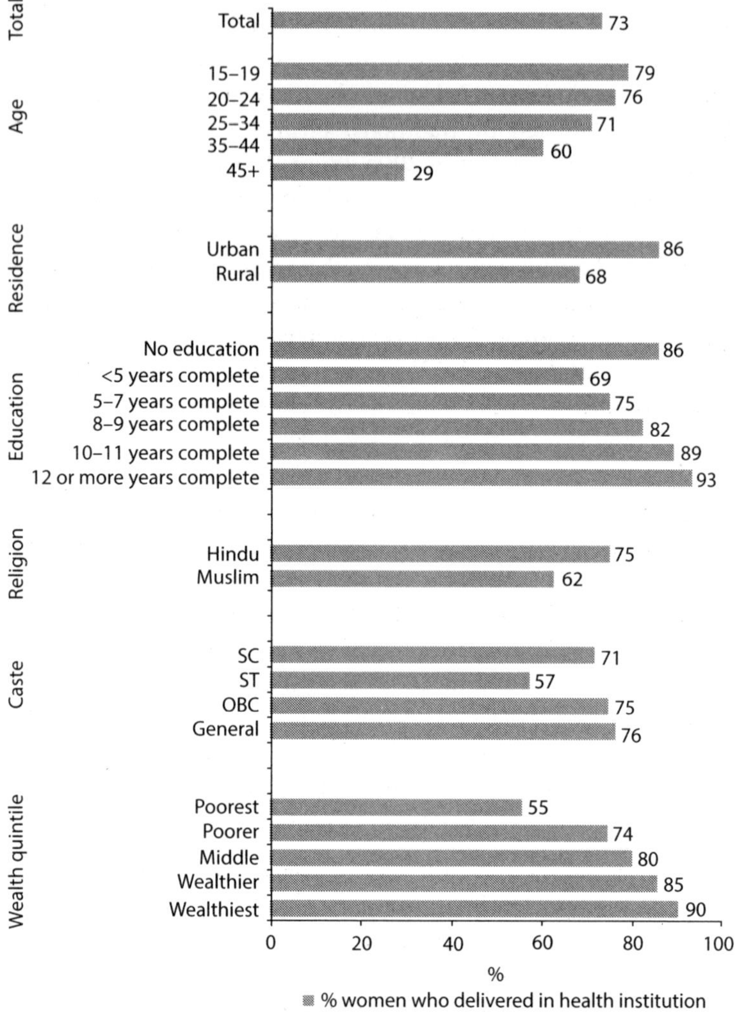

Figure 3.3 Percentage of Women Who Delivered in a Health Institution by Selected Background Characteristics, India, 2009
Source: United Nations Children's Fund (2010).

compared to 17 per cent of their urban counterparts reported a C-section; just 2 per cent of women in the lowest wealth quintile had a caesarean section delivery, compared to 26 per cent of those in the uppermost quintile. Findings suggest, moreover, a strong association between private sector deliveries and caesarean section rates: almost twice as many women who underwent their last delivery in the private sector reported a C-section delivery as did those whose delivery occurred in a public sector facility (28 per cent versus 15 per cent) (International Institute for Population Sciences and Macro International 2007). Small-scale studies have noted that the risk of undergoing a caesarean section was four or more times higher in private facilities than in public sector facilities (Mishra and Ramanathan 2002; Sreevidya and Sathiyasekaran 2003).

Postpartum care Postpartum care remains limited, although percentages of women receiving care appears to have increased. Strictly comparable indicators are not available: for example, in 2005–06, just 41 per cent of women who had delivered in the five years prior to the interview reported a check-up within two months of the delivery of their most recent birth, and only 37 per cent received a check-up in the critical first two days (International Institute for Population Sciences and Macro International 2007). In the 2009 survey, the reference period was 10 days following delivery and we find that 60 per cent of women received a check-up during this period (United Nations Children's Fund 2010). State-wise and socio-demographic differences are not available for 2009, but 2005–06 data suggest that differences were stark: experience of a postpartum check-up and a postpartum check-up in two days of delivery ranged from 12–15 per cent and 11–13 per cent, respectively, in Nagaland and Uttar Pradesh to 87–91 per cent and 85–87 per cent, respectively, in Kerala and Tamil Nadu. As in indicators of antenatal and delivery care, better educated, economically better off and urban women fared far better than their uneducated, poor and rural counterparts, respectively.

Care of the newborn Findings suggest that even as of 2009, far fewer than 90 per cent of newborns received essential care. Just two-thirds of newborns received a check-up within 24 hours of delivery (66 per cent), ranging from 61 per cent in rural areas to 78 per cent in urban areas (United Nations Children's Fund 2010). Even so, improvements in practices are evident. For example, 73 per cent of women began breastfeeding within a day of birth in 2009, compared to many fewer in 2005–06 (55 per cent); only 12 per cent had provided the infant a prelacteal feed, compared to 57 per cent in 2005–06.

Care-seeking practices for complications experienced by neonates have not been extensively documented. What is available suggests that danger signals are poorly understood, providers from whom care is sought are often untrained, and there is a care-seeking bias against girls. For example, a focused ethnographic study in slum areas of Meerut suggests that although mothers cited a number of important danger signals based on perceived severity and combinations of signs of illness, they failed to recognize the significance of such symptoms as fever and umbilical stump swelling, unless accompanied with signs like difficult breathing and blood, respectively. Care was uniformly sought from informal private practitioners (Balsara et al. 2009). Gender disparities in neonatal care seeking are observed: for every two male neonates, only one female neonate was found to have been admitted to a health facility (Paul et al. 2011). Yet another study of neonatal morbidity and care-seeking behaviours of slum and non-slum dwellers at Lucknow that recruited neonates within 48 hours of birth and followed them up at 6 weeks (+/- 15 days) reports that care seeking was significantly more likely to have been undertaken for a male than female neonate (OR = 1.24, 95 per cent CI = 1.24 to 91.99; P = 0.03) and male neonates were almost four times as likely as female neonates to have been seen by a qualified provider (OR = 3.8, 95 per cent CI = 1.05 to 13.94; P = 0.04) (Srivastava, Awasthi, and Mishra, 2008).

Family planning practices and unmet need

Contraceptive use has been increasing in India. However, there continues to be substantial unmet need for contraception, particularly among the young, the method mix remains skewed towards sterilization and the shift towards non-terminal methods is not yet apparent.

FP Use and Method Mix Nationally, both the NFHS and the District Level Household Survey, conducted in 2005–06 and 2007–08, respectively, concur that 55–60 per cent of currently married women were using some method of contraception and almost half were using a modern method of contraception (International Institute for Population Sciences and Macro International 2007; International

Table 3.3 Trends in contraceptive use, 1992–93 to 2005–06

	1992–93	1998–99	2005–06	2005–06 married men (with wife)
Any method	40.7	48.2	56.3	50.9
Any traditional method	4.2	5.4	7.8	6.8
Any modern method	36.5	42.8	48.5	44.1
Female sterilisation	27.4	34.2	37.3	30.6
Male sterilization	3.5	1.9	1.0	0.9
Oral contraceptives	1.2	2.1	3.1	3.7
IUCD	1.9	1.6	1.7	1.4
Injectables	0.0	NA	0.1	0.0
Condoms	2.4	3.1	5.2	7.3
Other	NA	NA	0.0	0.1
% non-terminal modern of all modern method use	15.1	15.9	17.9	28.3

Source: International Institute for Population Sciences (1995); International Institute for Population Sciences and ORC Macro (2000); International Institute for Population Sciences and Macro International (2007).

Institute for Population Sciences 2010). As seen in Table 3.3, although modern method use has increased substantially—from 37 per cent to 49 per cent—over the period 1992–93 and 2005–06, the increase is no more than one percent per year (International Institute for Population Sciences and Macro International 2007).

Notwithstanding the greater programme emphasis on non-terminal methods than before, the leading method of contraception continues to be female sterilization; indeed, the increase in modern method use in the 13 years between NFHS-1 and 3 is almost entirely attributable to increases in sterilization. Non-terminal method use remains limited. Indeed, just 10 per cent of married women were using a non-terminal method in 2005–06, and trends in non-terminal method use suggest little change in the share of non-terminal methods in overall modern contraceptive use in the period between 1992–93 and 2005–06 (from 15.1 per cent to 17.9 per cent).

Use of contraceptive male methods is limited. For the first time in 2005–06, direct evidence on contraception is available from both women and men. By and large, patterns reported by men resemble those reported by women (Table 3.3). Overall, contraceptive prevalence reported by men was somewhat lower than that reported by women (44 per cent versus 49 per cent reported modern method use, for example). Male sterilization and condom use were reported by just 1 per cent and 5 per cent, respectively, of women, and by 1 per cent and 7 per cent, respectively, of men. Women's reports highlight that over the 13 years between NFHS-1 and NFHS-3, male method use remained fairly constant at 5–6 per cent.

Contraceptive prevalence varied considerably by state. Percentages of women reporting any form of contraception ranged from 34 per cent in Bihar to more than 65 per cent in Andhra Pradesh, Gujarat, Himachal Pradesh, Kerala, and Maharashtra. As seen in Table A3.3, modern contraceptive use ranged, at the same time, from less than 33 per cent in such states as Assam, Bihar, Jharkhand, and Uttar Pradesh to 60 per cent or more in such states as Andhra Pradesh, Himachal Pradesh, Karnataka, Maharashtra, and Tamil Nadu.

Although female sterilization continued to be the leading modern method used in every state, the method mix also varied considerably across states. In Andhra Pradesh, for example, just 2 per cent of all women used a non-terminal or traditional method. In contrast, in West Bengal, 17 per cent of all women used a non-terminal method and 21 per cent used a traditional method; and in Punjab 24 per cent and 7 per cent, respectively, used a non-terminal and a traditional method. Among those reporting male-method use, while male sterilization rates hardly varied across states (2–6 per cent) variation was wide in the case of condom use: condom use was reported by fewer than 5 per cent of married women in most states, but reached 16 per cent in such states as Punjab and Uttarakhand, and 23 per cent in Delhi.

Differentials in contraceptive use patterns (modern and traditional) are evident with regard to socio-demographic factors as well (Figure 3.4). Percentages of women practising contraception increased steadily with age, as well as with education and wealth status. Muslim women and women from tribal households were somewhat less likely than Hindu women and those from general caste households, respectively, to have practised contraception.

Also notable is the extent to which differentials have narrowed over time. For example, in NFHS-1, there was a 25 point difference between percentages of uneducated women and those with

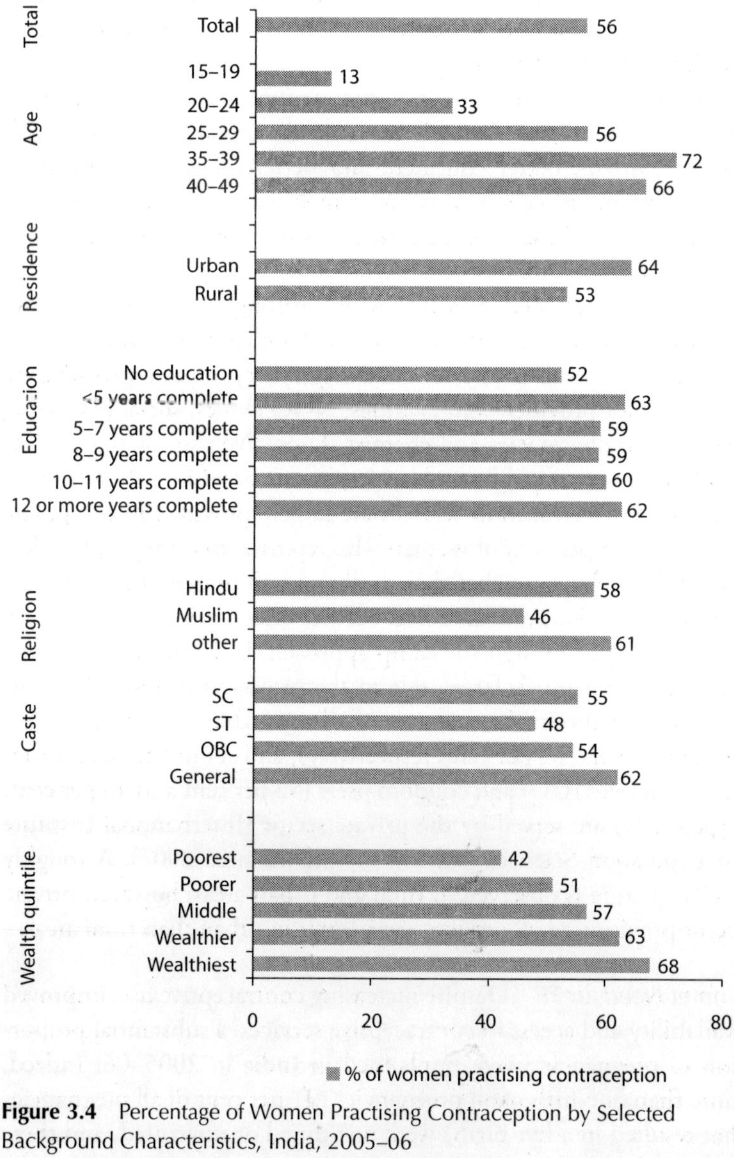

Figure 3.4 Percentage of Women Practising Contraception by Selected Background Characteristics, India, 2005–06

Source: International Institute for Population Sciences and Macro International (2007).

more than secondary schooling who were practising contraception (34 per cent and 59 per cent, respectively, not shown in figure); by 2005–06, there was just a 10 point difference (52 per cent and 62 per cent, respectively). Similar narrowing of differences were observed in the case of rural-urban residence. However, differences continued to remain wide in the case of wealth status and other indicators (see Jain and Jain 2010 for a full analysis).

The proportion of women using contraception (using a non-terminal method) also varied by socio-demographic factors, with younger, urban, better educated, and better off women practising contraception, as well as Muslim women who were practising contraception and those from general castes more likely to report non-terminal methods than others (Figure 3.5).

Contraceptive services are provided through a network of government hospitals and urban family welfare centres in urban areas, and PHCs and sub-centres in rural areas. They are also provided by private sector providers and facilities, NGO clinics, social marketing outlets, and pharmacies and chemist shops. Even so, there is a clear divide in terms of public and private sector provision of contraceptive services. Sterilization services are largely provided in the public sector: 84–85 per cent of women who reported that they had undergone tubal ligation or that their husband had undergone vasectomy reported that the procedure had been conducted in the public sector, most often through the camp approach. In contrast, the private sector played a much larger role in the provision of reversible contraceptive methods: the majority of all injectable and oral pill users (83 per cent and 64 per cent, respectively), and about half of all Intrauterine device (IUD) and condom users (52 per cent and 46 per cent, respectively) are served by the private sector (International Institute for Population Sciences and Macro International 2007). A roughly similar picture is observed in rural and urban areas; however, private sector provision of all services was greater in urban than rural areas.

Unmet Need for FP Despite increasing contraceptive use, improved availability and access to contraceptive services, a substantial proportion of pregnancies were unplanned in India in 2005–06. Indeed, more than one-fifth of all pregnancies (21 per cent of all pregnancies that resulted in a live birth) were mis-timed or unwanted, and there

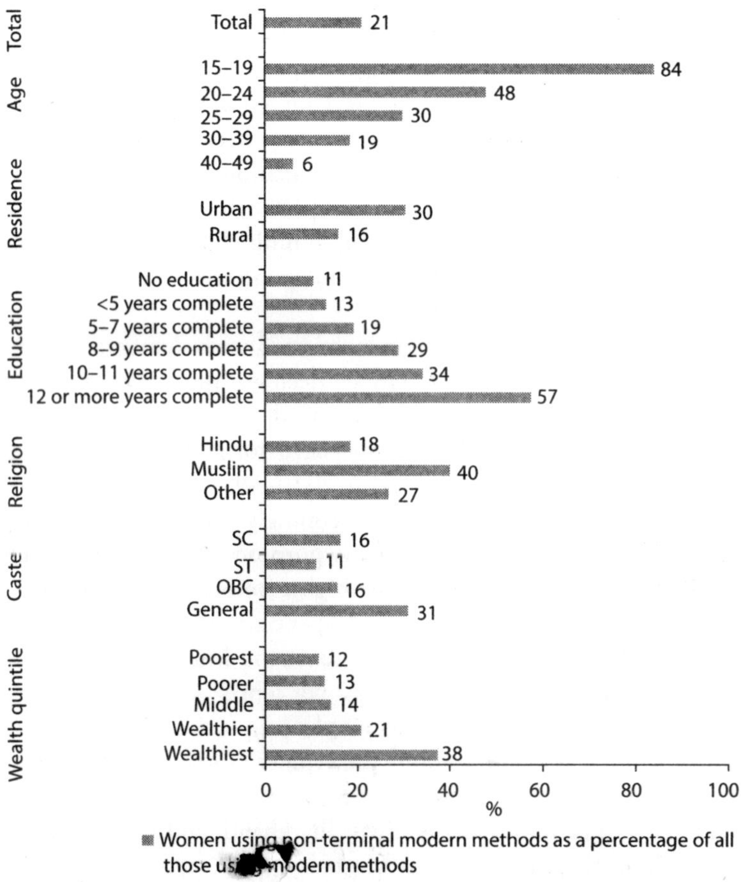

Figure 3.5 Among Currently Married Women Practising Contraception, Percentage Using a Non-Terminal Method of Contraception by Selected Background Characteristics, India, 2005–06

Source: International Institute for Population Sciences and Macro International (2007).

is no evidence that this percentage had declined over the preceding seven years (International Institute for Population Sciences and Macro International 2007; Santhya 2004). It is estimated that if all unwanted births had been eliminated, the TFR would have dropped to below replacement levels of fertility (1.9 births per woman). Moreover, several studies of abortion seekers report that a key reason for the abortion was to postpone or limit childbearing (see for example, Jejeebhoy, Zavier, and Kalyanwala 2010), clearly highlighting that there is a substantial unmet need for contraception in India.

Findings from NFHS-3 also suggest that 13 per cent of currently married women had an unmet need for contraception, a decline of 3 percentage points in the seven years between NFHS-2 and NFHS-3 (International Institute for Population Sciences and Macro International 2007). Findings suggest that while the needs of the large majority of women who wished to limit childbearing are being satisfied (89 per cent), the needs of those who wished to delay pregnancy were not (just 44 per cent).

Unmet need for contraception by selected socio-demographic factors is presented in Figure 3.6. Unmet need was most evident among young women: 27 per cent of those aged 15–19 and 21 per cent of those aged 20–24 had an unmet need for contraception, compared with 3–9 per cent of those aged 30–49. As expected, unmet need among the young was overwhelmingly for spacing methods, and that of older women for limiting purposes. Aside from age differentials, unmet need tends to be higher among rural than urban married women (14 per cent versus 10 per cent), the poorest than the wealthiest (18 per cent versus 8 per cent) and Muslim women than Hindu women (19 per cent versus 12 per cent).

Pronounced regional differences in the proportion of women with an unmet need for contraception are evident (Table A3.3). NFHS-3 shows that the level of unmet need was over 20 per cent in such northern and eastern states as Bihar, Jharkhand, and Uttar Pradesh, and such north-eastern states as Meghalaya and Nagaland. It was, in contrast, less than 10 per cent in the four southern states, in Gujarat and Maharashtra in the west, Haryana, Himachal Pradesh, and Punjab in the north, and West Bengal in the east.

Abortion

An estimated 6.7 million abortions take place in India each year. It is estimated, moreover, that most of these abortions are conducted by uncertified providers or in unregistered facilities, that is, they violate the provisions of the MTP Act (Chhabra and Nuna 1994). Indeed, just 0.62 million abortions are reported to have been performed in 'institutions approved for MTP work' (Ministry of

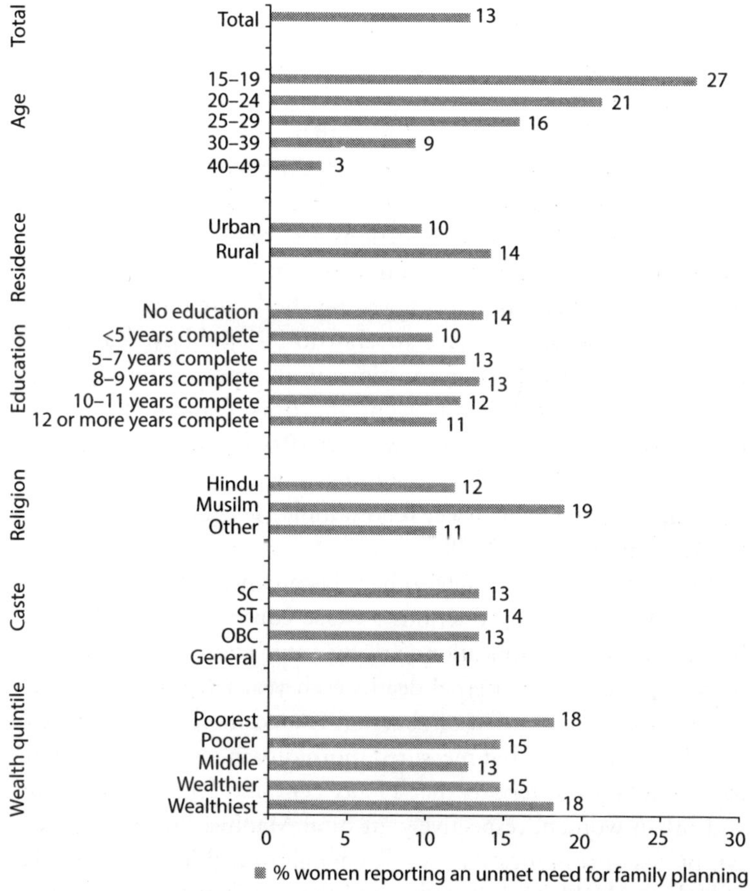

Figure 3.6 Percentage of Currently Married Women Reporting an Unmet Need for Family Planning, by Selected Background Characteristics, India, 2005–06
Source: International Institute for Population Sciences and Macro International (2007).

Health and Family Welfare, 2011a). However, evidence from rural areas of two districts each of Maharashtra and Rajasthan shows that 13 per cent and 11 per cent of married women aged up to 39 had experienced an abortion, and 7 per cent and 4 per cent, respectively, had so experienced in the five years prior to the interview (Jejeebhoy, Zavier, and Kalyanwala 2010). Abortion ratios, the number of abortions per 100 live births, has been found to be in the range of 5 to 11 per 100 live births in a range of studies in Maharashtra,

Madhya Pradesh, and Rajasthan (Elul et al. 2004; Ganatra et al. 2008; Jejeebhoy, Zavier, and Kalyanwala 2010; Malhotra et al. 2003). Among those who experienced abortion, moreover, second trimester abortion were frequently reported. In the district level study in rural Maharashtra and Rajasthan, for example, 21 per cent and 24 per cent of women who had experienced an abortion in the five years prior to the interview reported a second trimester abortion. Second-trimester abortions are more likely to take place among the less educated, the poor, the young and the unmarried than among other women, suggesting the limited access, in practice, that these groups have to abortion (Jejeebhoy, Zavier, and Kalyanwala 2010). Repeat abortions were reported by 18–25 per cent of women reporting a recent abortion (Ganatra et al. 2008; Jejeebhoy, Zavier, and Kalyanwala 2010). In addition, the large majority of abortion clients seek to terminate their pregnancy from a private sector facility (see, for example, Jejeebhoy et al. 2011a; 2011b; Ganatra et al. 2008).

Many abortions are likely to have been conducted in unsafe conditions, with potentially serious adverse consequences for women's health. Indeed, complications arising from abortion contribute to some 8 per cent of maternal deaths each year (Registrar General of India 2006). The burden of abortion-related morbidity is also considerable: one study that measured morbidity in terms of both symptoms and bed-rest reports that 17 per cent and 13 per cent of rural and urban women, respectively, in rural Madhya Pradesh, reported symptoms of complications severe enough to require 8 or more days of bed rest (Nyblade, Edmeades, and Pearson 2010).

The availability of MA and MVA has resulted in a welcome shift away from dilation and curettage (D&C). A recent study noted that the use of D&C fell from 56–62 per cent to 32–37 per cent between 2007 and 2010 in districts of Maharashtra, and correspondingly, from 56–88 per cent to 38–43 per cent in districts of Rajasthan. At the same time, the use of MVA increased from 20–22 per cent to 28–29 per cent, and of medical abortion from 7–17 per cent to 33–38 per cent in districts of Maharashtra, and, correspondingly, from 4–20 per cent to 31–32 per cent and 4–16 percent to 23–27 percent in districts of Rajasthan (Jejeebhoy et al. 2011a; 2011b). Evidence points to the increasing use of mifepristone-misoprostol without a prescription (Ganatra, Manning, and Pallipamulla 2005; Tank 2011). The studies described above in districts of Maharashtra and Rajasthan suggest, for example, that among those whose pregnancy was not terminated by a certified provider, three-quarters had purchased mifepristone-misoprostol directly from a chemist without a prescription (Jejeebhoy et al. 2011a; 2011b). Although the evidence suggests that such a practice has not necessarily resulted in complications, there is a risk that in the absence of information, the method will be used incorrectly or by women who have crossed the effective gestational limit.

Abortions take place largely among married women, and largely because of unintended pregnancy, because the last child was too young, for health reasons or because of foetal problems (Ganatra 2000). Delayed abortion—that is, into the second trimester—among rural women is, moreover, associated with poverty, lack of agency and lack of access to an appropriate facility. For example, a recent study attributed second trimester abortion to women's exclusion from abortion-related decision making, unsuccessful prior attempts to terminate the pregnancy, and distance from the facility in which the abortion was performed; to a lesser extent, it was also attributed to selective abortion of female foetuses and following prenatal sex detection (Zavier, Jejeebhoy, and Kalyanwala 2012). A number of community-based studies provide evidence of sex selective abortion: 3–18 per cent of abortions reported in these studies were estimated to have been sex-selective of female foetuses (Ganatra et al. 2008; Elul et al. 2004; Malhotra et al. 2003). The distortion of the sex ratio at birth, estimated to be 904 girls per 1,000 boys in 2006–08 (United Nations Population Fund 2010) and the decline in the child (ages 0–6) sex ratio from 927 girls per 1,000 boys in 2001 to 919 in 2011 (Office of the Registrar General and Census Commissioner, India 2013) are clearly indicators of the pervasiveness of the practice of sex-selective abortion. Women attempting sex selective abortions may not opt for legal services, and since sonography can detect foetal sex only in the second trimester, women opting for sex-selective abortion are exposed to greater risks than other abortion seekers (Ganatra 2000: Johnston 2002; Santhya and Verma 2004).

Post-abortion contraceptive counselling is not routinely provided, and many women fail to adopt a method of contraception following their abortion. The study in rural Maharashtra and Rajasthan noted that 37–40 per cent were counselled about post-abortion contraception, and that just half of those whose abortion had taken place in the five years preceding the survey had adopted post-abortion contraception. Significantly more of those counselled than not counselled had adopted a method post-abortion (Jejeebhoy, Zavier, and Kalyanwala, 2010; Zavier, Jejeebhoy, and Kalyanwala 2012). A recent study has noted huge inequities in access to post-abortion contraception. Poor and socially excluded women were less likely to use any contraceptive method after abortion, particularly non-terminal methods; in addition, the socially excluded were considerably more likely than others to discontinue using a method of contraception (Zavier and Padmadas 2012).

Infertility Evidence on the prevalence of infertility in India is sparse. It is estimated that about 8–10 per cent of couples experience infertility, primary as well as secondary (Ministry of Health and Family Welfare 2010a). According to the NFHS-3, 2 per cent of currently married women aged 40–49 were childless, a good proxy for primary infertility (International Institute for Population Sciences and Macro International 2007); higher rates were observed in a community-based study in one district of Andhra Pradesh — 12 per cent—among women aged 20–49 (Unisa 2008). While several epidemiological factors are responsible for infertility, such reproductive health factors, notably unhygienic obstetric practices, including at the time of abortion and delivery, and STIs are also responsible (Widge 2004). Consequences of infertility for women's life remain dire in India. Childless women are often stigmatized, suffer violence, and face abandonment (Unisa 1999).

Infertility care and management are not a public health priority and treatment-seeking practices are poorly studied. A recent study of 86 women seeking treatment in facilities in three states (Odisha, Tamil Nadu, and Uttar Pradesh) reports that about half had sought treatment for more than five years (SAMA–Resource Group for Women and Health 2010). The study in rural Andhra Pradesh notes that almost three in five (59 per cent) of women who experienced infertility had sought treatment for their infertility, and proportions who sought treatment increased with marital duration, education and standard of living. Contrary to the belief that women first approached providers of Indian systems of medicine, 73 per cent of women who had sought treatment had gone directly to an allopathic provider, and the vast majority of these (90 per cent) opted for a provider in the private sector. Costs were high: among women who had sought at least one type of treatment, the average cost was nearly Rs 7,000 (Unisa 2008).

There is now an increasing trend towards the use of assisted reproductive techniques (ARIs), such as artificial insemination by the husband or donor, in vitro fertilization, surrogate mothers and other techniques. Their success rates vary, and the take-home baby rate is estimated by clinics as 30–40 percent. ART services are rarely available at public sector facilities (Widge 2004; SAMA — Resource Group for Women and Health 2010). Where services are provided, they are largely restricted to diagnosis and testing services, and in some cases, artificial insemination by the husband, but no other ART services; public sector gynaecologists do not consider infertility services a priority (Widge and Cleland 2008). Studies show that treatment is increasingly sought by rural women, counselling is largely absent, expenses are considerable, and often there are hidden costs not quoted to the client at the start of the treatment; also, consent taking procedures are not consistently followed, women seeking ART services are less than fully informed about procedures, success rates and alternatives, and had no more than a vague understanding of the treatment they were receiving (SAMA — Resource Group for Women and Health 2010).

STIs/RTIs and Other Gynaecological Morbidities

It is estimated that 14–16 per cent and 15–18 per cent, respectively, of the adult population of India residing in low-medium and high HIV prevalence states, respectively, suffer from STIs or RTIs, and that STI prevalence ranged from 4.7 per cent per cent in rural areas of low-moderate HIV prevalence states to 6 per cent in urban and rural areas of high prevalence states (National AIDS Control Organisation 2006b). Overall, therefore, roughly 5 per cent of the adult population in India suffers from STIs.

Smaller studies have observed higher rates of infection. A study in Goa reports that 28 per cent of almost 3,000 women tested suffered from any RTIs (bacterial vaginosis, candida, trichomonas vaginalis, chlamydia trachomatis, neisseria gonorrhoea); endogenous infections were relatively common (BV, 18 per cent; candida, 9 per cent), and 4 per cent tested positive for a STIs (Patel et al. 2006). A study of gynaecological morbidity in a Delhi slum found higher rates of infection: of 301 women tested, 42 per cent tested positive for bacterial vaginosis, 29 per cent for chlamydia, and 4 per cent each for trichomoniasis and syphilis (Garg et al., 2008). Among men aged 15–49 in these slums, 9 per cent reported urethral discharge, 6 per cent reported itching, 3 per cent reported a genital ulcer, and one per cent reported swelling of the groin; a seroprevalence rate of 1.5 per cent and 3.6 per cent for trichomoniasis and syphilis, respectively were found (Garg et al. 2007).

Reports of other gynaecological morbidities, including pelvic inflammatory disease, prolapse, and fistulae have been less frequently studied. A synthesis of six community-based studies of gynaecological morbidity in India reported prolapse among 1 to 7 per cent of all women surveyed (Koenig et al. 1998). More recently, a study in a New Delhi slum found that 26 per cent of slum women were clinically diagnosed with pelvic inflammatory disease, and 14 per cent reported prolapse (Garg et al. 2008).

Clinic based studies suggest that trends in the profile of STIs observed among clinic attendees has been changing. A comparison of female attendees at a large hospital in Delhi over the period 1990–93 to 2002–04 reports that over this 15 year period, there was a significant rise in viral STIs and syphilis, and a reduction in other STIs (Ray et al. 2006). Among men, clinic-based studies indicate genital ulcer disease, particularly syphilis. Among those attending STI clinics, the prevalence of syphilis ranges between 13 and 57 per cent (Chaudhary et al. 1988; Chopra et al. 1990; Singh et al. 1990; Kamat and Banker, 1993; George et al. 1997; Risbud et al. 1999). There are, however, variations in diagnostic criteria used in all these studies, and therefore it is difficult to make comparisons.

Few studies have explored care seeking practices for symptoms of infection. A study of household use of health services in rural areas of two districts of Andhra Pradesh found that while almost all women sought ANC services from the public sector (96 per cent), few did so for STI symptoms (16 per cent), and just 4 per cent sought STI related services from a PHC (Mitchell, Mahal, and Bossert 2011).

HIV Scenario and Implications for Reproductive and Sexual Health

An estimated 2.4 million Indians were HIV+ in 2009, with overall rates declining from 0.45 per cent in 2002 to 0.31 per cent in 2009 (NIMS and NACO 2012). The estimated number of new infections has declined to approximately 120,000 new HIV infections in 2009 from an estimated 270,000 new infections in 2000. The epidemic continues to be concentrated in high-risk populations, that is, sex workers, men who have sex with men, transgenders, injecting drug users, and clients of sex workers. HIV prevalence is estimated to be 12.2 per cent among IDUs, 6.8 per cent among men who have sex with men, and somewhat lower among female sex workers (5.9 per cent). Of the HIV+ population, 39 per cent are female and 4 per cent are children. In contrast, HIV prevalence rates are low in the general population; for example, estimates for the year 2008 suggest that the prevalence among ANC clinic attendees is 0.6 per cent (National AIDS Control Organisation 2010c). Unprotected sex is the major route of HIV transmission, accounting in total for 89 per cent of infections (87 per cent heterosexual and 2 per cent homosexual). Other routes include parent to child transmission (5 per cent), use of infected syringes and needles (2 per cent) and use of infected blood and blood products (1 per cent) (National AIDS Control Organisation 2010c).

Socio-demographic disparities in HIV prevalence may be gleaned from Table 3.4, drawing on data from the NFHS 3 in which HIV testing covered just six states, namely the high prevalence states of Andhra Pradesh, Karnataka, Maharashtra, Manipur, and Tamil Nadu, and the low prevalence state of Uttar Pradesh (International Institute for Population Sciences and Macro International 2007). HIV prevalence is observed among the young, and female rates are as high as or higher than corresponding rates among males in the ages 15–24. In addition, well educated and better off men and women, those residing in rural areas, and Muslims were less likely than others to be HIV+; caste differentials were not evident.

Table 3.4 HIV Prevalence by Background Characteristics, India, 2005–06

	Women	Men
Age		
15–19	0.07	0.01
20–24	0.17	0.19
25–29	0.28	0.43
30–39	0.35	0.59
40–49	0.18	0.44
Residence		
Urban	0.29	0.41
Rural	0.18	0.32
Education		
No	0.27	0.50
<5 yrs	0.49	0.36
5–7 years	0.20	0.47
8–9 years	0.11	0.40
10–11 years	0.14	0.23
12 or more years	0.07	0.16
Religion		
Hindu	0.25	0.37
Muslim	0.06	0.21
Other	0.48	0.18
Caste		
Scheduled caste	0.23	0.34
Scheduled tribe	0.12	0.39
Other backward caste	0.24	0.36
General caste	0.18	0.34
Wealth		
Poorest	0.18	0.39
Poorer	0.20	0.31
Middle	0.24	0.31
Wealthier	0.34	0.52
Wealthiest	0.12	0.24

Source: International Institute for Population Sciences and Macro International (2007).

Regional variation in prevalence rates persists: as of 2009, the six high prevalence states (Andhra Pradesh, Karnataka, Maharashtra, Mizoram, Nagaland, and Tamil Nadu) accounted for 57 per cent of people living with HIV/AIDS (NIMS and NACO 2012). HIV prevalence has declined at the all-India level and in the high prevalence states; however, it has increased in some low and moderate prevalence states (Arunachal Pradesh, Assam, Jharkhand, Kerala, Meghalaya, and Odisha (NIMS and NACO 2012)).

In light of advances in anti-retroviral therapy, the availability of highly effective treatment regimens for the prevention of parent-to-child transmission and of ARTs that allow sero-discordant couples to bear children without infecting the uninfected partner, it is becoming increasingly important to address the fertility preferences of persons living with HIV/AIDS. Two studies, conducted in Karnataka and Tamil Nadu respectively, have explored the fertility desires, intentions, and fertility decision-making of people living with HIV/AIDS and the barriers they face in fulfilling their desires. Findings suggest that many women and men had modified their pre-HIV family size preference downwards once they learned about their status: some had decided to limit childbearing altogether, while others opted to go ahead and have at least one child. Key factors preventing People Living with HIV and AIDS (PLHA) from opting to have a child following disclosure were health related fears, the fear of losing a pregnancy or a child, lack of a supportive environment and limited awareness of and access to PPTCT and ARV. PLHA who opted to have a child were, in contrast, far more likely to report a supportive environment, awareness of available therapies, and favourable perceptions about the quality of care received (Kalyanwala, Iyengar, and Janardha 2007; Kanniappan, Jeyapaul and Kalyanwala 2008).

Sexual and Reproductive Health Problems Experienced by Menopausal Women

Very little is currently known about the sexual and reproductive health needs of women in the post-reproductive age groups. The few studies that are currently available suggest that a sizeable proportion of older women experience gynaecological problems, including vaginal discharge, bleeding PV, uterine prolapse and so on. For example, a study of 197 women aged 45 years and above in Kerala shows that such conditions as uterine prolapse, vaginal bleeding, and bleeding PV were reported by 25 per cent, 13 per cent, and 6 per cent of women, respectively (Aswathy et al. 2006). Another study of some 100 of women in the age group 45 and above in Tamil Nadu found that one in eight women reported one or more gynaecological problems; vaginal discharge was the most commonly reported problem among them (Christian Medical College and Population Council 2000).

Individual Level Factors Underlying Poor Sexual and Reproductive Health

Several factors at individual level are observed to have compromised sexual and reproductive health in India. Notably, the evidence highlights such factors as a lack of awareness of health promoting behaviours, limited female agency and persistent traditional notions of masculinity and femininity, inadequate male involvement, and limited spousal communication.

Limited awareness

Awareness of health promoting behaviours in the area of sexual and reproductive health remains far from universal in India. For example, in the area of maternal and newborn health, recent research from Rajasthan observed that although women who had availed of JSY benefits were significantly better informed than non-beneficiaries about best practices related to the care of women during pregnancy, delivery, and the postpartum period and of the newborns, overall levels of awareness remained moderate. Just 30 per cent of women had comprehensive awareness of best practices in the antenatal period, 40 per cent were aware of essential birth preparations, 35 per cent were aware of the need for postpartum care even if the mother felt well, and 16 per cent had comprehensive awareness of best practices for newborn care (Santhya et al. 2011b). Awareness of danger signals is also limited: a study of delivery and postpartum morbidity in the Delhi slums observed that even among women experiencing excessive bleeding and high grade fever, just 28 per cent and 13 per cent, respectively, recognized the condition as a severe morbidity (Goyal and Bhandari, 2008).

In the area of contraception, while awareness of at least one contraceptive method is virtually universal (99 per cent) among currently married men and women, awareness of non-terminal method is not universal, especially among women. For example, just 74 per cent, 76 per cent, and 87 per cent of currently married women were aware of IUCDs, condoms and oral pills, respectively. Moreover, percentages aware of specific methods increased only marginally over time: for example, awareness about condoms increased from 71 per cent in 1998–99 to 76 per cent by 2005–06, and of oral pills from 80 per cent to 87 per cent (International Institute for Population Sciences and Macro International 2007).

Awareness about the legality of abortion is also limited (see for example, Elul et al. 2004, Ganatra et al. 2008; Jejeebhoy, Zavier, and Kalyanwala 2010; Malhotra et al. 2003). For example, a community-based study found that while three quarters of rural women were aware that abortion is legal in at least one situation, misconceptions were widespread: about half believed that it is illegal in the case of unmarried women or contraceptive failure; almost all women, 88 per cent and 97 per cent in Maharashtra and Rajasthan respectively, believed that women who undergo abortion must have their husband's consent (Jejeebhoy, Zavier, and Kalyanwala 2010). Conflicting messages also prevail: the perception that abortion is illegal in India has been partly fuelled by conflicting messages about the illegality of one type of abortion, that is, abortion following prenatal sex detection, and the legality of abortions for other reasons (Nidadavolu and Bracken 2006).

Misconceptions about HIV transmission routes and means of protection against HIV are evident. For example, findings from NFHS-3 show that just 17 per cent of all women and 33 per cent of all men had comprehensive awareness of HIV, that is, they rejected common misperceptions about transmission and were aware of the importance of consistent condom use and single-partner relations as means of avoiding infection (International Institute for Population Sciences and Macro International 2007).

Limited female agency and wide gender power imbalances

Within the age and gender-stratified family systems prevailing in India, women's agency is hugely constrained. There is considerable evidence of the extent to which limited agency—in terms of decision-making, freedom of movement, control over economic resources and experience of violence—has compromised health promoting behaviours and timely care-seeking. As discussed in Chapter 5, agency is particularly constrained among young women.

Almost 40 per cent of women interviewed in NFHS-3 did not participate in decisions relating to their own health care and more than half (52 per cent) were not permitted to attend a health facility unescorted (International Institute for Population Sciences and Macro International 2007). Moreover, 62 per cent of women who participated in most decisions, compared to 44 per cent of those who did not participate in any, had practised contraception; 37 per cent versus 30 per cent of those who did and did not make decisions had received postpartum care, and 52 per cent versus 46 per cent of those who did and did not make decisions had been delivered by a skilled attendant. Neonatal mortality was, moreover, lower among women reporting decision-making authority than those denied the authority to make decisions (36 versus 43 per 1,000 live births).

Gender power imbalances are evident in the persistence of marital violence, experienced by almost two in five women (39 per cent). Its negative effects on sexual and reproductive health are considerable: a significant and consistent association is observed between the experience of spousal violence and unintended pregnancy, pregnancy-related care, foetal and infant mortality, symptoms of RTIs/STIs and mental health disorders. These associations were observed, moreover, from an early age, suggesting that women are at risk of ill-health from early married life (Jejeebhoy, Santhya, and Acharya 2010; Kostick et al. 2010; Patel et al. 2006).

Women's inability to refuse marital sex, even if they suspect their husband has engaged in extra-marital relations, and gendered attitudes that condone pre- and extra-marital sex for men but not women also have the potential to compromise women's health. Several studies have noted that as a result, many women, including the newly married, are at risk of acquiring infections from their husbands (see, for example, Santhya and Jejeebhoy 2007). Links between a husband's extramarital relationship and women's experience of vaginal discharge and symptoms of STIs have also been observed (Patel et al. 2006). Indeed, a case study of factors underlying the slow progress in reproductive health indicators in Andhra Pradesh has pointed to, among other factors, the fact that the low status of women, and limited community commitment to realizing their rights, have compromised timely care seeking (Prakasamma 2009).

Limited male involvement and traditional notions of masculinity

Men's attitudes and behaviours influence not only their own sexual and reproductive health outcomes but also those of their wives or partners. However, the health system response has stressed men's needs only in terms of HIV and related practices, and has neglected measures to include them in reproductive and child health programmes or implement, among them, programmes intended to change traditional notions of masculinity and build greater respect for women.

We have seen, in earlier sections, that just six percent of couples practising contraception were using a male method, even as recently as 2005–06; consistent condom use among men reporting high risk behaviours has also been found to be limited. Male involvement in their wife's pregnancy-related care is also limited. Of men whose youngest living child was less than three years old at the time of NFHS-3, and whose wife had received antenatal care, as many as one quarter (26 per cent) had never accompanied their wife for an antenatal check-up. Moreover, two in five husbands of women who had not received any antenatal care, and 45 per cent of husbands whose wife did not deliver institutionally reported that it was because the husband did not think it necessary or did not allow his wife to seek care (International Institute for Population Sciences and Macro International 2007).

Limited spousal communication

Spousal communication about sexual and reproductive matters is limited. While NFHS–3 did not collect information on spousal communication, evidence from NFHS-2 indicates that less than one in five currently married women had discussed family planning with their husbands (International Institute for Population Sciences and ORC Macro 2000). A study of pregnant women who attended an antenatal clinic in Delhi found that 45 percent of the husbands reported that they had discussed family planning with their wife (Mishra and Ramanathan 2002). A study of men in Madhya Pradesh reports that one-third of men who responded to a survey questionnaire and most of those participating in focus group discussions reported themselves to be the sole decision maker about reproductive health (Char, Saavala, and Kulmala 2009). Limited communication is also evident among the young: the *Youth Study* found, for example, that just one-third (34 per cent) of married men aged under 30 and half (54 per cent) of married young women aged 15–24 had ever discussed contraception with their spouse (International Institute for Population Sciences and Population Council 2010). Where communication occurs, moreover, it is selective: A study of young men and women in Guntur district (Andhra Pradesh) and Dhar and Guna districts (Madhya Pradesh) found that topics discussed frequently included antenatal care seeking but rarely included contraception (Santhya, Jejeebhoy, and Ghosh 2008).

Spousal communication on reproductive illnesses, especially STIs, is also limited. For example, a community-based study of married men and women in rural Tamil Nadu showed that only 37 per cent of women with symptoms of possible RTIs and one-fifth (20 per cent) of men with symptoms had informed their spouse about their illness experience (Santhya and Dasvarma 2002). Facility-based studies at STI clinics confirm this finding: only 18 percent of married and unmarried men attending clinics in Gujarat had informed their wife or partner about their illness, as had less than one-third of husbands of women attending antenatal clinics in Delhi (Mishra and Ramanathan 2002) and two-fifths of married males at a clinic in Maharashtra (Sahasrabuddhe et al. 2002).

Programme Challenges

Although many programmatic innovations have been implemented to improve reproductive health care delivery—the JSY programme, the ASHA scheme, upgrading of skills of health care providers, task shifting to intermediate cadres of health workers, 24 hour transport response, subcontracting the private sector, providing for birth companions and so on—gaps remain. These gaps threaten the likelihood that India will meet all the goals set in the NRHM, the Population Policy and the Five Year Plans. Overarching obstacles inhibiting the successful implementation of programmes include poor governance and weak technical leadership, with frequent changes in the health sector hierarchy; undue prioritisation of some aspects of reproductive health to the disadvantage of others; and limited resources, with just 1–1.3 per cent of India's GDP allocated to health against a target of at least 2 per cent recommended in the XIth Five Year Plan (see, for example, Paul et al, 2011; Planning Commission 2011a). More specifically, inadequate infrastructure and human resources, inadequate attention to provider capacity and training, poor quality of services, and gaps in the delivery of a range of reproductive health services have seriously compromised the pace of improvement in sexual and reproductive health outcomes.

Infrastructure and Human Resources

Limitations with regard to infrastructure and human resources play a key role in compromising access to and the quality of health services in general, including reproductive health services.

As far as infrastructure and trained personnel are concerned, as of 2010, there were a total of 147,069 subcentres, 23673 PHCs, and 4,535 CHCs in rural areas (Ministry of Health and Family Welfare, 2011a); and an estimated shortfall of 19,590 sub-centres, 4,252 PHCs and 2,115 CHCs in the country (Planning Commission 2011b).

In addition, equipment is not always available or in working condition, the supply chain management remains poor and procurement systems are limited (Ministry of Health and Family Welfare 2011b). Stock-out of drugs is frequent, and essential drugs, such as magnesium sulphate, oxytocin and misoprostol were not available in many CHCs and even District Hospitals (Ministry of Health and Family Welfare 2011c). Inadequate blood storage facilities have also been noted (see, for example, Vora et al. 2009). Even the Midterm Appraisal of the Eleventh Five Year Plan reported that beneficiaries are often required to purchase gloves, syringes, and drugs, and that facilities are understaffed, poorly run and poorly maintained. Subcentres are particularly poorly equipped.

Lack of human resources poses as severe a constraint to health service delivery as does the poor infrastructure. The density of doctors, nurses and midwives in India is 1.9 per 1,000 population, against a minimum requirement of 2.5 health workers per 1,000 population (Planning Commission 2011b) suggesting an acute shortage of resources for health, notably in rural areas. Indeed, the Planning Commission has acknowledged while there is a need for 205,000 ANMs, 72,150 nurses, 31,948 doctors (at PHC level) and 18142 specialists for rural areas, not all posts have been filled and there is a shortage of seven per cent of ANMs, nine per cent of nurses, 19 per cent of doctors at PHC level, and 63 per cent of specialists in rural areas (Planning Commission, Health Division 2012). Smaller case studies suggest even more serious shortages: for example, a study in Gujarat showed a shortfall of 22 per cent, 20 per cent and 15 per cent among ANMs, female health assistants, and PHC doctors (Mavalankar et al. 2009).

These shortages in human resources are attributed to a number of factors, including difficulties in recruiting and retaining doctors and nurses in rural areas, especially in the high focus states, delays in sanctioning posts, and limited investment in building a cadre of midwives (Ministry of Health and Family Welfare, 2011c; Prakasamma, 2009). Indeed, findings that access to emergency obstetric care has not increased as rapidly as expected, and that the volume of complications addressed within the public health system remains sub-optimal (Ministry of Health and Family Welfare 2011c) may be attributed to the lack of obstetricians and anaesthetists willing to be posted in rural facilities. While the inclusion of contractual staff has significantly improved the availability of staff at health centre level, contractual employment is fraught with problems, including delayed renewal of contracts, poor service conditions, high turnover, and disparities between contractual and permanent staff including in terms of salary (Ministry of Health and Family Welfare 2011c).

Provider Capacity and Training

Significant measures have been taken, under the NRHM, to strengthen provider capacity. For example, a national training strategy has been devised that addresses the needs of a wide array of health care providers and health system managers (Ministry of Health and Family

Welfare 2008). Manuals have been developed that address not only different cadres of providers (from ASHAs to MOs) but also different thematic areas (adolescent reproductive and sexual health, maternal and newborn health, child health and nutrition for example). Efforts have been made, moreover, to clearly define the tasks and responsibilities of cadres at various levels of the health system. Guidelines are now available to be used at state and district levels that specify the package of services that each level of the health system is expected to provide and related quality parameters, supervisory structures, institutional linkages, community support mechanisms and assessment systems (Ministry of Health and Family Welfare 2010d).

The reach of provider training has been variable. For example, ASHA training comprises a 23 day package spread over a year, and this is continued with on the job training, and supportive supervision from the ANM and PHC medical officers (Ministry of Health and Family Welfare 2006). Some seven modules have been prepared that cover the role of the ASHA (Module 1) maternal and child health (Module 2), family planning, RTI/STI, HIV/AIDS and ARSH (Module 3), national health programmes, AYUSH and management of minor ailments (Module 4), reading materials, including a focus on leadership skills (Module 5), maternal and child health (Module 6) and child health and nutrition (Module 7); modules 6 and 7 have not been widely rolled out as of mid-2011. A large number of ASHAs have been trained; however, while a total of 8.3 lakh ASHAs have been selected to date, not all of these ASHAs have undergone training in all five modules. For example, while 94% have been trained in the first module, this percentage fell to 77–81 for Modules 2, 3 and 4; just 44% of all ASHAs were fully trained, that is had been trained in all five modules (Planning Commission 2011c; Ministry of Health and Family Welfare 2011d).

Training in skilled birth attendance (SBA) is also observed to be variable. The 6th JRM of the RCH Programme-2 observed that although SBA training that includes a newborn care component is already in place and states are actively rolling this out, guidelines/protocols available for skilled attendance at birth are not always followed. Many SBAs lack skills for newborn care (such as for resuscitation, management of sick newborns, and use of equipment such as, for example, baby warmers) and this remains a major obstacle to the provision of newborn care services (Ministry of Health and Family Welfare 2009).

Although the programme has expanded to include new components, for example, the ASHA programme or the Adolescent Reproductive and Sexual Health Strategy, corresponding inputs into provider training have lagged, and it is not clear that all providers are fully trained prior to the rollout of these new aspects. As discussed above, not all ASHAs have been trained in all the modules relating to their activities. Moreover, although new tasks have been added to providers' activities—such as, for example, requiring ANMs and MOs to provide reproductive and sexual health information and services to adolescents, including the unmarried—training has neither been universal, nor has it covered both the content of information to be imparted and strategies for imparting the information in ways that resonate with the target audience. Finally, it is not clear that training has succeeded in enabling providers to clarify values and address discomfort about imparting information and services relating to sexual and reproductive life, or on sensitizing providers about gender issues, respect for reproductive rights, and the importance of providing respectful services.

Provider awareness is also of concern. For example, awareness of health promoting behaviours was limited among many ASHAs (Santhya, Jejeebhoy, and Zavier 2011a; Ministry of Health and Family Welfare 2011d; CORT 2007a; 2007b; 2007c; 2007d; 2007e; 2007f; 2008a; 2008b); an eight-state evaluation found that just 26 per cent of ASHAs recognized foul-smelling vaginal discharge as a danger signal during the postpartum period and 34 per cent knew that a newborn should not be bathed immediately (Ministry of Health and Family Welfare 2011e). Medical officers at PHCs in selected districts of Maharashtra and Rajasthan were ill-informed about abortion-related issues: for example, just half were aware that the consent of the husband or guardian is not required in order for an adult woman to undergo abortion, and just 83–87 per cent were aware that MBBS doctors are not permitted to provide medical abortion unless they have been specifically certified to provide MTPs (Jejeebhoy et al. 2011a; 2011b).

Training does not always translate into enhanced knowledge or the practice of new skills. Under the NRHM, staff nurses and ANMs have been permitted to initiate treatment of pregnancy related complications, including intravenous fluids and injectable oxytocins, antibiotics, and magnesium sulphate, and there has been a focus on

ANM training to enhance their skills as SBAs. The limited evidence available suggests that many ANMs are not using these skills. A recent study of some 96 ANMs in two districts in Rajasthan reports that 36 per cent had conducted deliveries in the last three months; of those who had conducted deliveries, just 6 per cent had always used the partograph while conducting the deliveries, and just 22 per cent gave oxytocin injections always or sometimes during the third stage of labour (Santhya and Jejeebhoy 2012). At the same time, multi-skilling of general doctors to provide comprehensive obstetric or anaesthetic services has not been widely undertaken.

Limited Attention to Raising Community Awareness of Available Services

Evidence suggests that programmes have failed to raise community-level awareness about, for example, the availability of services in the public sector, people's entitlements or the eligibility criteria for availing of various programmes. Awareness about the availability of programmes intended to promote reproductive health (JSY, ASHA, 24×7 facilities, for example), and the location of services (for example, for abortion) is, therefore, not universal. For example, of recently delivered women in Rajasthan, just 46% had heard of the ASHA, and while almost all (98 per cent) knew about JSY, many fewer were aware of the eligibility conditions for availing of benefits; just 60 per cent and 62 per cent, respectively, were aware that all women were eligible for benefits, irrespective of their age and parity, and just 49 per cent were aware of the exact amount of cash provided to women under the programme (Santhya et al. 2011b). The study exploring abortion related awareness and experience found, similarly, that no more than 72 per cent and 80 per cent of women in districts of Maharashtra and Rajasthan, respectively, were aware that abortion is available in public sector facilities (Jejeebhoy, Zavier, and Kalyanwala 2010).

Inequitable Reach of Services

Several studies have highlighted that, not with standing the RCH–2 programme, the reach of sexual and reproductive health services remains limited and inequitable. For example, contact with a health worker (ANM, AWW, ASHA, MPW, other) in the three months prior to the NFHS-3 interview was reported by just 17 per cent of women. Twice as many rural as urban women (21 per cent and 10 per cent, respectively) had contact with a health worker (International Institute for Population Sciences and Macro International 2007). An analysis of who benefitted most from improvements in maternal health care seeking over the periods covered by NFHS-1, NFHS-2 and NFHS-3 suggests that increments in antenatal care and skilled attendance at delivery were more likely to have been experienced by non-poor than poor mothers (Pathak, Singh, and Subramanian 2010).

Several programme assessments, including of the JSY, have also noted the inequitable reach of programmes. JSY assessments have noted that the poorest, the least educated women, and those belonging to socially and economically excluded groups were less likely than other women to have benefitted from the programme (Lim et al. 2010; Santhya et al. 2011b;. Sidney et al. 2012). Similarly, very young mothers were less likely than others to have availed of the JSY (Santhya et al. 2011b, Santhya 2009). There are also indications that the urban poor have been relatively neglected in reproductive health programming.

In short, while the reach of sexual and reproductive health services has increased, particularly as a result of the JSY, inequities persist, and the poor, the socially excluded, the poorly educated, the young, and those in urban slums—the neediest—are disproportionately excluded from the ambit of services.

Poor Quality of Services

The poor quality of sexual and reproductive health services in the public sector has been widely observed, and such issues as lack of cleanliness, long waiting times, shortages of drugs, lack of visual and auditory privacy, demands for unauthorized payments, and absence of respectful treatment documented. For example, NFHS-3 reports that among women who had made a visit to a public, NGO or private sector health facility or attended a health camp for themselves or their children in the three months preceding the NFHS-3 interview, half (48 per cent) of those who had attended a public sector facility compared to almost three-quarters of those who had attended a private sector facility found the facility to be very clean. Moreover, of those whose problem required privacy, just 82 per cent of those who attended a public sector facility, compared to 91 per cent of those who attended a private sector one, reported that privacy was provided; and average waiting time was almost twice as long for those seeking care at a public sector facility as a private one. Likewise, information provided tended to be incomplete: the leading topic discussed was immunisation, and even among pregnant women, such topics as delivery care and preparedness and postpartum care were discussed with fewer than five per cent. Likewise, even among non-pregnant women who were not practising contraception, family planning was discussed with just 8 per cent. Poor quality of services was also expressed in terms of concerns about the absence of a provider or a female provider (20 per cent and 23 per cent respectively), lack of availability of drugs (23 per cent) and distance to a health facility (25%) (International Institute for Population Sciences and Macro International 2007).

Provider and facility level studies have also pointed to lacunae affecting the quality of services: a lack of supplies, skewed prioritization of responsibilities, delays in payments and inadequate mentoring or supervision, for example. An evaluation of the ASHA programme, has shown, for example, that just 68 per cent, or 5.7 lakh ASHAs were in position with drug kits (Ministry of Health and Family Welfare 2010a). Moreover, because of their focus on JSY, ASHAs were found to pay far less attention to the provision of antenatal and postpartum care, and the promotion of breastfeeding and family planning than they did to facilitating institutional deliveries (Ministry of Health and Family Welfare 2011e; Planning Commission 2011d; Santhya, Jejeebhoy, and Zavier 2011a; United Nations Population Fund 2009). An eight-state evaluation of ASHAs corroborates this observation: although 90 per cent of ASHAs were engaged in promoting institutional delivery, over 20 per cent of pregnant women were not met by ASHAs even in the best performing districts and this percentage was as high as 50 per cent in poor performing districts where ASHAs' support is needed most (Ministry of Health and Family Welfare 2011e).

The quality of services is also hampered by the uneven use of best practices. For example, the active management of the third stage of labour was practised infrequently; instead, as observed earlier, unmonitored intrapartum oxytocin has been observed even in hospital deliveries (Iyengar et al 2009a; 2009b; Sharan, Strobino, and Ahmed 2005). A study of delivery related practices among women delivering in Rajasthan shows that only 29 per cent of women reported that the health care provider had conducted all essential examinations when they were admitted in the hospital for delivery and 8 per cent of women reported that the provider had used oxytocin for the management of the third stage of labour. The study also found that harmful practices during labour and delivery were widespread. For example, 36 per cent of women reported that the health care provider applied strong fundal pressure before they delivered; 74 per cent reported that the provider gave them an oxytocin injection to speed up the delivery. Only 61 per cent of the women reported that the facility was clean, that visual privacy was ensured at the facility and that they were allotted a bed and was not asked to share it with other women (Santhya et al., 2012). Even in deliveries conducted in PHCs, labour was monitored through repeated unhygienic vaginal examinations and drying and wrapping of the baby were delayed.

Recent assessments indicate a mixed picture with regard to the practice of discharging women from the facility soon after delivery. The CES observed, for example, that over half of all women who were delivered institutionally remained in the facility for at least 48 hours (United Nations Children's Fund 2010). The recent assessment in Rajasthan, discussed above, of maternal health services reports that 60 per cent of recently delivered women remained at the facility at least for 24 hours after delivery (Santhya et al. 2012). Others have observed, in contrast, that large proportions are discharged within 24 hours of delivery (Iyengar et al. 2008; 2009a; Devadasan et al. 2008). Indeed, a survey in Rajasthan reports that 14 per cent of mothers were discharged within six hours of delivery and 70 per cent in less than 24 hours of delivery (Iyengar et al 2008; 2009a). Findings are mixed, also, with regard to the practice of allowing the escort to remain with the woman during delivery. A small study in Tamil Nadu observed providers overriding government orders to permit women to have a birth attendant in the labour room (Subha Sri 2009). The study in Rajasthan, discussed above, reports that 47 per cent of women were allowed to have the escort to remain with them during delivery (Santhya et al., 2012). Poor quality of other aspects of pregnancy related care has also been documented, including requiring 2–3 pregnant women to occupy a single bed at PHC level (for example, Sharma 2008). There is, moreover, little evidence of improvements in the quality of postpartum care: the study in Rajasthan of women who had recently delivered shows that postpartum check-ups received by mothers were far from comprehensive; similarly, information received on self-care and newborn care was limited (Santhya et al. 2011b).

Concerns about the quality of care characterise HIV/AIDS/STI/RTI services as well. The mid-term review of NACP-III observed, for example, that while remarkable progress has been achieved on most indicators, there is a need for significant quality improvements, especially in areas with high HIV prevalence (National AIDS Control Organisation 2010a). Health care providers are not always adept at communicating messages linking HIV and reproductive health: for example, about the prevention of STIs, unintended pregnancy and vertical transmission of HIV, promotion of a healthy sexual life and relationships free from stigma and discrimination. They are also not necessarily well-informed about HIV and sexual and reproductive health and rights, or have the skills to provide good quality care (Bharat and Mahendra 2007).

Continued Unmet Need for Family Planning

A number of factors may be responsible for the programme's inability to satisfy the demand for family planning reported earlier. Various assessments have, for example, noted a flagging commitment to the provision of family planning services (Ministry of Health and Family Welfare, 2009). The 6th Joint Review Mission (JRM) of RCH Programme-2 observed that family planning service provision has not received due attention, especially at FRUs and 24×7 PHCs. Similar concerns were expressed in the review meeting of state nodal officers of the RCH Programme (Ministry of Health and Family Welfare 2011b). The report highlighted the lack of provider motivation, inadequate attention to postpartum contraception, and the continued focus on the camp mode for sterilization as continuing concerns affecting the uptake of contraception.

Moreover, although the programme is said to provide a cafeteria of contraceptive methods, choices offered are, in practice, limited. In fact, only six methods are offered in the programme: tubal ligation and vasectomy, and oral contraceptives, IUCDs, condoms and emergency contraceptive pills (Ministry of Health and Family Welfare 2010; annual report). Methods that are perceived as less effective, such as spermicides and diaphragms, are not available in the public sector. Methods that have aroused controversy, such as implants and injectables (Net-En, Depo Provera) are also not available to women from the public health system, even though studies in India have found injectables to be safe, effective, and acceptable to significant percentages of women (Indian Council for Medical Research 2008; Jejeebhoy and Zavier 2012). Emergency contraceptive pills, although available, are not being provided, reportedly due to the lack of training for providers on ECP (Ministry of Health and Family Welfare 2009).

Service delivery issues have also been noted. Although a large number of facilities are reported to be offering sterilization services, efforts to promote fixed day/fixed site services appear to have failed, and services continues to be camp based (Ministry of Health and Family Welfare 2009). Counselling at facilities continues to be weak; and counselling for postpartum and post-abortion contraception particularly limited (Ministry of Health and Family Welfare 2009). Community-based family planning services, including counselling, distribution of contraceptives and referral services through ASHAs, VHNDs, and VHSCs have not yet been operationalized effectively (Ministry of Health and Family Welfare 2010a). At the same time, public private partnerships for the delivery of family planning services have not been effectively forged across most states in India and there remains a reluctance to accredit private providers at state and district level (Ministry of Health and Family Welfare 2009).

Finally, client choice is constrained because providers do not involve women in the selection of contraceptive methods or provide them information that could help them arrive at a decision for themselves. For example, in 2005–06, of women using modern contraceptives at the time of the interview and who had initiated use in the previous five years, just 28% were informed about more than one method of contraception (International Institute for Population

Sciences and Macro International 2007); while far from universal, this represents a considerable increase, from 15 per cent, reported seven years earlier (NFHS-2). Private sector health care providers were more likely to inform clients about alternative methods of contraception (33 per cent) than were public or NGO sector providers (25–29 per cent). Also far from universal was the experience of contraceptive counselling with regard to how the method works, what likely side effects are and how side-effects can be managed. Indeed, at the time of NFHS-3, of women who were practising contraception and had adopted a method in the previous five years, just 32 per cent were informed about side-effects or problems relating to the method they had adopted, and just 26 per cent were told what to do if they experienced side effects (IIPS and Macro International 2007). NGO sector providers were, however, more likely than public and private sector providers to inform women about side-effects (46 per cent versus 31–35 per cent) and action to take in case side-effects were experienced (43 per cent versus 25–28 per cent).

In short, the persistence of unmet need is attributable to the limited basket of contraceptives, and notably, non-terminal methods, that are effectively available. Some methods, such as injectables, are not yet available in the public sector; efforts to ensure the regular and wide availability of popular non-terminal methods and emergency contraceptives have not been sustained. Counselling, correspondingly, has not encouraged non-terminal method use, postpartum or post-abortion contraceptive practice, and quality of care practices have not always respected clients' right to make contraceptive choices. Finally, it is not clear that efforts have been made to reach the most vulnerable, including the newly married who may wish to postpone the first pregnancy.

Limitations in Meeting Women's Need for Abortion Services

The NRHM Operational Guidelines stipulate that MVA and MA should be provided at PHC level for women up to 8 and 7 weeks of gestation, respectively, and these, along with second trimester abortion and management of post-abortion complications should be available at all facilities from the CHC level (those identified as FRUs) upward (Ministry of Health and Family Welfare, 2010c). These guidelines have not been realized, and abortion services are typically unavailable and inadequate in the public health system at levels below the District Hospital in most states, as noted by many, including the 6th JRM of the RCH Programme (Ministry of Health and Family Welfare 2009). The JRMs' assessment acknowledged that the availability of services varies by state and is particularly of concern at the peripheral levels of care: safe abortion services are reportedly provided by just 73 per cent of FRUs and 28 per cent of PHCs.

Other assessments have suggested an even bleaker picture. For example, a study assessing the effects of a comprehensive abortion care intervention in districts of Maharashtra and Rajasthan found that prior to the implementation of the intervention, abortion services were provided in just one (1 per cent) of the 87 PHCs located in Aurangabad and Jalna districts of Maharashtra and none of the 69 PHCs in Bundi and Tonk districts of Rajasthan; and in just five of the 19 RHs (CHCs) in the selected districts of Maharashtra districts, and seven of the 11 CHCs in the selected districts of Rajasthan (Jejeebhoy et al., 2011a; 2011b). Leading reasons for this lack of availability were the facts that most PHCs and even some CHCs lacked trained staff, necessary certification, and/or the required equipment and supplies for providing safe abortions (Barge et al. 1998; 2004; Duggal and Barge 2004; Kalyanwala, Zavier, and Jejeebhoy 2010).

Other obstacles have also been noted. Cumbersome procedures for the accreditation of providers and certification of sites permitted to provide abortion services have inhibited providers from opting to conduct abortions. Moreover, while abortions take place largely in the private sector, private sector providers face difficulty, at district level, in becoming accredited. MTP Committees in several states and districts do not exist or do not function and reporting of MTPs is uneven (Action Research and Training for Health (ARTH) and Dept of Medical, Health and Family Welfare, Rajasthan, 2009). At the same time, updated and comprehensive abortion care training and service delivery guidelines have not been put into practice in all states, compromising efforts to upgrade provider skills and familiarize providers with comprehensive abortion care (Ministry of Health and Family Welfare 2010e).

Where services are available, their quality is of concern. Invasive methods such as D&C continue to be widely used for induced abortions (Ministry of Health and Family Welfare, 2009). Despite the fact that medical abortion is an approved method of abortion, drugs are not available through the public health system (Ministry of Health and Family Welfare 2009). Providers themselves are poorly informed about the MTP Act, and women's right to obtain services from the public sector (Jejeebhoy et al. 2011a; 2011b). Indeed, the Midterm Appraisal of the Eleventh Five Year Plan Appraisal noted that ASHAs are unaware of the facilities that the rural poor could access for safe abortion.

Violations of women's right are also evident. Poor quality of care, lack of confidentiality, and the frequent insistence by providers on concurrent family planning deter women from seeking abortion in public sector facilities (Barua and Apte 2007; Elul et al. 2004; Ganatra 2000). Providers in almost all the facilities in the district-level study in Maharashtra and Rajasthan required the husband's written consent and many refused abortion to minors and the unmarried. Quality of care reported by women who had undergone abortion was indifferent, with relatively few women counselled about post-abortion contraception (Jejeebhoy et al. 2011a; 2011b; Jejeebhoy, Zavier, and Kalyanwala 2010).

Attempts to clarify the differences between the MTP Act and the PCPNDT Act have been limited. As a result, there continues to be confusion, among women, about whether all abortion and not simply sex selective abortion is against the law (Nidadavolu and Bracken 2006). This confusion, resulting from the relative emphasis on the illegality of sex selective abortion and the relative silence about the legality of abortion in general, may also have inhibited women from seeking abortion in the public sector. Following the dismal findings of the 2011census with regard to the child sex ratio, this confusion between the right to abortion and the illegality of sex selective abortion has taken on new proportions. At national and state levels, measures to curb sex selective abortion have been proposed—such as restricting second trimester abortions on the one hand, and denying abortion to women whose gestation age is 10 weeks and who seek abortion for reasons of contraceptive failure on the other—that will succeed, if implemented, in making access to legal abortions even more difficult.

Limited Emphasis on Engaging Men in Reproductive Health

Health system biases persist against involving men in reproductive health. There has been, effectively, a bifurcation of services for men and women, with HIV/AIDS related activities focused on men, and sexual and reproductive health services focused on women. The ASHA programme and other periphery-level services overwhelmingly cater to women. For example, efforts to make men welcome during their wife's antenatal check-ups, at the time of delivery or sterilization are rare. Of men whose youngest living child was aged under three years, only 21–25 per cent reported that they had ever been informed by a health care worker about such specific signs of pregnancy complication as vaginal bleeding, convulsions and prolonged labour, and just 37 per cent had been told what to do in case of complications (International Institute for Population Sciences and Macro International, 2007). Family planning services are also more focused on women than men, and couple counselling is rarely reported. At the same time, men's written consent, while not required by law, is fairly widely required in practice for women undergoing sterilization or MTP.

Gaps in Policies and Laws

Goals set in policy documents have not been met and accountability mechanisms to probe factors underlying the nation's inability to meet the goals set by such instruments as the Population Policy 2000 and the XIth Five Year Plan are not in place. For example, the Population Policy 2000 set itself 14 goals to be achieved by 2010, several of which were measurable, including a goal of achieving a maternal mortality ratio of below 100 per 100,000 live births and an IMR below 30 per 1,000 live births by the year 2010. The XIth Plan moved the goalpost, and set similar goals (an MMR of 100 per 100,000 live births and an IMR of 28 per 1,000 live births) to be achieved now by 2012. While improvements have been noted, goals were far from met by 2010, and are unlikely to be met by 2012 as this chapter has shown, and as has been acknowledged by the Steering Committee on Health for the XIIth Plan (Planning Commission 2012). Indeed, this committee has moved the goalpost again; now, its report suggests that an MMR of 109 and an IMR of 27 will not be attained till 2015. Clearly, commitment to meeting these goals has been limited, and leading reasons may include wide state-wise differences in operationalizing programmes to ensure their achievement on the one hand, and inadequate public spending on health (1 per cent of GDP).

The lax enforcement of laws that have a bearing on sexual and reproductive health issues and limited awareness of these laws among the population is another concern. For example, as shown in greater detail in Chapter 4, the marriages of large proportions of young women continue to be undertaken in childhood in violation of the law, few such marriages have been prosecuted, and awareness of the law remains far from universal, even among the young (International Institute for Population Sciences and Population Council 2010). Likewise, while the MTP Act and its amendments have protected women's right to terminate an unwanted pregnancy, including with the use of non-surgical methods, the law remains restrictive in many ways. Safe abortion services, and abortion services in the public sector remain limited (Jejeebhoy et al. 2011a; 2011b) for a variety of reasons, including over-medicalized, tedious and unnecessary certification procedures that permit only obstetricians-gynaecologists and MBBS physicians trained and certified to provide abortion to conduct even medical abortions and MVA. Research has documented, for example, the safety and efficacy of medical abortion and MVA conducted by nurses and Ayurveds trained to provide these methods of abortion (Jejeebhoy, Kalyanwala, Zavier et al. 2011; 2012); yet, the Act denies this category of health care professionals the right to provide first trimester abortion. While efforts to amend the MTP Act are ongoing and have been endorsed by many, including the Federation of Obstetric and Gynaecological Societies of India (FOGSI) and a South Asia Regional Consultation on expanding access to safe abortion and post-abortion care (Population Council 2011), the law remains restrictive. Also of concern is the limited awareness among women about their right to avail of the MTP Act in public sector facilities, and their right to demand services without the consent of their husband (Jejeebhoy et al., 2011a; 2011b).

Notwithstanding the increasing use of ARTs and the potential for misuse that this represents, there does not exist, to date, a law that regulates its use. A Bill, namely, the Assisted Reproductive Technologies (Regulation) Bill, 2010, has been drafted, that addresses the accreditation and supervision of ART clinics and certification procedures, quality of care including confidentiality, restrictions on the sale of gametes, zygotes, and embryos, the rights and duties of parents and donors, and the rights of the child (Ministry of Health and Family Welfare 2010e). However, this Bill has been criticized by civil society groups as falling short on several issues, including that it does not sufficiently protect women from unethical provider practices and does not sufficiently address the regulation and monitoring mechanisms to be undertaken in hospitals offering ARTs (Sama Resource Group for Women and Health 2010). Indeed, as of today, there exist no requirements that a clinic must fulfil in order to provide ART services, and questions have been raised about the exploitation of childless couples, the high costs of treatment, and poor quality of care (SAMA Resource Group for Women and Health 2010; Widge, 2004). There is concern, moreover, that the technology is being misused for prenatal sex detection or selection. Also of concern is the absence of a national registry that collates information systematically, or standard protocols that outline the need for counselling and consent, and for the mandatory provision of information on likely costs, realistic success rates, and available alternatives (SAMA Resource Group for Women and Health 2010).

* * *

Findings of this overview of India's sexual and reproductive health situation suggest that although significant strides have been made, there has been repeated under-achievement of reproductive health goals set, and the achievement of reproductive rights remains, in practice, limited. Pregnancy related outcomes, both in terms of maternal and neonatal mortality and morbidity, remain unacceptably high. At the same time, access to services, notwithstanding the flagship JSY, is far from universal, and postpartum services are particularly poorly accessed. Quality of services and care is also limited; best practices are not used and traditional harmful practices persist. Contraception does not reflect informed choice. The continued focus on female sterilization suggests that neither men's involvement nor non-terminal methods have been adequately incorporated into the programme. Unmet need for contraception persists, and is concentrated among the young and the rural. Notwithstanding the law, an overwhelming majority of abortions continue to take place outside of the legally sanctioned provider and facility structures, and abortion-related mortality plays an important role in the sluggish decline of maternal mortality in the country. Infertility is experienced by considerable minorities of Indian couples, and misuse of ARTs is increasingly observed. Symptoms of gynaecological morbidity and RTIs/STIs are observed among considerable proportions of women and men, but treatment seeking remains compromised. Finally, while rates of HIV have declined, the epidemic has become increasingly feminised, and unprotected sex remains the key route of transmission.

Progress has been uneven and differentials remain wide. Adverse sexual and reproductive health outcomes are far more likely to be observed in some regions, including many northern and eastern states, than in others. In many instances, outcomes are particularly compromised among the rural population, the poor, the socially excluded, the poorly educated and the young as compared to other groups, suggesting persistent inequitable access to services and inability to take protective actions.

This review has outlined a number of barriers at the individual, family, and community level as well as gaps in policies, laws, and programmes that may account for the sluggish pace of improvement in sexual and reproductive health. At the individual level, these include limited awareness of health promoting behaviours and facilities from which counselling, care and supplies may be obtained, limited health care seeking practices, limited female agency and wide gender power imbalances, limited male involvement and the persistence of traditional notions of masculinity, and limited spousal communication about sexual and reproductive health matters. At programme level, poor infrastructure and limited human resources remain a severe constraint to health service delivery. Provider capacity remains variable, as does the reach and quality of provider training. The reach of services remains limited and inequitable, and often miss those most in need, that is, the poorest, the least educated, the socially excluded and those residing in remote areas. Quality of care is variable, and women's or clients' rights are frequently violated: information and counselling provided is cursory, best practices are not always employed. Clients' rights—for example, to confidentiality, to choose a contraceptive method, to have an attendant in the labour room, or to decide on post-abortion contraception—are not always respected.

In conclusion, our review clearly shows that while improvements are evident, much remains to be accomplished in the area of sexual and reproductive health and rights. Challenges are evident both at the individual level and at the programme implementation level, and while programme promises are well-conceived, follow-through has been, in many instances, disappointing. Indeed, what is needed is a continued monitoring of the extent to which policies and laws need to be modified on the one hand, and greater commitment to and more effective realization of policy goals and programme recommendations on the other.

Appendix

Table A3.1 Maternal Mortality Ratio, and Neonatal, Postneonatal and Perinatal Mortality Rates, by State, India

	Maternal mortality ratio[1]	Neonatal mortality rate[2]	Postneonatal mortality rate[2]	Perinatal mortality rate[2]
	2007–09	2005–06	2005–06	2005–06
India	**212**	**39.0**	**18.0**	**48.5**
North	NC	35.1	17.9	42.0
Delhi	NA	29.3	10.5	35.0
Haryana	153	23.6	18.1	36.7
Himachal Pradesh	NA	27.3	8.9	30.2
Jammu and Kashmir	NA	29.8	14.9	37.6
Punjab	172	28.0	13.7	33.2
Rajasthan	318	43.9	21.4	49.4

	Maternal mortality ratio[1]	Neonatal mortality rate[2]	Postneonatal mortality rate[2]	Perinatal mortality rate[2]
Uttarakhand	NA	27.6	14.3	38.1
Central	**NA**	**47.0**	**23.9**	**56.7**
Chhattisgarh	NA	51.1	19.7	63.5
Madhya Pradesh	269[a]	44.9	24.7	46.1
Uttar Pradesh	359[b]	47.6	25.0	59.5
East	**NA**	**41.2**	**17.7**	**54.7**
Bihar	261[c]	39.8	21.9	58.7
Jharkhand	NA	48.6	20.2	57.6
Odisha	258	45.4	19.3	55.6
West Bengal	145	37.6	10.4	46.8
Northeast	**NA**	**38.3**	**19.8**	**52.5**
Arunachal Pradesh	NA	34.0	26.7	40.2
Assam	390	45.5	20.6	63.3
Manipur	NA	18.7	11.1	26.3
Meghalaya	NA	23.6	21.0	23.4
Mizoram	NA	16.3	17.7	26.6
Nagaland	NA	19.8	18.5	22.5
Sikkim	NA	19.4	14.3	16.0
Tripura	NA	33.1	18.3	42.0
West	**NC**	**30.8**	**10.2**	**37.2**
Goa	NA	8.8	6.5	12.4
Gujarat	148	33.5	16.2	40.2
Maharashtra	104	31.8	5.7	35.8
South	**127**	**28.7**	**12.1**	**36.2**
Andhra Pradesh	134	40.3	13.2	47.3
Karnataka	178	28.9	14.3	35.3
Kerala	81	11.5	3.8	10.8
Tamil Nadu	97	19.1	11.2	33.0
Other states	**160**	—	—	—

[a]Includes Chhattisgarh; [b]Includes Uttarakhand; [c]Includes Jharkhand; Source: [1]Office of Registrar and Census Commissioner (2013); [2]International Institute for Population Sciences and Macro International (2007); Regional estimates for neonatal, postneonatal and perinatal mortality rates are calculated from individual data from NFHS-3 (2005–06); NA: not available.

Table A3.2 Percentage of Women by Maternal Health Indicators and State, India, 2005–10

	Maternal health indicators (%)					
	Ever-married women severely anaemic[1] (%)	Women who had three or more ANC visits (%)[2]	Women who received two or more TT injections during pregnancy (%)[2]	Women who received all recommended types of antenatal care (%)[2]	Women who delivered in a health/institution[2]	Women whose delivery was attended by trained health personnel[2]
India	1.8	68.7	86.9	26.5	72.9	76.2
North	1.9	NA	NA	NA	NA	NA
Delhi	0.3	83.4	92.4	41.6	83.6	84.6
Haryana	1.9	68.6	88.9	42.9	63.3	69.3
Himachal Pradesh	1.2	67.4	83.1	39.2	50.3	53.7
Jammu and Kashmir	1.8	87.0	94.5	43.5	80.9	82.9
Punjab	1.4	73.4	92.6	29.4	60.3	66.7
Rajasthan	2.5	55.2	81.0	14.6	70.5	75.8
Uttarakhand	1.6	54.8	84.9	17.0	53.5	58.7
Central	1.5	NA	NA	NA	NA	NA
Chhattisgarh	1.8	71.4	88.4	19.9	44.9	56.4

	Maternal health indicators (%)					
	Ever-married women severely anaemic[1] (%)	Women who had three or more ANC visits (%)[2]	Women who received two or more TT injections during pregnancy (%)[2]	Women who received all recommended types of antenatal care (%)[2]	Women who delivered in a health/institution[2]	Women whose delivery was attended by trained health personnel[2]
Madhya Pradesh	1.0	60.0	87.2	11.1	81.0	82.9
Uttar Pradesh	1.6	38.2	80.6	12.4	62.1	64.2
East	1.1	NA	NA	NA	NA	NA
Bihar	1.0	33.8	85.9	4.5	48.3	53.2
Jharkhand	1.3	57.5	89.8	10.9	40.1	47.3
Odisha	1.3	77.0	95.2	37.5	75.5	79.1
West Bengal	0.9	83.2	94.6	17.4	69.5	72.6
Northeast	2.9	NA	NA	NA	NA	NA
Arunachal Pradesh	1.8	50.4	64.1	16.3	69.9	71.9
Assam	3.5	66.4	90.1	21.3	64.4	65.5
Manipur	0.5	85.0	86.9	28.4	80.0	82.7
Meghalaya	2.3	71.0	76.6	28.1	63.6	65.2
Mizoram	0.6	79.0	73.7	21.7	83.0	85.1

(Continued)

Table A3.2 *(Continued)*

	Maternal health indicators (%)					
	Ever-married women severely anaemic[1] (%)	Women who had three or more ANC visits (%)[2]	Women who received two or more TT injections during pregnancy (%)[2]	Women who received all recommended types of antenatal care (%)[2]	Women who delivered in a health/institution[2]	Women whose delivery was attended by trained health personnel[2]
Nagaland	—	29.4	46.6	3.5	30.4	43.8
Sikkim	2.0	87.3	86.5	27.7	68.9	69.9
Tripura	1.5	83.1	90.9	21.5	82.6	83.1
West	2.2	NA	NA	NA	NA	NA
Goa	0.7	97.7	87.4	53.4	99.8	99.8
Gujarat	2.9	83.2	79.7	45.7	78.1	85.2
Maharashtra	1.8	82.6	79.4	27.0	81.8	85.5
South	2.4	NA	NA	NA	NA	NA
Andhra Pradesh	3.3	97.0	93.9	46.2	94.2	95.6
Karnataka	2.2	91.3	91.3	40.2	86.4	88.4
Kerala	0.4	90.8	90.0	77.9	99.9	99.9
Tamil Nadu	2.3	92.6	92.5	44.1	98.4	98.6

Source: [1]International Institute for Population Sciences and Macro International (2007), Regional estimates are calculated for severe anaemia from NHFS-3 (2005–06); [2]United Nations Children's Fund, 2010. NA: not available.

Table A3.3 Percentage of Women Practising Contraception and Reporting an Unmet Need for Family Planning by State, India, 2005–06

	Contraceptive use			Currently married women with unmet need for family planning		
	Any method	Any modern method	Per cent non-terminal method	Spacing	Limiting	Total
India	56.3	48.5	20.8	6.2	6.6	12.8
North	56.3	51.4	32.9	5.0	6.2	11.2
Delhi	66.9	56.5	57.9	3.3	4.5	7.8
Haryana	63.4	58.3	33.3	3.1	5.2	8.3
Himachal Pradesh	72.6	71	22.1	2.4	4.9	7.3
Jammu and Kashmir	52.6	44.9	35.4	5.8	8.7	14.5
Punjab	63.3	56.1	43.0	2.6	4.7	7.3
Rajasthan	47.2	44.4	21.2	7.3	7.3	14.6
Uttarkhand	59.3	55.5	38.9	4.4	6.5	10.9
Central	47.7	37.2	27.1	7.8	9.8	17.6
Chhattisgarh	53.2	49.1	10.4	5.3	4.8	10.1
Madhya Pradesh	55.9	52.8	13.6	5.4	5.9	11.3
Uttar Pradesh	43.6	29.3	40.6	9.1	12.1	21.2
East	50.6	39.4	26.4	7.7	8.5	16.2

(*Continued*)

Table A3.3 *(Continued)*

	Contraceptive use			Currently married women with unmet need for family planning		
	Any method	Any modern method	Per cent non-terminal method	Spacing	Limiting	Total
Bihar	34.1	28.9	15.6	10.7	12.1	22.8
Jharkhand	35.7	31.1	23.5	11.3	11.9	23.2
Odisha	50.7	44.7	23.7	6.8	8.1	14.9
West Bengal	71.2	49.9	34.1	4.0	4.0	8.0
Northeast	54.2	29.3	51.7	5.2	7.7	12.9
Arunachal Pradesh	43.2	37.3	39.4	8.3	10.6	18.9
Assam	56.5	27	51.5	3.5	7.1	10.6
Manipur	48.7	23.6	62.7	5.0	7.4	12.4
Meghalaya	24.3	18.5	49.2	23.2	11.8	35
Mizoram	59.9	59.6	28.0	12.3	5.0	17.3
Nagaland	29.7	22.5	55.6	10	16.1	26.1
Sikkim	57.6	48.7	47.2	5.6	11.2	16.8
Tripura	65.7	44.9	59.7	3.8	6.5	10.3
West	66.6	61.8	19.6	5.1	3.9	9.0
Goa	48.2	37.2	30.4	7.4	5.7	13.1

	Contraceptive use			Currently married women with unmet need for family planning		
	Any method	Any modern method	Per cent non-terminal method	Spacing	Limiting	Total
Gujarat	66.6	56.5	22.8	4.3	3.7	8.0
Maharashtra	66.9	64.9	18.0	5.4	3.9	9.3
South	65.2	62.9	6.3	4.4	3.1	7.5
Andhra Pradesh	67.6	67	2.1	3.0	1.7	4.7
Karnataka	63.6	62.5	8.0	6.0	3.6	9.6
Kerala	68.6	57.9	14.2	6.0	2.9	8.9
Tamil Nadu	61.4	60	7.7	4.0	4.5	8.5

Source: International Institute for Population Sciences and Macro International (2007), Regional estimates are calculated from NHFS-3 (2005–06).

References

Action Research and Training for Health (ARTH) and Department of Medical, Health and Family Welfare, Rajasthan. 2009. Implementation of the Medical Termination of Pregnancy Act in Rajasthan, India: Status Report 2007–08. Udaipur, ARTH.

Agarwal, S., V. Sethi, K. Srivastava, P.K. Jha, and A.H. Baqui. 2010. 'Birth Preparedness and Complication Readiness Among Slum Women in Indore City, India', *Journal of Health Population Nutrition,* 28(4): 383–391.

Aswathy, S., S. Sumithra, L.S. Valsala, S. Sandheep, V. Lohidas, P. Shobha. et al. 2006. 'Self-Reported Morbidity and Awareness Regarding Common Cancers in Elderly Women', *Journal of Community Medicine,* 38(1): 106–11.

Bang, A.T., R.A Bang, S. Baitule, M. Deshmukh, and M. Hanimi Reddy. 2001. 'Burden Of Morbidities and the Unmet Need for Health Care in Rural Neonates: A Prospective Observational Study in Gadchiroli, India', *Indian Pediatrics,* 38: 952–65.

Bang, A. T., H.N. Reddy, S.B. Baitule, M.D. Deshmukh, and Rani A. Bang 2005. 'The Incidence of Morbidities in a Cohort of Neonates in Rural Gadchiroli, India: Seasonal and Temporal Variation and a Hypothesis About Prevention', *Journal of Perinatology,* 25: S18–S28.

Baqui, A.H., G. L. Darmstadt, E. K. Williams, V. Kumar, T.U. Kiran, D. Panwar et al. 2006. 'Rates, Timing and Causes of Neonatal Deaths in Rural India: Implications for Neonatal Health Programmes', *Bulletin of the World Health Organization, September* 2006, 84(9).

Barge, S., M.E. Khan, S. Rajagopal, N. Kumar, S. Kumber et al. 1998. 'Availability and Quality of MTP Services in Gujarat, Maharashtra, Tamil Nadu and Uttar Pradesh', Paper presented at the Global Meeting on Post-abortion Care and Operations Research, organised by Population Council, New York.

Barge, S., H. Bracken, B. Elul, N. Kumar, W.U. Khan, S. Verma et al. 2004. *Formal and Informal Abortion Services in Rajasthan, India: Results of a Situation Analysis.* New Delhi: Population Council.

Barnes, L. 2007. 'Women's Experience of Childbirth in Rural Jharkhand', *Economic and Political Weekly,* 41(48): 62–70.

Barua, A. and H. Apte. 2007. 'Quality of Abortion Care: Perspectives of Clients and Providers in Jharkhand', *Economic and Political Weekly,* 42(48): 71–80.

Bharat, S. and V.S. Mahendra. 2007. 'Meeting the Sexual and Reproductive Health Needs of People Living with HIV: Challenges for Health Care Providers', *Reproductive Health Matters,* 15(29) Supplement: 93–112.

Balsara, Zohra Patel, P. Winch, G. Darmstadt, S. Agarwal, and A. Baqui. 2009. Care Seeking for Neonatal Morbidity in the Urban Slums of Uttar Pradesh, India. Presented at the APHA meetings.

Chhabra, R. and S.C. Nuna. 1994. *Abortion in India: An Overview*. New Delhi: Ford Foundation.

Char, Arundhati, M. Saavala, and Teija Kulmala. 2009. 'Male Perceptions on Female Sterilization: A Community-Based Study in Rural Central India', *International Perspectives on Sexual Health,* 35(3): 131–138.

Chopra, A., R.R. Mittal, P. Singh, and P. Sharma. 1990. 'Patterns of Sexually Transmitted Diseases at Patiala', *Indian Journal of Sexually Transmitted Diseases* 11: 43–45.

Chaudhary, S.D., K.K. Bhattia, R.K. Bansal, and V.K. Jain. 1988. 'Pattern of Sexually Transmitted Diseases in Rohtak', *Indian Journal of Sexually Transmitted Diseases*, 9: 4–7.

Christian Medical College and Population Council. 2000. *Understanding Health Needs in the Post-Reproductive Age Group* (unpublished report).

CORT. 2007a. *Assessment of Janani Suraksha Yojana in Assam*. Vadodara: Centre for Operations Research and Training.

———. 2007b. *Assessment of Janani Suraksha Yojana in Himachal Pradesh*. Vadodara: Centre for Operations Research and Training.

———. 2007c. *Assessment of ASHA and Janani Suraksha Yojana in Madhya Pradesh*. Vadodara: Centre for Operations Research and Training; New Delhi: UNICEF.

———. 2007d. *Assessment of ASHA and Janani Suraksha Yojana in Orissa*. Vadodara: Centre for Operations Research and Training; New Delhi: UNICEF.

———. 2007e. *Assessment of ASHA and Janani Suraksha Yojana in Rajasthan*. Vadodara: Centre for Operations Research and Training; New Delhi: UNICEF.

———. 2007f. *Assessment of Janani Suraksha Yojana in West Bengal.* Vadodara: Centre for Operations Research and Training.

———. 2008a. *Assessment of Janani avam Bal Suraksha Yojana in Bihar*. Vadodara: Centre for Operations Research and Training; New Delhi: UNICEF.

———. 2008b. *Assessment of Janani Suraksha Yojana in Uttar Pradesh*. Vadodara: Centre for Operations Research and Training; New Delhi: UNICEF

Devadasan N., M.A. Eliasa, D. John, S. Grahacharya, and L. Ralte. 2008. 'A Conditional Cash Assistance Programme for Promoting Institutional Deliveries Among the Poor in India: Process Evaluation Results', *Studies in Health Services Organisation & Policy*, 24: 257–74.

Duggal, R. and S. Barge. 2004. 'Abortion Services in India: Report of a Multicentric Enquiry', *Abortion Assessment Project-India*. Mumbai: CEHAT/Healthwatch.

Elul, B., S. Barge, S. Verma, R. Ved, R. Singhi, and K. Lockwood 2004. *Unwanted Pregnancy and Induced Abortion: Data from Men and Women in Rajasthan, India*: Report. New Delhi: Population Council.

Ganatra, B. 2000. 'Abortion Research in India: What We Know and What We Need To Know', in R. Ramasubban and S.J. Jejeebhoy eds, *Women's. Reproductive Health in India*. Jaipur: Rawat Publications.

Ganatra, B., V. Manning, and S.P. Pallipamulla. 2005. 'Availability of Medical Abortion Pills and the Role of Chemists: A Study from Bihar and Jharkhand, India', *Reproductive Health Matters*, 13(26): 65–74.

Ganatra, B., S. Hirve, S.L. Garda, and V.N. Rao. 2008. 'Induced Abortions in Rural Western Maharashtra: Prevalence and Patterns', in M. Koenig, S.J. Jejeebhoy. J. Cleland, and B. Ganatra eds, *Reproductive Health in India: New Evidence*. New Delhi: Rawat Publications.

Garg, S., M.M. Singh, A. Nath, P. Bhalla, V. Garg, and V.K. Gupta. 2007. 'Prevalence and Awareness about Sexually Transmitted Infections among Males in Urban Slums in Delhi', *Indian Journal of Medical Sciences*, 61: 269–77.

Garg, S., P. Bhalla, N. Sharma, R. Sahay, A Puri, R. Saha et al. 2008. *Comparison of Self-reported Symptoms of Gynaecological Morbidity with Clinical and Laboratory Diagnosis in a New Delhi Slum*. In M.A. Koenig, S. Jejeebhoy, J. Cleland, and B. Ganatra eds, *Reproductive Health in India New Evidence* Jaipur: Rawat Publications.

George, S., M. Jacob, T.J. John, M.K. Jain, N.S. Nathan, P.S. Rao, et al. 1997. 'A Case-Control Analysis of Risk Factors in HIV Transmission in South India', *Journal of Acquired Immune Deficiency Syndromes and Human Retrovirology*, 14: 290–93.

Government of India. 1971. *The Medical Termination of Pregnancy Act (Act. No. 34)*. New Delhi: Government of India.

———. 2003. *The Medical Termination of Pregnancy Rules (Amendment)*. New Delhi: Government of India.

Goyal, S.M and N. Bhandari. 2008. *Delivery and Postnatal Morbidity among Women in Urban Slums in New Delhi*. In M.A. Koenig, S.J. Jejeebhoy, J. Cleland, and B. Ganatra eds, *Reproductive Health in India: New Evidence* Jaipur: Rawat Publications.

Indian Council for Medical Research (ICMR). 2008. *Study on 2 Monthly Injectable Contraceptive Norethisterone Enanthate (200mg): Summary Report*. Accessed at http://www.mohfw.nic.in/dofw%20website/Final_Net-En_Report.pdf on 18.02.2011.

International Institute for Population Sciences (IIPS). 1995. *National Family Health Survey (MCH and Family Planning), India, 1992–93*. Mumbai: IIPS.

———. (IIPS) and ORC Macro. 2000. *National Family Health Survey (NFHS-2), 1998–99; India*. Mumbai: IIPS.

International Institute for Population Sciences (IIPS) and Macro International 2007. *National Family Health Survey (NFHS-3), India, 2005–06*. Mumbai: IIPS.

International Institute for Population Sciences (IIPS). 2010. *District Level Household and Facility Survey (DLHS-3), 2007–08: India*. Mumbai: IIPS.

International Institute for Population Sciences (IIPS) and Population Council. 2010. *Youth in India: Situation and Needs 2006–2007*. Mumbai: IIPS.

Iyengar, S.D., K. Iyengar, J.C. Martines, K. Dashora, and K.K. Deora. 2008. 'Childbirth Practices in Rural Rajasthan, India: Implications for Neonatal Health and Survival', *Journal of Perinatology*, 28: S23–S30.

Iyengar, Kirti, S. D. Iyengar, V. Suhalka, and K. Dashora. 2009a. 'Pregnancy-related Deaths in Rural Rajasthan, India: Exploring Causes, Context, and Care-seeking Through Verbal Autopsy', *Journal of Health Population and Nutrition,* 27(2): 293–302.

———. 2009b. 'Comparison of Domiciliary and Institutional Delivery-care Practices in Rural Rajasthan, India,' *Journal of Health, Population and Nutrition*, 27(2): 303–312.

Jain, A. and A. Jain. 2010. *Family Planning and Fertility in India. Paper presented at UNFPA-ICOMP Regional Consultation on Family Planning in Asia and the Pacific Addressing the Challenges*. Bangkok: Thailand.

Jeffery, Patricia, A. Das, J. Dasgupta, and R. Jeffery. 2007. 'Unmonitored Intrapartum Oxytocin Use in Home Deliveries: Evidence from Uttar Pradesh, India'. *Reproductive Health Matters*, 15(30): 172–178.

Jejeebhoy, S.J. and A.J.F. Zavier. 2012. *Injectable Contraceptives: Perspectives and Experiences of Women and Health Care Providers in India*. New Delhi: Population Council.

Jejeebhoy, S.J., A.J.F. Zavier, and S. Kalyanwala. 2010. *Assessing Abortion-Related Experiences and Needs in Four Districts of Maharashtra and Rajasthan, 2006*. New Delhi: Population Council.

Jejeebhoy, S.J., K.G. Santhya, and R. Acharya. 2010. *Health and Social Consequences of Marital Violence: A Synthesis of Evidence from India*. New Delhi: Population Council.

Jejeebhoy, S.J., A.J. Francis Zavier, R. Acharya, and S. Kalyanwala. 2011a. *Increasing Access to Safe Abortion in Rural Rajasthan: Outcomes of a Comprehensive Abortion Care Model*. New Delhi: Population Council.

Jejeebhoy, S.J., S. Kalyanwala, A.J. Francis Zavier, R. Kumar, S. Mundle, J. Tank et al. 2011b. 'Can Nurses Perform Manual Vaccum Aspiration (MVA) as Safely and Effectively As Physicians? Evidence from India', *Contraception*, 84(2011): 615–621.

Jejeebhoy, S.J., S. Kalyanwala, S. Mundle, J. Tank, A.J. Francis Zavier, R. Kumar et al. 2012. 'Feasibility of Expanding the Medical Abortion Provider Base in India to Include Ayurved Physicians And Nurses', *International Perspectives on Sexual and Reproductive Health*, 38(3): 133–142.

Johnston, H.B. 2002. *Abortion Practice in India: A Review of the Literature*. Mumbai: CEHAT.

Kalyanwala, S., S. Iyengar, and S. Janardhan. 2007. *Factors Underlying the Fertility Intentions of People Living with HIV/AIDS in Karnataka*. New Delhi: Population Council.

Kalyanwala, S., A.J.F. Zavier, and S. Jejeebhoy. 2010. *Public Health Facilities and Women's Access to Abortion: A Situation Analysis in Maharashtra and Rajasthan*. New Delhi: Population Council (unpublished report).

Kamat, H.A. and D.D. Banker. 1993. 'Human Immunodeficiency Virus-1 Infection Among Patients with Sexually Transmitted Diseases in Bombay', *National Medical Journal of India,* 6(1): 11–13.

Kanniappan, S., M.J. Jeyapaul., and S. Kalyanwala. 2008. 'Desire for Motherhood: Exploring HIV-positive Women's Desires, Intentions and Decision-Making in Attaining Motherhood', *AIDS Care,* 20(6): 625–30.

Koenig, M., S. J. Jejeebhoy, S. Singh, and S. Sridhar. 1998. 'Investigating Gynaecological Morbidity in India', *Reproductive Health Matters*, 6(11): 84–97.

Kostick, K.M, S.L. Schensul, K. Jadhav, R. Singh, A. Bavadekar, and N. Saggurti. 2010. 'Treatment Seeking, Vaginal Discharge and Psychosocial Distress Among Women in Urban Mumbai', *Culture, Medicine and Psychiatry,* 34: 529–547.

Lahariya, C. and V.K. Paul. 2010. 'Burden, Differentials and Causes of Child Deaths in India', *Indian Journal Paediatrics,* 77: 1312–1321.

Lim, S.S., L. Dandona, J. A. Hoisington, S.L. James, M.C. Hogan, and E. Gakidou. 2010. 'India's Jananki Suraksha Yojana, a Conditional Cash Transfer Programme to Increase Births in Health Facilities: An Impact Evaluation', *Lancet,* 375(9730): 2009–23.

Malhotra, A., L. Nyblade, S. Parasuraman, K. MacQuarrie, N. Kashyap, and S. Walia 2003. *Realizing Reproductive Choice and Rights: Abortion and Contraception in India, Report*. Washington DC: International Council for Research on Women.

Marfatia, Y.S., S. Barge, S. Parmar et al. 2000. 'Treatment Seeking Behaviours of STD Cases Attending Skin and VD Department and Private Clinics in Vadodara', unpublished.

Mavalankar, D.V., K.S. Vora, K.V. Ramani, P. Raman, B. Sharma, and M. Upadhya. 2009. 'Maternal Health in Gujarat, India: A Case Study', *Journal of Health, Population and Nutrition*, 27(2): 235–248.

Ministry of Health and Family Welfare (MOHFW). 1994. The Pre-conception and Pre-natal Diagnostic Techniques (Prohibition of Sex Selection) Act, 1994. New Delhi: MOHFW, Government of India.

———. 2000. *National Population Policy 2000*. New Delhi: Department of Family Welfare, MOHFW, Government of India.

———. 2005a. *National Rural Health Mission (2005–2012). Mission Document*. New Delhi: MOHFW, Government of India. Accessed on 25 March, 2012 at http://www.mohfw.nic.in//NRHM/Documents/Mission_Document.pdf.

———. 2005b. *RCH Phase II: National Program Implementation Plan*. New Delhi: MOHFW, Government of India.

———. 2006. *ASHA Support Mechanism*. New Delhi: MOHFW, Government of India. Accessed on 22 June 2011 at http://mohfw.nic.in/NRHM/asha.htm#abt.

———. 2007. *National Guidelines on Prevention, Management and Control of Reproductive Tract Infections Including Sexually Transmitted Infections*. New Delhi: MOHFW, Government of India.

———. 2008. *National Training Strategy for In-Service Training Under National Rural Health Mission*. New Delhi: MOHFW, Government of India.

———. 2009. *National Rural Health Mission Reproductive & Child Health Program Phase II, 6th Joint Review Mission*. New Delhi: Donor Coordination Division, MOHFW, Government of India.

———. 2010a. *National Rural Health Mission, State Wise Progress As on 30.09.2010*. New Delhi: Department of Family Welfare, MOHFW, Government of India.

———. 2010b. *Annual Report 2010–2011*. New Delhi: MOHFW, Government of India.

———. 2010c. *Operational Guidelines on Maternal and Newborn Health*. New Delhi: MOHFW, Government of India. Accessed on 5 June 2011 at http://nhsrcindia.org/search_resources_data.php

———. 2010d. The *Assisted Reproductive Technologies (Regulation) Bill-2010*. New Delhi: MOHFW, Government of India.

———. 2010e. *Comprehensive Abortion Care: Training and Service Delivery Guidelines*. New Delhi: MOHFW, Government of India.

Ministry of Health and Family Welfare (MOHFW) 2011a. *Family Welfare Statistics in India 2011*. New Delhi: MOHFW, Government of India.

———. 2011b. *Agenda Note: Review Meeting of State Nodal Officers, RCH programme*. New Delhi: RCH Division, MOHFW, Government of India.

———. 2011c. *Fourth Common Review Mission Report 2010*. New Delhi: MOHFW, Government of India.

———. 2011d. *Update on the ASHA Programme*. New Delhi: MOHFW, Government of India.

———. 2011e. *ASHA: Which Way Forward? Evaluation of ASHA Programme*, New Delhi: MOHFW, Government of India.

———. n.d. *Operational Guidelines for Implementation of Integrated Management of Neonatal and Childhood Illness (IMNCI)*. New Delhi: MOHFW, Government of India.

———. 2010. *Annual Report 2010–2011*. New Delhi: MOWCD, Government of India.

Mishra, U.S. and M. Ramanathan. 2002. 'Delivery-related Complications and Determinants of Caesarean Section Rates in India', *Health Policy and Planning*, 17(1): 90–98.

Mitchell, A., A. Mahal, and T. Bossert. 2011. 'Healthcare Utilisation in Rural Andhra Pradesh', *Economic and Political Weekly*, 46(5): 15–19.

National AIDS Control Organisation (NACO). 2006a. *National AIDS Control Programme Phase III (2006–2012)*. New Delhi: MOHFW, Government of India.

National AIDS Control organisation (NACO) 2006b. *HIV/AIDS Epidemiological Surveillance and Estimation Report for the year 2005*. New Delhi: MOHFW, Government of India.

———. 2010a. *Annual Report 2009–10*. New Delhi: NACO.

———. 2010b. *Condom Promotion, National AIDS Control Programme, Phase-III, India*. New Delhi: NACO.

———. 2010c. *National AIDS Control Programme, Response to the HIV Epidemic in India*. New Delhi: NACO.

Nidadavolu, V. and H. Bracken. 2006. 'Abortion and Sex Determination: Conflicting Messages in Information Materials in a District of Rajasthan, India', *Reproductive Health Matters*, 14(27): 160–171.

National Institute of Medical Statistics (NIMS) and National AIDS Control Organisation (NACO). 2012. *Technical Report: India HIV Estimates 2010*: NACO. New Delhi: NACO. Accessed at 07 June 2012 at <http://www.nacoonline.org>.

Nyblade, L., J. Edmeades, and E. Pearson. 2010. 'Self-reported Abortion-related Morbidity: A Comparison of Measures in Madhya Pradesh', India. *International Perspectives on Sexual and Reproductive Health*, 36(3): 140–148.

Office of Registrar General, India. 2009. *Special Bulletin on Maternal Mortality in India, 2004–06, Sample Registration System*. New Delhi: Office of the Registrar General and Census Commissioner.

———. 2011. *Special Bulletin on Maternal Mortality in India 2007–09, Sample Registration System*. New Delhi: Office of the Registrar General.

Office of the Registrar General and Census Commissioner, India. 2013. *Census of India 2011: Primary Census Abstract: Data Highlights, India, Series 1*. New Delhi: Controller of Publications.

Patel, V., M. Rodrigues and N. DeSouza. 2002. 'Gender, Poverty and Postnatal Depression: A Study of Mothers in Goa, India', *American Journal of Psychiatry*, 159(1): 43–47.

Patel, V., H.A. Weiss., D. Mabey, B West, S. D'Souza, V. Patil et al. 2006. 'The Burden and Determinants of Reproductive Tract Infection in India: A Population Based Study of Women in Goa, India', *Sexually Transmitted Infections*, 82: 243–249.

Pathak, P., A. Singh, and S.V. Subramanian. 2010. 'Economic Inequalities in Maternal Health Care: Prenatal Care and Skilled Birth Attendance in India', *PLoS ONE*, 5(10): e13592. Doi:1-.1371/journal.pone.0013593.

Paul, V.K., H.S. Sachdev., D.V. Mavalankar, P Ramachandran, M.J. Sankar, N. Bhandari et al. 2011. 'Reproductive Health, and Child Health and Nutrition in India: Meeting the Challenge', *Lancet*, 377: 332–49.

Planning Commission, Health Division. 2012. *Report of the Steering Committee on Health for the 12th Five-Year Plan*. Planning Commission, New Delhi.

Planning Commission. 2011a. *Approach to the Twelfth Five Year Plan*. New Delhi: Planning Commission. Accessed on 25 April, 2012 at http://www.pib.nic.in/archieve/eec/2011/planning2011.pdf.

———. 2011b. *Faster, Sustainable and More Inclusive Growth: An Approach to the Twelfth Five Year Plan*. New Delhi: Planning Commission.

———. 2011c. *Mid-Term Appraisal Eleventh Five Year Plan 2007–2012*. New Delhi: Oxford University Press.

———. 2011d. *Report of the Working group on National Rural Health Mission (NRHM) for the 12th Five Year Plan*. New Delhi: Planning Commission.

Prakasamma, M. 2009. 'Maternal Mortality-reduction Programme in Andhra Pradesh', *Journal of Health, Population and Nutrition*, 27(2): 220–234.

Population Council. 2011. *Expanding Access to Safe Abortion and Post-abortion Care: Recommendations of a South Asia Regional Consultation*. New Delhi: Population Council.

Rajan, V., V.K. Machanda, and S. Nagarajan. 2010. *Quality of Obstetric Care in India: Will We 'Deliver' in Time? in India Health Beat Supporting Evidence-based Policies and Implementation*. Volume 3(5).

Ray, K., M. Bala., S.M. Gupta, N. Khunger, P. Puri, S. Muralidhar et al. 2006. 'Changing Trends in Sexually Transmitted Infections at a Regional STC centre in North India', *Indian Journal of Medical Research,* 124: 559–568.

Registrar General, India (RGI). 2000. *Sample Registration System Bulletin,* April. New Delhi: Office of Registrar General.

———. 2001. *Census of India, Provisional Population Totals, Series I, Paper I. 2001.* New Delhi: Office of Registrar General.

———. 2006. *Maternal Mortality in India: 1997–2003, Trends, Causes and Risk Factors.* New Delhi: Office of Registrar General.

———. 2011. *Sample Registration System Bulletin, Volume 45 No. 1.* New Delhi: Office of the Registrar General.

Risbud, A., K. Chan-Tack., D. Gadkari, R.R. Gangakhedkar, M.E. Shepherd, R. Bollinger et al. 1999. 'The Etiology of Genital Ulcer Disease by Multiplex Polymerase Chain Reaction and Relationship to HIV infection Among Patients Attending Sexually Transmitted Disease Clinics in Pune, India', *Sexually Transmitted Diseases;* 26(1): 55–62.

Sahasrabuddhe, V. V., T. A. Gholap., Y.S. Jethava, N.S. Joglekar, R.G. Brahme, B.A. Gaikwad et al. 2002. 'Patient-led Partner Referral in a District Hospital Based STD clinic', *Journal of Postgraduate Medicine,* 48(2): 105–08.

SAMA—Resource Group for Women and Health. 2010. *Constructing Conceptions: The Mapping of Assisted Reproductive Technologies in India.* New Delhi: SAMA—Resource Group for Women and Health.

Santhya, K.G. and G.L. Dasvarma. 2002. 'Spousal Communication on Reproductive Illness Among Rural Women in Southern India', *Culture, Health and Sexuality,* 4(2): 223–26.

Santhya, K.G. 2004. 'Contraceptive Use Dynamics', in S.J. Jejeebhoy ed. *Looking Back Looking Forward: A Profile of Sexual and Reproductive Health in India.* New Delhi: Rawat Publications.

———. 2009. *Understanding Pregnancy-related Morbidity and Mortality Among Young Women in Rajasthan.* New Delhi: Population Council.

Santhya, K.G and S. Verma. 2004. 'Induced Abortion', in S.J. Jejeebhoy ed. *Looking Back Looking Forward: A Profile of Sexual and Reproductive Health in India.* New Delhi: Rawat Publications.

Santhya, K.G and S.J. Jejeebhoy. 2007. 'Early Marriage and HIV/AIDS Risk Factors Among Young Women', *Economic and Political Weekly,* 52(14): 1291–1297.

Santhya, K.G., S.J. Jejeebhoy and S. Ghosh. 2008. *Early Marriage and Sexual and Reproductive Health Risks: Experiences of Young Women and Men in Andhra Pradesh and Madhya Pradesh, India.* New Delhi: Population Council.

Santhya, K.G., S.J. Jejeebhoy and A.J. Francis Zavier. 2011a. *Implementing the Janani Suraksha Yojana: Perspectives and Experiences of Accredited Social Health Activists in Rajasthan*. New Delhi: Population Council.

Santhya, K.G., S.J. Jejeebhoy, R. Acharya, and A.J.F. Zavier. 2011b. *Effects of the Janani Suraksha Yojana on Maternal and Newborn Care Practices: Women's Experience in Rajasthan*. New Delhi: Population Council.

Santhya, K.G. and S.J. Jejeebhoy. 2012. Providing Maternal and Newborn Health Services: Experinces of Auxiliary Nurse Midwives in Rajasthan. New Delhi: Population Council.

Santhya, K.G., S.J. Jejeebhoy, R. Acharya, and A.J.F. Zavier. 2012. 'Conditional Cash Transfers and Quality of Delivery Care: Women's Experience of the Janani Suraksha Yojana in Rajasthan, India', (unpublished paper).

Sharan, M., D. Strobino and S. Ahmed. 2005. 'Intrapartum Oxytocin Use for Labor Acceleration in Rural India', *International Journal of Gynaecology and Obstetrics*, 90: 251–57.

Sharma, R. 2008. *Janani Suraksha Yojana: A Study of the Implementation Status in Selected Districts of Rajasthan*. Udaipur: Population Research Centre, Mohanlal Sukhadia University.

Sidney, Kristi, V. Diwan, Z. El-Khatib, and Ayesha de Costa 2012. 'India's JSY Cash Transfer Program for Maternal Health: Who Participates and who Doesn't—A Report from Ujjain district', *Reproductive Health*, 9 (2): 1–7.

Singh, K.G., M.K. Joshi, and A. K. Bajaj. 1990. 'Pattern of Sexually Transmitted Diseases in Allahabad', *Indian Journal of Sexually Transmitted Diseases*, 11: 6–8.

Singh, M. and V.K. Paul. 1997. 'Maternal and Child Health Services in India with Special Focus on Perinatal Services'. *Journal of Perinatology*, 17(1): 65–69.

Sreevidya, S. and B.W.C. Sathiyasekaran. 2003. 'High Caesarean Rates in Madras (India): A Population-based Cross-sectional Study', *British Journal of Obstetrics and Gynaecology*, 110: 106–10.

Srivastava, N.M., S. Awasthi and R. Mishra. 2008. 'Neonatal Morbidity and Care-seeking Behavior in Urban Lucknow *Indian Paediatrics*', 45(3): 229–32.

Subha, Sri. B. 2009. Translating Medical Evidence into Practice—Working with Communities and Providers to Promote Active Management of the Third Stage of Labour. *Health and Population Innovation Fellowship Programme Working Paper No. 11*. New Delhi: Population Council.

Tank, J. 2011. Provision of Abortion by AYUSH and Nurses in India: FOGSI Perspectives on What Next. Presentation made at the 'Consultation on

Expanding Access to Safe Abortion and PAC in South Asia: Is Provision of Services by Midlevel Providers a Feasible Option?' 07–08 March 2011, New Delhi, India.

Unisa, S. 2008. 'Sequence of Fertility Treatments Among Childless Couples in Ranga Reddy District, Andhra Pradesh', In M. A. Koenig, S. Jejeebhoy, J. Cleland, and B. Ganatra eds, *Reproductive Health in India: New Evidence*. Jaipur: Rawat Publications.

———. 1999. 'Childlessness in Andhra Pradesh, India: Treatment-Seeking and Consequences', *Reproductive Health Matters*, 7–13: 54–64.

United Nations Population Fund. 2009. *Concurrent Assessment of Janani Suraksha Yojana (JSY) in Selected States: Bihar, Madhya Pradesh, Orissa, Rajasthan, Uttar Pradesh*. New Delhi, UNFPA.

United Nations Population Fund, (UNFPA). 2010. *Trends in Sex Ratio at Birth and Estimates of Girls Missing at Birth in India*. New Delhi. UNFPA:

United Nations Children's Fund (UNICEF). 2010. *Coverage Evaluation Survey 2009*. New Delhi: UNICEF.

Vora, K.S., D.V. Mavalankar, K.V. Ramani, M. Upadhyaya, B. Sharma, S. Iyengar et al. 2009. 'Maternal "Health Situation in India: A Case Study"', *Journal of Health, Population and Nutrition*, 27(2): 184–201.

World Health Organization. 2012. *Trends in Maternal Mortality: 1990 to 2010, WHO, UNICEF, UNFPA and The World Bank Estimates*. Geneva: World Health Organisation. Accessed on 25 March, 2012 at http://whqlibdoc.who.int/publications/2012/9789241503631_eng.pdf.

Widge. A. 2004. 'Infertility', in S.J. Jejeebhoy eds. *Looking Back Looking Forward: A Profile of Sexual and Reproductive Health in India*. New Delhi: Rawat Publications.

Widge, A. and J. Cleland. 2008. 'The Public Sector's Role in Infertility Management in India', *Health Policy and Planning*, 24(2): 108–115.

Zavier, A. J.F., S.J. Jejeebhoy, and S. Kalyanwala. 2012. 'Factors Associated with Second Trimester Abortion in Rural Maharashtra and Rajasthan, India', *Global Public Health*, 7(8): 897–908.

Zavier, A.J.F. and Sabu S. Padmadas. 2012. 'Post-abortion Contraceptive Use and Method Continuation in India', *International Journal of Gynecology and Obstetrics*, 118(1): 65–70.

4

Adolescents and Youth in India

Challenges and Opportunities

K.G. Santhya

Shireen J. Jejeebhoy

Today, about 358 million people in India–nearly one-third of the country's population—are young people aged 10–24 (Office of the Registrar General and Census Commissioner, India 2006). It is increasingly recognized that whether India achieves the Millennium Development Goals, whether it achieves its population stabilization objectives and whether it can realize the advantage of its demographic dividend will depend on the nation's investment in its young people. Compared to earlier generations, the situation of young people in India has undoubtedly improved: they are healthier and better educated than ever before, and gender disparities in child mortality, school enrolment, and educational attainment have narrowed. Nonetheless, many obstacles exist that inhibit young people from making informed life choices and from adopting egalitarian notions of masculinity and femininity, limit young women's exercise of agency, and compromise young people's health, notably in the sexual and reproductive health arena.

There are, however, some encouraging signals. One of these is political commitment for meeting the health and development needs of young people. For example, India has articulated its commitment to promoting and protecting the sexual and reproductive health and rights as well as meeting the development needs of adolescents and youth through numerous policies and programmes, and particularly over the last decade and a half. The National Population Policy, the National AIDS Prevention and Control Policy (NACP), the National Youth Policy, and the National Skill Development Policy are key examples of the recognition that the sexual and reproductive needs and rights of adolescents and young people require urgent attention. Likewise, the National Adolescent Reproductive and Sexual Health Strategy, the National Skill Development Initiative, the Adolescence Education Programme (AEP), and the Rashtriya Madhyamik Shiksha Abhiyan (RMSA) are notable examples of the country's commitment to addressing the development needs of adolescents and young people.

This chapter synthesizes key programmes in India that focus on or have implications for the sexual and reproductive health and rights, and development of young people, summarizes what is known about the sexual and reproductive health, and development situation of young people and maps the challenges in and opportunities for meeting the sexual and reproductive health needs and rights as well as development needs of young people.

Programme Initiatives to Address Young People's Health and Development Needs

Since the 1990s, several programmes with considerable focus on health and development needs of youth have been initiated in India. This section describes the six broad areas of youth programming: raising young people's awareness about reproductive and sexual health matters, facilitating their access to reproductive and sexual health counselling and services, supplementing nutrition, addressing gender disparity, enabling young people to acquire educational levels and marketable skills, and building a supportive environment.

Programmes to Raise Awareness About Sexual and Reproductive Issues

A number of programmes have been implemented to raise awareness about sexual and reproductive matters among young people. While some of these programmes have targeted young people in school, others have focused on those out of school. Some programmes have targeted the population more generally, but have acknowledged young people as a group requiring special attention.

For those in school

India has had a long history of programmes intended to provide information to school- and college-going youth on sexual and reproductive matters: programme content has, however, evolved considerably, from a focus on population and development issues to one on sexual and reproductive health, safe sex, and skill-building to ensure health promoting practices (see Santhya and Jejeebhoy 2007). This latter focus was underscored in the AEP launched in 2005 by the Ministry of Human Resource Development and the National AIDS Control Organisation (NACO). The AEP seek to empower young people with accurate, age-appropriate, and culturally relevant information, promote healthy attitudes and develop skills to enable them to respond to real life situations effectively. The programme focuses on young people in Classes 9 and 11. During 2005–06, the AEP was implemented in 112,000 schools and some 288,000 teachers were trained (National AIDS Control Organization n.d.).

Unfortunately, since 2006, serious reservations have been expressed in India about the sexuality component of the programme, and several states have banned the provision of AEPs in state-run schools. Indeed, a Committee on Petitions formed to evolve a consensus on the implementation of the AEP, comprising Rajya Sabha members from several political parties, recommended that 'there should be no sex education in schools' (Rajya Sabha Committee on Petitions 2009). Following the concerns raised, efforts have been made by several stakeholders including the civil society organizations, researchers, UN agencies and concerned government departments to generate support for implementing culturally sensitive, holistic AEP (Jaya, 2010). NACO and NCERT, for example, established an expert committee that reviewed the original curriculum. The committee reiterated the need to continue AEP in Classes IX and XI and provided state education departments greater flexibility to modify the existing programme if necessary. A revised curriculum was developed by NACO in collaboration with the Ministry of Human Resource Development and comprises a 16-hour programme in four sections: (a) the passage from childhood to adolescence; (b) adolescent reproductive and sexual health (ARSH); (c) mental health and substance use; and (d) life skills and HIV prevention (National AIDS Control Organization, 2008a; 2008b). The NACP-III proposes to consolidate and upscale the AEP (National AIDS Control Organization, 2006). The NCERT with support from UNFPA has further revised training and resource materials to be used under the AEP (National Council of Educational Research and Training, 2011). The revised curriculum, under such broad headings as the process of growing up, prevention of HIV/AIDS and prevention of substance/drug abuse, covers such themes as understanding changes during adolescence and being comfortable with them, establishing and maintaining positive and responsible relationships, understanding and challenging stereotypes and discrimination, understanding and reporting abuse and violations, and the prevention of HIV/AIDS and substance abuse.

The AEP is implemented through State Councils of Educational Research and Training/State Boards with the support of State AIDS Control Societies. During 2009–10, the AEP was implemented in 47,000 of over 145,000 high schools and higher secondary schools across the country (National AIDS Control Organization 2010). It is also being implemented, with the support of UNFPA, by such national-level agencies as the Central Board of Secondary Education (CBSE), the Navodaya Vidyalaya Samiti (NVS), the Kendriya Vidyalaya Sangathan (KVS), the National Institute of Open Schooling and the Council of Boards of Secondary Education (Jaya and Yadav 2010; National Council of Educational Research and Training, 2011). By the end of 2010, with the support of UNFPA, at least two nodal teachers from 3,000 CBSE schools, all the 919 KV schools and all the 583 NVS schools had received orientation on adolescence education issues. The NCERT has integrated adolescent concerns in such mainstream subjects as science, psychology and social sciences; this process of integration is acknowledged to require further strengthening. Moreover, a life skills component has been integrated in the secondary curriculum of the National Institute of Open Schooling that enrols some 400,000 students each year. Drawing on a pilot experiment in which life skills were integrated in 17 lessons across the subjects of Hindi, English, Science, Social Sciences, and Home Science, the NIOS is currently in the process of integrating life skills in all the lessons pertaining to these five subjects (approximately 130 lessons) for the academic year 2011–12 (Narayan and Jaya, 2011). The AEP is also being implemented by civil society organizations in partnership with state education departments and state AIDS control societies. For example, the CEDPA has reached some 300,000 students in 1,485 government secondary schools in Jharkhand; some 87 master trainers and 2,161 nodal teachers from government schools have been trained to impart AEP curriculum (CEDPA, 2011). The AEP has also been endorsed in the RMSA (Ministry of Human Resource Development 2009a).

Other programmes intended to provide information to school- and college-going youth on sexual and reproductive matters include the School Health Programme launched in 2008 under the National Rural Health Mission (NRHM), Red Ribbon Clubs (RRCs) established under NACP-II and NACP-III, the University Talk AIDS Programme and the Youth Unite for Victory on AIDS campaign. The School Health Programme comprises interventions to improve in-school adolescents' awareness of health, hygiene, and nutrition matters through curricular formats, and of growing up issues and sexual and reproductive matters through co-curricular approaches (Ministry of Health and Family Welfare, n.d.). The University Talk AIDS Programme, initiated for college students to spread awareness of HIV and safe sex in 1991, has reached over seven million young people in the country (National AIDS Control Organization, 2004). Additionally, while the current status is not known, Yuva, a network of seven youth organizations, the Nehru Yuva Kendra Sangathan, the National Service Scheme, the Indian Red Cross Society, the National Cadet Corps, Bharat Scouts and Guides, the

Youth Hostels Association of India and the Association of Indian Universities, under the auspices of the Ministry of Youth Affairs and Sports and NACO is working towards equipping young people with prevention, education and life skills for promoting healthy and safe behaviour and practices amongst them (National AIDS Control Organization, n.d.).

Programmes for out-of-school youth

Fewer activities have been conducted to raise awareness about sexual and reproductive matters among out-of-school youth till relatively recently. However, with the spread of HIV/AIDS, a number of programmes have been initiated for out-of-school youth. Again, the key programmes emanate from the NACP and the Ministry of Health and Family Welfare's thrust on young people.

The NACP-II conducted the Village Talk AIDS Programme to reach out-of-school youth. The Nehru Yuvak Kendra Sangathan, likewise, has undertaken awareness campaigns, including on sexual and reproductive matters and HIV/AIDS. However, as noted in the strategy and implementation plan document of NACP-III, the reach of these activities remains limited (National AIDS Control Organization, 2006). Under NACP-III, RRCs were established in villages to provide youth oriented counselling, life skill education, recreation and guidance in a confidential and enabling environment. The RRC serves as a complementary and comprehensive prevention intervention to support and reinforce youth initiatives conducted by community volunteers and link workers. Additionally, vulnerable young people in districts characterized by large concentrations of sex workers, injecting drug users, or men having sex with men, significant outmigration or high HIV prevalence, are to be reached by link workers who are entrusted with the task of implementing behaviour change communication strategies using life-skills based participatory learning processes. Moreover, with support from the MOWCD, RRCs will be established for adolescent girls (National AIDS Control Organization 2006).

The National Adolescent Reproductive and Sexual Health Strategy also recognizes that out-of-school youth have special information needs. It advocates that awareness raising activities for youth are implemented at least once a month by Auxiliary Nurse Midwives (ANMs), *Anganwadi* workers, Accredited Social Health Activists (ASHAs), youth group coordinators and male health workers. Themes covered are to range from the importance of delaying marriage and first pregnancy to sexual risk reduction strategies, gender relations, and the role of men (Ministry of Health and Family Welfare 2006a).

The Ministry of Youth Affairs and Sports, with the support of the UNFPA, has formed 3,824 teen clubs in 64 Districts in 31 States; these teen clubs offer a platform for providing adolescents opportunities for life skills focused experiential learning on reproductive and sexual health issues in a gender sensitive matter, imparting information on education and skills building for better employability and improving access to youth friendly and gender sensitive services in the public and private sectors (Ministry of Youth Affairs and Sports 2011; Narayan and Jaya 2011).

Programmes that Facilitate Access to Sexual and Reproductive Health Counselling and Services

Although policies and programmes in India have underscored the right of young people to sexual and reproductive health counselling and services, service delivery has not been youth-friendly or responsive to their unique needs. Compared to awareness raising programmes, sexual and reproductive health counselling and services are provided overwhelmingly through the National Adolescent Reproductive and Sexual Health Strategy outlined in the RCH Programme; AIDS control programmes play a smaller role in providing services to young people.

The Adolescent Reproductive and Sexual Health Strategy focuses on reorganizing and strengthening the existing public health system to meet young people's needs, mobilizing communities to create an enabling environment and encourage young people to access services, and providing preventive, promotional, curative, and referral services to them (Ministry of Health and Family Welfare 2006a). It notes that 'friendly services are to be made available for all adolescents, married and unmarried, girls and boys'. The ARSH programme advocates care at two levels for young people: routine sub-centre clinics run by female health workers and weekly 2-hour teen clinics organized at primary health centre (PHC)/CHC/district level run by the health worker and medical officer. At sub-centre level, the health worker will provide non-terminal contraceptive methods, routine antenatal care services, abortion related referrals, RTI/STI/HIV related education, nutritional counselling, information on menstrual hygiene, and immunisation of pregnant adolescents. At the teen clinics, such services as the provision of contraceptive supplies, management of menstrual disorders, provision of RTI/STI preventive education and management, pregnancy termination and related counselling, nutritional counselling and counselling for sexual problems will be provided.

Also proposed in the National Adolescent Reproductive and Sexual Health Strategy were initiatives to orient medical officers, ANMs and lady health visitors (LHVs) on the provision of sexual and reproductive health services. Orientation programmes underscore the need to address both the married and the unmarried, as well as adolescent girls and boys. They also highlight the significant obstacles that young people may face in seeking information and counselling, including young married women's lack of autonomy, perceptions of poor quality of care and judgemental services at health centres, and young people's own reluctance to discuss sexual matters (Ministry of Health and Family Welfare 2006b; 2006c).

Other schemes under the NRHM that have relevance for young people include the ASHAs scheme, the *Janani Suraksha Yojana* (JSY) and the School Health Programme. One of the themes included in the training package for ASHAs is adolescent health, orienting ASHAs about pregnancy risks that very young mothers may suffer, the vulnerability of adolescent girls to HIV/AIDS and so on (Ministry of Health and Family Welfare 2006d). A more recently prepared module on skills that save lives, not yet rolled out, also touches upon adolescent sexual and reproductive health (Ministry of Health and Family Welfare 2010). The JSY, launched in 2005, provides cash assistance to women who undergo institutional deliveries (Ministry of Health and Family Welfare 2006e). With revisions in its eligibility criteria in October 2006, all pregnant women in low performing states, irrespective of age, parity and economic status, who undergo institutional delivery in a government health facility or an accredited private facility are entitled to receive JSY benefits. The School Health programme, launched in 26 states from 2008, offers a range of screening and referral services to school-going adolescents. For example, anaemia screening and height and weight monitoring activities are incorporated in the programme. Additionally, medical officers from primary health centres are expected to conduct health check-ups once in six months in schools and inform adolescents about the availability of services (Ministry of Health and Family Welfare n.d.)

Several states have begun innovative programs to address the multi-faceted needs of adolescents. In Assam, an adolescent anaemia initiative is being implemented in three districts, which will benefit 67,000 girls approximately. An outreach health programme for adolescents is also being piloted in an additional district in Assam with support from MNGOs and field-level NGOs. In Punjab, the state has planned to socially market sanitary napkins for school-going adolescent girls and will also operationalize adolescent-friendly health centres in selected districts. In Rajasthan, a social marketing pilot project on sanitary napkins is being initiated in selected blocks of four districts. Further, the state has also initiated counselling sessions for adolescent girls through ASHA *Sahayoginis* (Ministry of Health and Family Welfare 2009a).

Key activities for youth envisaged under NACP-III include the establishment of youth-friendly linkages for referrals and follow-ups between health services and infection related services, and the promotion of social marketing of condoms through RRCs. Condom promotion efforts are to be undertaken by various youth groups including NYKS, NSS, and NCC units (National AIDS Control Organization 2006).

Programmes That Address Gender Disparities and Young People's Rights

Almost every policy has articulated a commitment to reduce gender disparities among young people. Correspondingly, programmes have advocated a range of measures to reduce gender imbalances among young people. The major programmes intended to address gender disparities are the ones supported by the Ministry of Women and

Child Development, Ministry of Youth Affairs and Sports and the Ministry of Human Resource Development.

Notable among the programmes designed to enhance the status of young women and address gender disparities are the Rajiv Gandhi Scheme for Empowerment of Adolescent Girls (RGSEAGs) (SABLA scheme) introduced in 2010 (Ministry of Women and Child Development, 2010) and the *Kishori Shakti Yojana* (KSY). The scheme merges two existing programmes, namely, the KSY and the Nutrition Programme for Adolescent Girls (NPAG) and was introduced in 200 districts, in which it replaces the KSY and the NPAG. The scheme focuses on both empowering adolescent girls aged 11–18 years and providing them nutritional supplementation. It provides adolescent girls a package of interventions including literacy and numeracy skills training, life skills education, vocational skills training, guidance on public resources, health check-ups and referral services, and nutritional supplementation. Implemented through existing *Anganwadi* centres, the scheme calls for the formation of *kishori samooh* (girls' groups), in which out-of-school adolescents will meet frequently (2 hours a day 3 day a week) and in-school girls will meet 1–2 times monthly; it also includes training camps, hands-on learning and sharing of experiences. The KSY continues as before in districts in which the SABLA is not implemented.

The National Programme for Youth and Adolescent Development (NPYAD) implemented by the Ministry of Youth Affairs and Sports is another notable scheme that pays special attention to providing opportunities for the holistic development of youth. A major component of the scheme is the development and empowerment of adolescents by providing them life skills education, counselling and career guidance and organizing residential camps that provide a second chance to acquire basic education and life skills to those left behind in the formal system. The scheme operates through NGOs and NYKS. Life skills education camps are held for batches of 40 for a one-week period (Ministry of Youth Affairs and Sports n.d.). The life skills approach has been emphasised in the AEP as well.

Several cash and non-cash transfer schemes have been proposed or implemented that focus on improving the status of girls (see, for a detailed review, Sekher 2010). A programme with national coverage is the *Balika Samridhi Yojana*, an investment scheme launched in 1997 to improve the status of the girl child by providing monetary incentives for completing schooling and postponing marriage till the age of 18 years.[1] Several state governments have also launched specific investment schemes to encourage schooling for girls, delay their marriage and change family and community attitudes towards girls. Yet another scheme introduced on a pilot basis in 2008 is the *Dhanalakshmi* Conditional Cash Transfer for Girl Child with Insurance Cover scheme (Ministry of Women and Child Development, 2010). Under this scheme, cash transfers are made to the family of the girl child (preferably the mother) on fulfilling certain specific conditionalities related to birth and registration, immunization, school enrolment and retention up to Class VIII and delay in marriage of the girl child till the age of 18 years. The Scheme is being implemented in eleven blocks across seven States (Andhra Pradesh, Bihar, Chhattisgarh, Jharkhand, Odisha, Punjab, and Uttar Pradesh) in the country. The Scheme was included in the Eleventh Plan and an Outlay of Rs 10 Crores was provided in the Annual Plan 2009–10. Several state governments have introduced state-specific conditional cash transfer programmes as well (Sekher 2010).

Programmes are also implemented by the Department of Education to address gender disparity in educational attainment, for example, the Kasturba Gandhi *Balika Vidyalaya, Mahila Samakhya* and the National Programme for Education of Girls at the Elementary Level, and the National Scheme of Incentive to Girls for Secondary Education. *Mahila Samakhya*, launched in the late 1980s and funded by the central government but implemented only in 83 districts in nine states, aims to educate and empower poor adolescent girls and build life skills among them; it is implemented through *Kishori Sangha*s in over 16,000 villages in nine states. Under this project, adolescent girls are given non-formal education in the

[1] Under the scheme, the central government deposits Rs 500 in a bank/post office in the name of the girl child, which is withdrawn to pay the insurance premium and incremental graded scholarship to the girl child as she graduates from different grades.

form of functional literacy, leadership and life skills training through *Mahila Shikshana Kendras*. Centres function in such states as Andhra Pradesh, Assam, Bihar, Gujarat, Jharkhand, Karnataka, Kerala, Uttar Pradesh, and Uttarakhand (Ministry of Human Resource Development, 2008).

Programmes that Enhance Nutrition Among Adolescent Girls

Recognizing the need of adolescent girls for nutritional supplementation, the NPAGs was initiated, on a pilot basis, in 2002 in two poorly developed districts of each of the major states and one in the remaining states. Under this programme, adolescent girls are identified and weighed by *Anganwadi* workers once a quarter, and all those weighing less than 35 kg are provided 6 kg of food grain per month free of cost for three months; and they and their families are provided nutrition education. The programme has been through many changes in terms of coverage, and since 2005–06, has been functioning in just 51 districts.

The SABLA programme discussed above provides nutritional supplementation to girls in the form of either cooked meals if feasible or take-home rations of at least 600 calories and 18–20 grams of proteins for 300 days of the year. At the same time, in conjunction with the NRHM programme, the programme will provide IFA tablets provided to adults to adolescent girls as well (Ministry of Women and Child Development 2010).

Programmes that Enable Young People to Acquire Educational Levels and Marketable Skills

The need to enable young people to acquire educational levels and marketable skills to compete in a globalizing world is increasingly recognised. Correspondingly, several programmes have been initiated in recent years to promote universal school enrolment and completion. Notable among these is the *Sarva Shiksha Abhiyan* (SSA), intended to universalize elementary education and to provide useful and relevant education to all children in the age group of 6–14 years by 2010. Recognizing that eight years of education are insufficient to prepare adolescents for a globalised world, efforts are underway, through the RMSA, to universalize access to and improve the quality of secondary education (Classes 9–12); plans are underway to provide secondary (Classes 9–10) and higher secondary schools (Classes 11–12) within 5 and 7–10 kilometres, respectively, of any habitation, ensure universal access to secondary education by 2017 and universal retention by 2020, and make special efforts to ensure that disadvantaged groups, including girls, are not deprived of this education (Ministry of Human Resource Development, 2009a). Efforts are also underway, through the recently announced *Saakshar Bharat* scheme (2009–12), to impart functional literacy and numeracy to those aged 15–35 years who are non-literate and non-numerate, enable the neo-literate to continue their learning and acquire equivalency to formal education, and impart relevant skills to improve their earning capacities (Ministry of Human Resource Development 2009b). Notably, the scheme does take note of the special needs of adolescents and young people.

In the area of skill development, the National Skills Development Initiative aims to empower individuals through improved skills, knowledge and qualifications to gain access to employment in an increasingly competitive global market (Ministry of Labour 2009). The initiative aims to meet, by 2022, the skilling needs of 500 million individuals. Objectives are to create opportunities for skill acquisition, with special attention to youth and women, and to school drop-outs. To achieve these ambitious goals, public private partnerships are envisaged, and outreach is to be expanded through a variety of mechanisms including skill development centres at village and block levels, mobile training and distance learning programmes; at the same time, the coverage of vocations will be expanded and soft skills, such as basic numeracy, literacy, rights, team work and confidence building will be folded into skill development curricula.

Programmes that Build a Supportive Environment

In order to build a supportive environment to enable youth to obtain information, seek counselling and services, and adopt safe practices, it is critical that communities in general, and young people's gatekeepers in particular, are sensitized to the unique needs of young people. Key gatekeepers include parents and parents-in-law, health care providers, teachers and other community-level functionaries, for example *Anganwadi* workers and organizers of self-help groups. Efforts on the ground to sensitise different gatekeepers have been limited. The National Adolescent Reproductive and Sexual Health Strategy proposes activities to reach a broad range of gatekeepers, including district officials, and members of panchayats, women's groups and civil society, with appropriate messages (Ministry of Health and Family Welfare 2006a).

The Health and Development Situation of Young People

Policies and programmes described above have aimed to address young people's needs in three distinct areas: education, livelihood skill building and provision of employment opportunities, and sexual and reproductive health. In this section we review the situation of young people in each of these three key areas.

Educational Attainment

While school attendance has increased from 59 per cent to 76 per cent among girls aged 6–14 and from 76 per cent to 83 per cent among boys between 1992–93 and 2005–06, educational attainment levels continue to be low in general, and particularly for females (International Institute for Population Sciences and Macro International, 2007). Achievement of milestones, for example

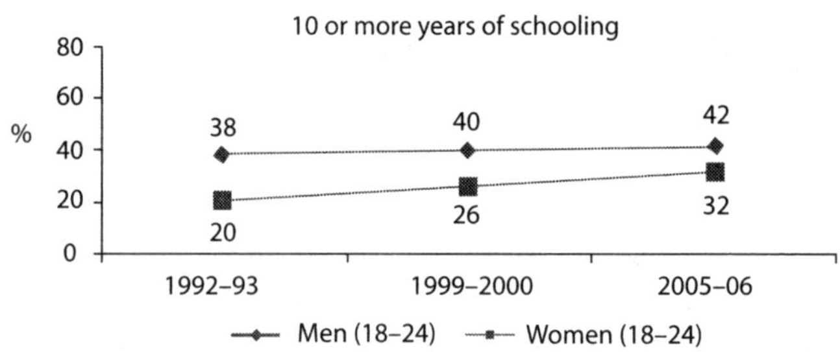

Figure 4.1 Percentage of Young People (18–24 year old) Who Had Completed Class 10, 1992–93 to 2005–06

Source: Calculated from household member data from NFHS-1, 2 and 3 surveys.

classes 8 and 10, remains far from universal: Just 42 per cent of young men and 32 per cent of young women aged 18–24 had completed Class 10. Moreover, the pace of increase in educational levels is modest, although it is faster for young women than men (Figure 4.1).

Considerable state-level differences exist in the proportion of young people who had completed high school (Table A4.1). The percentage of young men and women aged 18–24 years who had completed high school ranged from 22 per cent in Arunachal Pradesh to 82 per cent in Himachal Pradesh (in the case of young men) and from 17 per cent in Rajasthan to 70 per cent in Himachal Pradesh (in the case of young women). In fact, half or more of young men and women aged 18–24 years had completed high school in just 10 (Delhi, Haryana, Himachal Pradesh, and Punjab in the north,

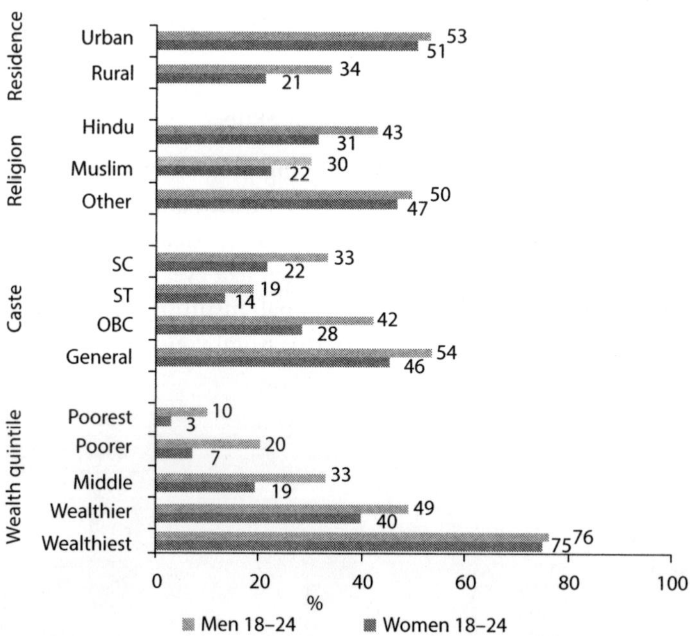

Figure 4.2 Percentage of Young Men and Women (18–24 Year Old) Who Had Completed High School by Selected Background Characteristics, 2005–06

Source: Calculated from individual male and female respondent data from NFHS-3 survey.

Manipur in the northeast, Goa and Maharashtra in the west and Andhra Pradesh, Kerala, and Tamil Nadu in the south) and 5 states (Delhi, Himachal Pradesh, Punjab, Goa, and Kerala), respectively, out of 29 states. Socio-demographic differentials indicate that rural youth, Muslim youth, those belonging to scheduled tribes and from poorest households were most disadvantaged than others (Figure 4.2). For example, just 10 per cent and 3 per cent of young men and women belonging to the poorest household had completed high school compared to 75–76 per cent of those belonging to the wealthiest household.

Not only that large proportion of young people failed to complete a high school, but many are getting poor quality education. For example, a recent evaluation of basic competencies of students in Class 8 in rural areas reports that as many as one in six children could not read standard text books for Class 2, one-third could not simple calculations, for example, division and about half could not perform simple tasks with regard to calculating area (Figure 4.3) (Pratham Resource Centre 2011).

Acquisition of Marketable, Vocational Skills

Although a number of vocational training programmes are available to youth through government, non-government, and private organizations, findings from the Youth Study indicate that just one-fifth of young men and a quarter of young women had ever attended a vocational training programme (International Institute for Population Sciences and Population Council 2010). Rural youth were consider-

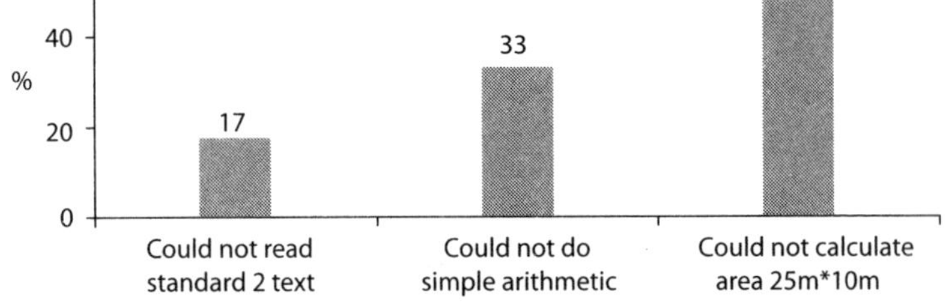

Figure 4.3 Quality of Education Received by Class 8 Students in Rural Areas, 2010

Source: Annual Status of Education Report (Rural) 2012.

ably less likely than their urban counterparts to have received training (16 per cent versus 32 per cent among young men; 17per cent versus 43 per cent among young women). Youth in Maharashtra and the southern states were more likely than their northern counterparts to

Table 4.1 Percentage of Youth Who Had Ever Attended a Vocational Training Programme by Background Characteristics

Background characteristics	Men 15–24	Women 15–24
Age		
15–19	15.5	20.9
20–24	26.0	28.9
Residence		
Urban	31.8	42.6
Rural	15.6	17.2
Education		
No education	6.7	4.1
<5 years complete	11.9	10.0
5–7 years complete	12.8	19.2
8–9 years complete	12.2	25.8
10–11 years complete	22.0	37.4
12 or more years complete	45.3	59.7
Religion		
Hindu	19.9	24.4
Muslim	24.1	24.0
Others	23.3	29.0
Caste/tribe		
Scheduled caste	18.2	19.9
Scheduled tribe	10.3	12.4
Other backward caste	20.8	23.8
General	26.2	35.6
Wealth index		
Poorest	8.3	6.6
Poorer	12.6	12.5
Middle	16.7	20.0
Wealthier	22.2	30.4
Wealthiest	35.0	47.2

Source: Calculated from Youth Study Data.

have ever attended a vocational training programme. The less educated, those belonging to scheduled tribes and those belonging to the poorest household were less likely than others to have ever attended a vocational training programme (Table 4.1).

Moreover, young men were more likely than young women to opt for marketable skills (computer training, auto mechanics, and driving for example). Leading skills acquired by young women–tailoring and handicrafts–are not attuned to market needs (Figure 4.4).

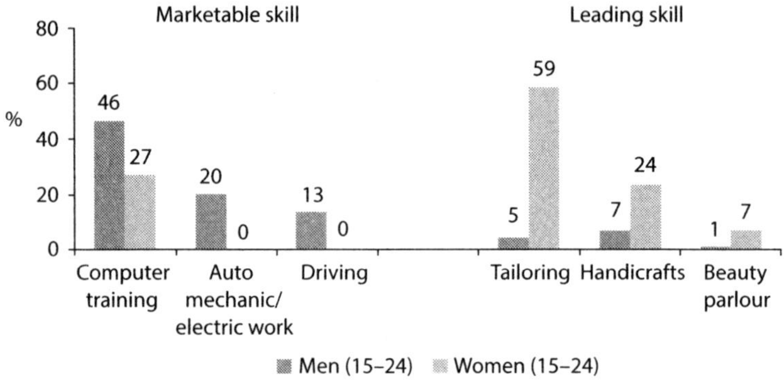

Figure 4.4 Type of Vocational Skills Acquired by Youth Who Had Ever Attended a Vocational Training Programme by Sex

Source: International Institute for Population Sciences and Population Council (2010).

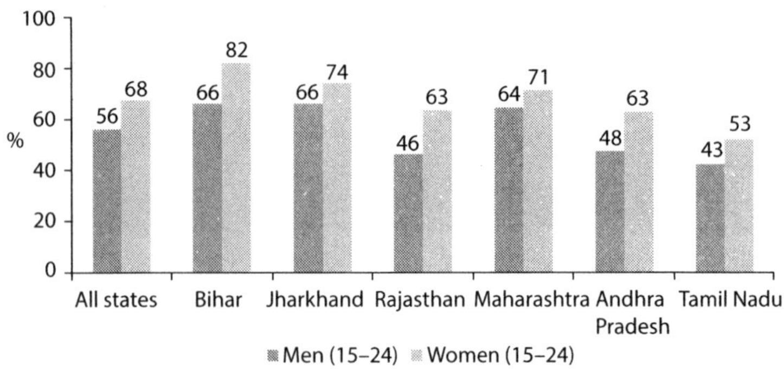

Figure 4.5 Percentage of Youth Who are Interested in Acquiring Vocational Skills by State

Source: International Institute for Population Sciences and Population Council (2010).

There remains a huge unmet need for vocational skill building; for example, large proportions of youth–56 per cent of young men and 68 per cent of young women–were interested in acquiring vocational skills (Figure 4.5). State-wise differences show that youth in the northern states were as likely as their counterparts in Maharashtra and more likely than their southern counterparts to report interest in attending vocational training programmes. However, larger proportions of youth in the southern states and Maharashtra than those in the northern states expressed a preference for training in new technologies, namely, computer skills.

Work Participation

Work profiles indicate considerable gend and rural-urban differences (National Sample Survey Organisation, 2006; 2010). In 2007–08, slightly over two-thirds of young men aged 15–29 years and one-third of young women in rural areas, and three-fifths of young men and one-seventh of young women in urban areas, were employed (principal and subsidiary). Findings, moreover, highlight that rates for both males and females have declined by 7 and 12 percentage points for males and females, respectively, in rural areas but remained basically unchanged in urban areas between 1993–94 and 2007–08 (Figure 4.6).

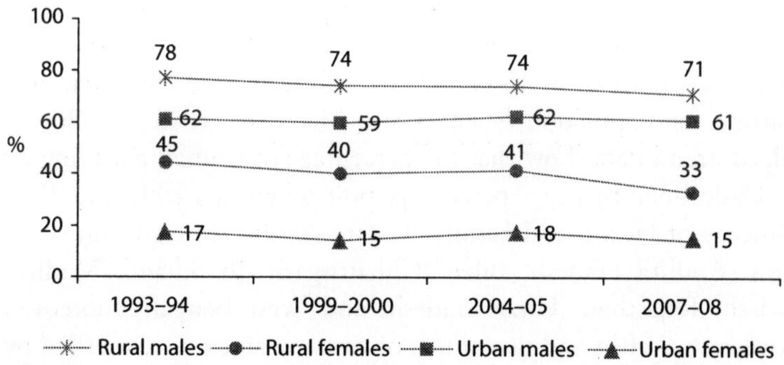

Figure 4.6 Work Force Participation Rate (usual status, principal and subsidiary) among Young People Aged 15–29 Years by Rural–Urban Residence and Sex, India, 1993–94 to 2007–08

Sources: National Sample Survey Organisation (2006, 2010).

State-wise differences were also evident (Table A4.2). In rural areas, work force participation rate ranged from 42 per cent in Manipur to 82 per cent in Gujarat among young men and from 2 per cent in Delhi to 61 per cent in Chhattisgarh among young women. In urban areas, the rate ranged from 27% in Nagaland to 74% in Gujarat among young men and 7 per cent in Delhi to 30 per cent in Sikkim among young women. Indeed, the rate registered three-quarters or more among young men in rural areas of 9 out of 29 states and in urban areas of just one state. It recorded half or more among young women in rural areas of just five states and in urban areas of not a single state.

The Sexual and Reproductive Health Situation of Young People

Evidence on the sexual and reproductive health situation of young people suggests that young people continue to have a wide array of unmet needs in the area of sexual and reproductive health.

Early entry into sexual life

Entry into sexual life occurs at a young age for many. Although India is committed to protecting adolescents from such harmful traditional practices as early marriage, and despite laws prohibiting marriage to young women before age 18 and to young men before age 21, marriage continues to take place in adolescence for significant proportions of young women. While the age at marriage for women has undergone a secular increase, the reality is that almost half of all women aged 20–24 were married by 18 years as recently as in 2006 (International Institute for Population Sciences and Macro International, 2007). Indeed, trend data show that the percentage of women marrying by age 18 declined by just 7 percentage points between 1992 and 2006 (Ministry of Health and Family Welfare 2009b). In eight out of 29 states (Andhra Pradesh, Bihar, Chhattisgarh, Jharkhand, Madhya Pradesh, Rajasthan, Uttar Pradesh, and West Bengal), moreover, between two-fifths and two-thirds of young women were married by 18 years (Table A4.3).

Wide disparities are evident in marriage age: poor, rural, and poorly educated young women and those from scheduled castes and

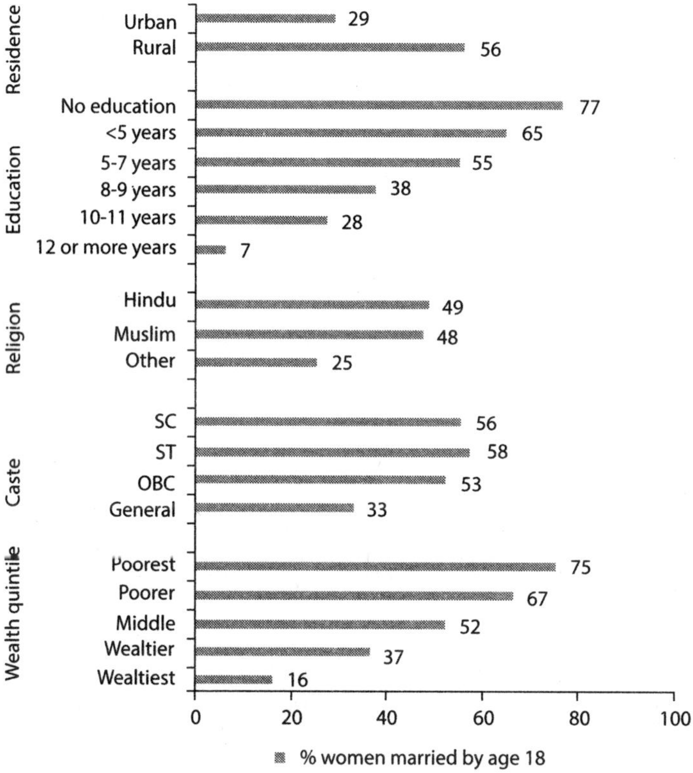

Figure 4.7 Percentage of Women (20–25 Year Old) Married by Age 18 by Selected Background Characteristics, 2005–06

Sources: Calculated from individual female respondent data from NFHS-3.

tribes are considerably more likely than other women to have experienced early marriage (Figure 4.7). While large proportions of young men were married before they were legally permitted to do so, just 10 per cent married before they were 18. The starkest difference is by schooling; 77 per cent of young women with no education were married before they were 18, compared to 7 per cent of those with 12 or more years of schooling

While marriage marks the onset of sexual activity among the large majority of young women, there is growing evidence of premarital onset of sexual activity in adolescence particularly among young

Table 4.2 Percentage of Youth Who Had Engaged in Pre-Marital Sex in Adolescence by Background Characteristics

Background characteristics	Men 15–24	Women 15–24
Residence		
Urban	5.1	2.5
Rural	13.7	6.4
Education		
No education	12.5	8.1
<5 years complete	13.1	9.7
5–7 years complete	15.5	7.7
8–9 years complete	14.4	5.0
10–11 years complete	9.8	4.0
12 or more years complete	4.9	0.9
Religion		
Hindu	10.7	4.8
Muslim	8.9	2.9
Others	19.3	8.2
Caste/tribe		
Scheduled caste	15.2	7.2
Scheduled tribe	18.0	15.3
Other backward caste	8.8	3.6
General	8.9	2.8
Wealth index		
Poorest	17.0	11.2
Poorer	15.3	8.6
Middle	11.4	5.6
Wealthier	9.7	3.2
Wealthiest	5.6	2.1

Source: Calculated from Youth Study Data.

men. Evidence from the Youth Study shows that 11 per cent of young men and 5 per cent of young women aged 15–24 had engaged in pre-marital sex in adolescence, that is, before age 20 (International Institute for Population Sciences and Population Council 2010). Differentials are apparent, with rural young women twice as likely (6 per cent vs. 3 per cent) and rural young men almost three times as likely (14 per cent vs. 5 per cent) to have experienced pre-marital sex in adolescence as their urban counterparts (Table 4.2). Differences were also apparent by other socioeconomic factors: for example, youth with 12 or more years of education and those who belonged to wealthier households were less likely than poorly educated and those from poorer households to report the experience of pre-marital sex. Young men and women from scheduled castes and tribes were considerably more likely than those from general castes and other backward castes to have so experienced.

Unsafe, unwanted, or forced sexual relations

Where sexual relations take place, they are often unsafe and for many young women, unwanted or forced. For example, the Youth Study reports that among young men and women who had engaged in pre-marital sex, 25 per cent and 21 per cent , respectively, had engaged in sex with more than one partner, with rural youth somewhat more likely than their urban counterparts to do so (International Institute for Population Sciences and Population Council 2010). Just 27 per cent and 7 per cent, respectively had ever used a condom, and even fewer, 13 per cent and 3 per cent , respectively, had used a condom consistently (Santhya, Jejeebhoy and Acharya 2011). Moreover, 18 per cent of young women (and 3 per cent of young men) were forced to engage in sex.

Socio-demographic differentials in multiple partnerships were narrow among young men (Table 4.3). Among young women, however, engaging in multiple partnerships before marriage declined with age (24 per cent of 15–19 year-olds versus 18 per cent of 20–24 year-olds). Differentials by religion and caste suggest that Muslim young women and those from general castes were less likely than others to have engaged in multiple partnerships (14 per cent versus 21–22 per cent and 11 per cent versus 19–29 per cent, respectively). Moreover, those who had completed 12 or more years were less likely than others to report multiple partnerships (13 per cent versus 22–23 per cent), while those in the poorest quintiles (first and second) were more likely than others to report pre-marital sex with multiple partners (24–31 per cent versus 15–18 per cent). Table 4.3 also show differentials in consistent condom use. Differences

Table 4.3 Percentage of Youth Who Had Pre-Marital Sex Reporting Multiple Partnerships and Consistent Condom Use by Background Characteristics

Background characteristics	Multiple partnerships		Consistent condom use	
	Men 15–24	Women 15–24	Men 15–24	Women 15–24
Age				
15–19	21.0	24.3	8.0	3.1
20–24	26.7	18.2	15.8	1.9
Residence				
Urban	20.3	15.9	21.2	1.9
Rural	25.5	22.9	10.6	2.7
Education				
No education	19.6	22.6	3.2	1.0
<5 years complete	19.4	22.5	11.1	2.2
5–7 years complete	27.6	22.5	9.8	4.0
8–9 years complete	24.0	27.8	14.5	3.1
10–11 years complete	26.7	11.9	14.3	1.0
12 or more years complete	24.0	13.0	18.4	2.9
Religion				
Hindu	25.0	21.9	11.9	2.1
Muslim	19.7	(14.0)	14.6	(2.3)
Others	23.6	21.4	19.5	4.3
Caste/tribe				
Scheduled caste	25.9	19.3	12.8	1.7
Scheduled tribe	26.5	29.0	8.9	4.2
Other backward caste	21.7	22.5	11.3	2.4
General	26.7	10.8	19.1	2.0
Wealth index				
Poorest	26.5	31.0	6.8	3.7
Poorer	25.3	23.5	5.3	2.7
Middle	23.0	14.8	11.4	2.3
Wealthier	23.0	16.0	19.1	0.6
Wealthiest	25.4	18.3	21.3	3.2

Source: International Institute for Population Sciences and Population Council (2010); based on 25–49 unweighted cases.

were uniformly negligible for young women, which is not surprising given that just 3 per cent of young women reported consistent condom use within pre-marital sexual relationships. Among young men, consistent condom use increased with age, education and wealth status. Differentials by religion and caste were less consistent.

Among the married too, NFHS-3 findings show that just 28 per cent of young women aged 15–24 were practising contraception; just 11 per cent were using a modern non-terminal method (Parasuraman et al., 2009). Fewer than one in five young women were currently practising contraception in 7 out of the 29 states (Bihar, Chhattisgarh, Jharkhand, Meghalaya, Nagaland, Odisha, and Rajasthan) (Table A4.4). Differentials were notable: adolescent girls were only one-third as likely as young women (20–24 year-olds) to currently use contraceptives; and young women from the poorest households only half as likely as those from the richest households to do so (Table 4.4).

Married young women were also likely, moreover, to face sexual violence; evidence from the Youth Study indicates that almost one-third (32 per cent) of married young women had ever experienced sexual violence perpetrated by their husband (International Institute for Population Sciences and Population Council 2010). Findings, moreover, indicate that sexual violence within marriage is more common in northern states (40–54 per cent) than in the western state of Maharashtra and the southern states (10–27 per cent).

Childbearing in childhood

Childbearing is initiated early and multiple pregnancies characterise the life of many young women. One in five young women aged 20–24 had their first baby before they were 18 years of age, and one in eight young women aged 20–24 had three children (International Institute for Population Sciences and Macro International, 2007). In 5 out of 29 states, between one-quarter and one-third of young women had their first birth by age 18 (Andhra Pradesh, Bihar, Jharkhand, West Bengal, Arunachal Pradesh) (Table A4.5). Rural young women were twice as likely as the urban to have their first birth by age 18. Differences by education, economic status, and caste were striking, with less educated young women, those belonging to poorest households and those belonging to scheduled tribes more

Table 4.4 Percentage of Married Young Women Currently Using Any Contraceptive Method and a Modern Non-Terminal Method by Background Characteristics

Background characteristics	Any method	Any modern non-terminal method
Age		
15–19	13.0	5.8
20–24	33.4	12.4
Residence		
Urban	35.0	18.3
Rural	25.2	8.1
Education		
No education	21.1	4.8
<5 years complete	30.5	9.6
5–7 years complete	30.0	10.7
8–9 years complete	32.5	13.8
10–11 years complete	32.1	17.5
12 or more years complete	35.9	25.6
Religion		
Hindu	27.1	9.8
Muslim	28.6	13.6
Others	38.0	15.7
Caste/tribe		
Scheduled caste	28.6	9.1
Scheduled tribe	20.4	6.1
Other backward caste	23.9	7.8
General	33.2	16.8
Wealth index		
Poorest	19.8	4.7
Poorer	24.4	6.8
Middle	27.8	8.1
Wealthier	32.3	14.7
Wealthiest	38.7	25.2

Source: Calculated from individual female respondent data from NFHS-3.

Table 4.5 Percentage of 20–24 Year Old Women Who Had Given Birth Before Age 18 and Married Young Women Aged 15–24 with Three or More Children by Background Characteristics

Background characteristics	Given birth before age 18 (20–24)	Three or more children (15–24)
Age		
15–19	–	1.4
20–24	21.7	17.5
Residence		
Urban	12.3	9.2
Rural	26.3	14.1
Education		
No education	39.3	20.6
<5 years complete	32.4	14.6
5–7 years complete	24.4	9.9
8–9 years complete	14.0	6.5
10–11 years complete	7.8	4.8
12 or more years complete	1.4	1.7
Religion		
Hindu	21.8	12.5
Muslim	24.6	15.9
Others	12.9	12.2
Caste/tribe		
Scheduled caste	26.6	14.5
Scheduled tribe	30.6	16.0
Other backward caste	22.8	13.7
General	14.3	9.3
Wealth index		
Poorest	38.9	18.6
Poorer	33.0	15.9
Middle	23.3	12.0
Wealthier	14.5	9.6
Wealthiest	5.4	4.4

Source: Calculated from individual female respondent data from NFHS-3.

likely than others to have given birth before they were 18 years of age (Table 4.5). For example, 39 per cent of young women with no education compared to 1 per cent of those with 12 or more years of schooling had their first birth before age 18. Socio-demographic differentials were notable with regard to the experience of multiple births as well. Young women from rural areas, those from the poorest households, and those with less education, were more likely than others to have three or more children before they transitioned out of young adulthood.

As a consequence, both maternal and neonatal mortality are higher among the young than among older women: 41 per cent of all maternal deaths take place among those aged 15–24 (Office of the Registrar General of India 2009) and neonatal mortality rates ranged from 54 per 1,000 live births among those aged 15–19 to 34 and 38, respectively among those aged 20–29 and 30–39 (International Institute for Population Sciences and Macro International 2007). Rural adolescents are particularly at risk: neonatal mortality among them is as high as 60/1,000 (compared to 31 among urban adolescents).

While the majority of adolescent girls bear children within a marital relationship, pre-marital pregnancy is indeed reported among significant minorities of sexually experienced unmarried youth. For example, the Youth Study reports that among young men and women who reported engaging in pre-marital sex with a romantic partner, 4 per cent of young men and 9 per cent of young women reported a pregnancy (Jejeebhoy, Santhya, and Acharya 2010). In a study among college students in Gujarat, 17 per cent of sexually experienced male students reported that they had made a girl pregnant and 8 per cent of sexually experienced female students reported that they had experienced a pregnancy (Sujay 2009).

Unintended pregnancy and abortion

Unwanted fertility is experienced by considerable proportions of young women. As many as 14 per cent and 18 per cent of births to adolescent mothers and young mothers in the five years preceding the NFHS-3 survey, respectively, were wanted at a later time or not wanted at all (International Institute for Population Sciences and

Table 4.6 Percentage of Births in the Five Years to Adolescent and Young Mothers That Were Unwanted by Background Characteristics

Background characteristics	Women 15–24
Age	
15–19	14.4
20–24	18.1
Residence	
Urban	17.4
Rural	16.7
Education	
No education	15.1
<5 years complete	18.3
5–7 years complete	17.4
8–9 years complete	19.6
10–11 years complete	19.2
12 or more years complete	16.8
Religion	
Hindu	16.2
Muslim	20.5
Others	14.8
Caste/tribe	
Scheduled caste	16.9
Scheduled tribe	13.5
Other backward caste	16.0
General	18.7
Wealth index	
Poorest	14.8
Poorer	17.9
Middle	17.9
Wealthier	17.5
Wealthiest	15.9

Source: Calculated from individual female respondent data from NFHS-3.

Macro International 2007). Births to young mothers (15–24) in the five years preceding the NFHS-3 survey that were unwanted ranged from 9 per cent in Delhi to 49 per cent in Mizoram. Indeed, over one-fifth or more of births were unwanted in 8 out of 29 states (Table A4.6). Socio-demographic differentials, however, were modest (Table 4.6).

While not much is known about abortion among the young, evidence suggests that young women—irrespective of marital status—are more disadvantaged than adult women, and that unmarried young women are particularly disadvantaged. It is estimated that between 1 and 10 per cent of abortion-seekers in India are adolescents (Ganatra 2000), though a few facility-based studies report that the proportion of adolescent abortion-seekers is as high as one in three (Chhabra et al. 1988; Solapurkar and Sangam 1985). A community-based study in rural Maharashtra reports that young women aged 15–24 constituted over half of married abortion-seekers in the area (Ganatra and Hirve 2002). In the study among college students in Gujarat referred to earlier, most pregnancies were aborted (Sujay 2009). Moreover, young women who seek abortion often tend to delay seeking it into the second trimester; for example, 25 per cent of unmarried and 9 per cent of married abortion seekers had delayed seeking abortion into the second trimester (Jejeebhoy et al. 2010).

RTI/STI and HIV

The Youth Study reports that significant proportions of youth had experienced symptoms of genital infection: 5 per cent and 17 per cent of young men and women, respectively reported symptoms of genital infection in the 3 months preceding the interview, with the married somewhat more likely than the unmarried to so report (International Institute for Population Sciences and Population Council 2010). Moreover, NFHS data suggest that young women were as likely as adult women to report STIs or symptoms of STIs (International Institute for Population Sciences and Macro International 2007). Data on HIV prevalence indicate that age-specific HIV prevalence rates are similar among young men and young women aged 15–24 (0.09 and 0.11 respectively) (Parasuraman et al. 2009).

Malnutrition

Malnutrition characterises the life of many youth, particularly young women; 11 per cent and 17 per cent of young men and women, respectively, were moderately or severely anaemic (Parasuraman et al. 2009). Adolescent girls and young women were equally likely to be anaemic, though adolescent boys were much more likely to be anaemic than young men. The prevalence of moderate or severe anaemia among young men ranged from 5 per cent or less in Goa, Kerala and Manipur to 15 per cent or more in Assam, Jharkhand, Meghalaya, Sikkim, Tripura, and West Bengal (Table A4.7). Among young women, it ranged from 10 per cent or less in Goa, Kerala, Manipur and Mizoram to 20 per cent or more in Andhra Pradesh, Assam, Gujarat, and Jharkhand. Differences by education and wealth status are notable; for example among young women, 22 per cent of those with no education compared to 13 per cent of those who had at least completed high school, and 22 per cent of those belonging to the poorest households compared to 13 per cent of those belonging to the richest households, were moderately or severely anaemic (Table 4.7).

Challenges and Opportunitiesin Meeting Youth Sexual and Reproductive Health Needs and Rights and Development Needs

A host of factors inhibits young people from achieving good sexual and reproductive health and realizing their rights, as well as from achieving education and marketable skills that would enable them to compete in a globalizing world. These factors span individual, family and community level challenges and gaps in policies, laws and programmes. These challenges, along with opportunities for overcoming these obstacles are outlined in the sub-sections below.

Individual-level Barriers

As described below, awareness of health-promoting behaviours, care-seeking for sexual and reproductive matters and social support remain limited among young people. Moreover, gender double standards

Table 4.7 Percentage of Youth Who Were Moderately or Severely Anaemic by Background Characteristics

Background characteristics	Men 15–24	Women 15–24
Age		
15–19	13.5	16.6
20–24	8.4	18.4
Residence		
Urban	7.7	16.2
Rural	13.0	18.1
Education		
No education	16.4	22.2
<5 years complete	15.6	20.6
5–7 years complete	15.0	18.0
8–9 years complete	10.9	15.7
10–11 years complete	8.8	14.9
12 or more years complete	5.3	11.8
Religion		
Hindu	11.3	17.7
Muslim	9.9	16.6
Others	10.5	17.2
Caste/tribe		
Scheduled caste	12.3	20.7
Scheduled tribe	18.3	24.3
Other backward caste	10.2	16.7
General	9.5	14.5
Wealth index		
Poorest	17.6	21.5
Poorer	14.2	19.4
Middle	12.0	18.4
Wealthier	8.7	16.0
Wealthiest	6.0	12.8

Source: Calculated from individual male and female respondent data from NFHS-3.

and power imbalances shape young people's lives. All these tend to compromise young people's health and development.

Table 4.8 Awareness of SRH Matters, Youth Aged 15–24

	Young men	Young women
Awareness of sex and pregnancy related matters		
% youth aware that a woman can get pregnant at first sex	36.5	45.1
% youth aware that a woman is most likely to become pregnant mid-cycle	38.5	38.4
Awareness of contraception		
% youth who had heard of at least one method of contraception	94.6	94.6
% youth aware that one male condom can be used just once	76.4	30.4
% youth aware that ECP can be taken up to 72 hours after sex	4.2	3.4
Awareness of HIV and STIs		
% youth who had ever heard of HIV/AIDS	90.7	72.5
% youth with comprehensive awareness of HIV/AIDS	45.4	28.4
% youth who had heard of STIs	19.0	14.9
Awareness of legal issues relating to SRH		
% youth aware of the legal minimum age at marriage for females	71.7	58.1
% youth aware that abortion is legal	25.7	22.9

Souce: International Institute for Population Sciences and Population Council (2010).

Limited Awareness of Health Promoting Behaviours

Notwithstanding commitments articulated in several national policies and programmes to raise young people's awareness of sexual and reproductive matters, the reality is that most young men and women continue to lack awareness. As Table 4.8 shows, fewer than half of young men and women were aware that a woman can become pregnant at first sex or is most likely to conceive midway through her cycle (37–45 per cent and 38–39 per cent, respectively). Likewise, although the large majority of young people had heard of contraception and HIV/AIDS, few had in-depth awareness about contraceptive methods or modes of HIV transmission. For example, 76 per cent of young men and 30 per cent of young women knew that one male condom can be used for just one sexual intercourse. Similarly, 45 per cent of young men and 28 per cent of young women had displayed comprehensive awareness of HIV/AIDS. Fewer than one in five had even heard of STIs other than HIV/AIDS. Similarly, despite laws on the minimum age at marriage and legal abortion, awareness of legal minimum age at marriage for females was far from universal among young men and women (58–72 per cent), and just one-quarter were aware that women are legally entitled to undergo abortion in India.

Limited healthcare-seeking practices

Although there are a host of policies and programmes that seek to improve young people's access to sexual and reproductive health services, many young people do not seek proper care for sexual and reproductive health problems. For example, few sexually experienced, unmarried youth had used condoms consistently in premarital relationships (13 per cent and 3 per cent of young men and women, respectively) (International Institute for Population Sciences and Population Council 2010). Contraceptive use, likewise, was limited within marriage. Not surprisingly, the unmet need for contraception is higher among married young women than adult women (23 per cent, compared to 11 per cent among those aged 30–34, International Institute for Population Sciences and Macro International 2007). Evidence suggests that adolescents are more likely than older women, and unmarried adolescents are more likely than their married counterparts, to seek abortions from unqualified or untrained providers, to have delayed abortions and to have undergo second trimester abortions (Ganatra and Hirve 2002; Jejeebhoy et al. 2010). Accessing pregnancy-related services is also limited among young women despite the fact that many of them are experiencing their first and most risky pregnancy at a young age. Just 54 per cent of young women had received three or more antenatal check-ups, 49 per cent of the deliveries of young women had been attended by a skilled attendant and 37 per cent of young women had received a postpartum check-up within two days of delivery (Parasuraman et al 2009). For symptoms of genital infection too, there is evidence that care-seeking is limited; just 56 per cent of young men and 40 per cent of young women who experienced symptoms of infection in the three months preceding the interview had sought care for such symptoms (International Institute for Population Sciences and Population Council 2010). The National Behavioural Surveillance Survey reports that 55 per cent of young men and 43 per cent of young women had sought care from a government or private health facility for symptoms of STIs experienced in the one year preceding the survey (National Institute of Medical Statistics and National AIDS Control Organisation 2008). Limited care seeking for symptoms of gynaecological morbidity has also been observed in other studies (Andrew and Patel 2002; Barua and Kurz 2001; Prasad et al 2005; Rani and Bonu 2003). Just 4 per cent and 11 per cent of young men and women had ever undergone an HIV test (International Institute for Population Sciences and Population Council 2010).

Also evident of young people's limited access to sexual and reproductive health services are findings from the Youth Study that a large proportion of youth–two-fifths of young men and half of young women–felt uncomfortable to approach health care providers for SRH services, including contraceptive supplies (International Institute for Population Sciences and Population Council 2010). Indeed, further analyses of these data suggest that among youth who had engaged in pre-marital sex, those who did not report discomfort in accessing services from a provider were twice as likely as those who did to have used condoms (Santhya, Acharya, and Jejeebhoy 2011a). Similarly, among married young women with symptoms suggestive of RTIs, those who did not report discomfort in accessing services from a provider were 1.3 times more likely than those who did to have sought treatment for such symptoms from formal providers (Sabarwal and Santhya 2012).

Gender power imbalances and limited female agency

Gender double standards and power imbalances shape young people's life and often undermine their ability—and notably young women's ability—to make sexual and reproductive choices both in marital and pre-marital partnerships. The Youth Study, for example, reports that just 27 per cent of young women (compared to 56 per cent of young men) made decisions independently on personal matters. Young women's mobility was also restricted: 73 per cent were permitted to visit a place in their own village unescorted (compared to almost all unmarried young men), and 24 per cent were permitted to visit a place outside their own village unescorted (compared to 82 per cent of unmarried young men). Finally, women's control over money was similarly more restricted than that of young men's (54 per cent of young women vs. 90 per cent of young men who owned a bank account controlled its operation) (International Institute for Population Sciences and Population Council 2010).

In the sexual and reproductive health arena, limited agency is evident from young women's lack of voice in decisions on when and whom to marry and on engaging in safe sex. The Youth Study reports that one-quarter of married young women (compared to 11 per cent of married young men) played no role in the determining the timing of their marriage or the selection of their spouse (International Institute for Population Sciences and Population Council 2010). Moreover, among those who had engaged in pre-marital sex, while about two in five young men and women reported that the decision to use contraception was made jointly, one half reported that the decision was made by the male partner on his own (46–54%). Also indicative of young women's limited agency is their experience of violence within marriage. A multivariate analysis of the correlates of physical and sexual violence, using data from the Youth Study, shows that young women who made decisions were significantly less likely than those who did not to have experienced each form of violence, and those who reported self-efficacy were considerably less likely than others to experience violence. The risk of experiencing physical and sexual violence was 20–25 per cent lower among young women who reported self efficacy than those who did not so report (Acharya et al. 2009).

Young people themselves often accept—and sometimes justify—double standards that condone and even encourage pre-marital relations for men but not for women. Findings from the Youth Study suggest that while 64–69 per cent of young men and women believed that a man's life would be ruined if he engaged in pre-marital sex, this percentage was considerably higher with regard to opinions about a woman's life (82–94 per cent; International Institute for Population Sciences and Population Council 2010). Other gender role attitudes held by both young women and men—for example that a woman must obtain her husband's permission for most things and that a man is justified in beating his wife on several matters—also have implications for women's ability to exercise choice in sexual and reproductive matters.

A different set of gender related factors underlie the vulnerability of young men. While young men are not subject to the stringent behavioural constraints imposed on young women, emerging evidence from a small number of studies indicates that the social construction of masculinity may undermine young men's decision-making abilities in SRH matters, their involvement in care and support of their wives in SRH matters and their ability to adopt protective behaviours. Studies that have explored the role of young husbands in decisions related to the use of contraception, timing of first pregnancy or care during pregnancy report that such decisions were beyond the control of a substantial proportion of both young women and their husband; for example, even where young women and their husband would have liked to delay pregnancy, the decision to practise contraception was often overruled by senior family members (Barua and Kurz 2001; Santhya et al 2003). They also suggest that prevailing norms about masculinity may inhibit married young men from playing a supportive role in the SRH of their wife, including in pregnancy-related care. Moreover, young men, married and unmarried, are affected by social pressure to have sex at an early age, as well as a sense of entitlement to sex in and outside of marriage, often under risky conditions, thereby putting young men and their partners at risk of STIs/HIV (Jejeebhoy and Sebastian 2004). Evidence from a study conducted by the Population Council in India suggests clear linkages between inequitable gender attitudes and masculinity norms on the one hand, and high-risk behaviours among men, including unprotected sex and gender-based violence, on the other (Verma et al. 2006).

Lack of a safe and supportive environment

Young people, in general, gain support from their peer networks, both informal and formal. However, findings from the Youth Study show that these social support networks are limited among young people, especially young women. For example, just 22 per cent of young women, compared to 42 per cent of young men reported at least five friends and just one-tenth reported membership in an organized group (International Institute for Population Sciences and Population Council 2010). Analysis of the associations between peer level factors and risky sex suggests that while young people reporting close peer connections were indeed more likely than others to report pre-marital sex (hazards ratios of 1.2–1.3); among the sexually experienced, those with close peer relations were significantly more likely than others to have used condoms (Santhya, Acharya, and Jejeebhoy 2011a). Qualitative data also indicate the influence of peers in informing youth about contraceptive methods and condom use, and among young men, even how to use condoms, where to get condoms, and help in procuring condoms (Santhya, Acharya, and Jejeebhoy 2011a).

Family-level Barriers

Young people, in general, lack a safe and supportive family environment, a shortcoming that is likely to pose major obstacles to their achievement of good sexual and reproductive health and the realisation of their rights. Parents often fail to serve as reliable sources of information for young people. A qualitative study with over 400 mothers and fathers of youth aged 15–24 in six states of India noted a number of factors that prevented parents from discussing sexual and reproductive matters with their children. For example, parents perceived that such discussion went against cultural norms and that youth today become aware of these matters on their own. Reasons cited by parents also included discomfort and embarrassment, both on the part of parents themselves and on the part of their children, about such discussion, and parental apprehensions that communicating about sexual matters would lead their children to engage in sexual activity (Jejeebhoy and Santhya 2011a). Other studies have also identified parents' own lack of awareness, their perception that their children were not at risk of HIV, and parental discomfort and perceptions that informing their children about sexual matters would lead youth to engage in sex as key factors limiting communication (Soletti et al. 2009; Mahajan and Sharma

2005; Garda and Alexander 2009; Shetty, Kowli, and Patil n.d.). Not surprisingly, the Youth Study reports that fewer than 10 per cent of young men and women had discussed growing up or pregnancy and reproduction-related matters with either of their parents; the exception was the finding that 77 per cent of young women had discussed growing up matters with their mother; this discussion was limited, however, to the mechanics of menstruation ('how to use the cloth') and behavioural dos and don'ts (International Institute for Population Sciences and Population Council 2010).

Authoritarian childrearing practices and parental violence characterize the life of many young people. For example, findings from the Youth Study show that as many as one-quarter of young men and women had observed their father beating their mother. Many reported experiencing a beating by a parent during adolescence (International Institute for Population Sciences and Population Council 2010). Although only a few studies in India have explored the links between parental closeness and sexual and reproductive health outcomes among young people, they reiterate the importance of the former. A study of youth in Pune reports that closeness to parents was negatively associated with pre-marital romantic and sexual relationships among young women (Alexander et al. 2007). Findings from the Youth Study, likewise, underscore the role that a supportive family environment plays: youth who reported a parent as confidant, were significantly less likely than others to initiate pre-marital sex early (hazards ratios of 0.782 and 0.875 for young women and men, respectively; Santhya et al. 2011d). In contrast, young women who had witnessed parental violence and experienced violence at the hands of parents were 1.3 times more likely than others to initiate pre-marital sex early. Moreover, young men who had witnessed parental violence and experienced violence at the hands of parents were more likely than others to perpetrate marital violence (Acharya et al. 2009).

Programme-related Challenges

Serious shortcomings in the implementation of programmes have compromised young people's achievement of good sexual and reproductive health and development.

Unmet need in educating youth

Current efforts to provide acceptable standards of schooling to the youth cohort fall short of what is required to enable the country to harness its demographic dividend and its youth to participate in and benefit from global development. These findings call for multi-pronged efforts.

The government has articulated its commitment to improving the schooling situation in the country in several policies and acts, but there has not been a strong commitment to ensuring that these programmes are effectively implemented and that these do indeed reach the most disadvantaged groups. Efforts have failed to address the economic pressures that dissuade parents from enrolling their children in school and from keeping them in school once enrolled. School-level barriers, notably, poor infrastructure, quality of education and academic failure, particularly among young women, have not been overcome, and efforts to incorporate livelihood skills building models within the school setting have not been established. The Working Group on Secondary and Vocational Education for the XIIth Five Year Plan observes that there has been slow progress on the implementation of various schemes during the XIth Plan period (Ministry of Human Resource Development 2011). Not all schemes have effectively reached the marginalised, and delays in the release of funds have also compromised the smooth implementation of various schemes. Chronic shortages in infrastructure were noted. Teacher training was found to be sub-optimal and therefore, had a limited impact on improving classroom dynamics.

Unmet need in providing marketable skills to youth

As observed by the Working Group on Secondary and Vocational Education for the XIIth Five Year Plan, vocational education in India continues to be characterised by several shortcomings: it is treated as distinct and separate from general education; vocational training institutes often do not have close linkages to employers or a sound understanding of their needs; the curriculum has remained static over the years and its quality remains uneven (Ministry of Human Resource Development 2011). The National Skills Development

Initiative that seeks to impart vocational skills training to 500 million persons by 2022 is a step in the right direction. As part of the initiative, 1,386 modules for employable skills covering 60 sectors have been developed; 36 assessing bodies have been empanelled for conducting assessments of these activities; some 1.1 million persons have been trained/tested (since inception); and 6,705 Vocational Training Providers (VTPs) have been registered (Ministry of Labour and Employment 2011). While it is too early comment on the progress of the initiative, it is important that the pace of implementation is accelerated without any delay.

Uneven and poor implementation of programmes intended to raise awareness of sexual and reproductive matters

Although a large number of programmes have been implemented to raise young people's awareness of sexual and reproductive matters, implementation of these programmes has been marred by several concerns. First, they have focused more on young people in schools and colleges than those outside the educational system. Moreover, the focus has been on students in Classes IX and XI; as a result, those who discontinue school prematurely—girls, the poor and the socially excluded—are not reached by school-based programmes. For example, further analyses of the Youth Study data indicate that those from economically poor households were less likely than those from wealthier households (3 per cent of those from the poorest quintile versus 24 per cent of those from the wealthiest quintile) and those belonging to scheduled castes and tribes were less likely than those belonging to general castes (10–11 per cent versus 19 per cent of those belonging to general castes) to have received family life or sex education from schools or colleges. Moreover, despite international evidence of the need to initiate such education at an earlier age, younger adolescents are excluded from age-appropriate education. Outside of the school system, programmes imparted through the Nehru Yuvak Kendras and youth clubs, and even the media, likewise, are likely to reach more males than females, given the gendered nature of youth participation in government and community-led programmes, and in exposure to the mass media (see Jejeebhoy and Santhya 2011b, for a review of programmes).

Second, of concern is the limited reach of the AEP and other similar programmes under the National Adolescent Reproductive and Sexual Health Strategy, that have held much promise for promoting awareness of sexual and reproductive health matters among the young. Unfortunately, reports suggest that they have been unevenly implemented and their reach remains limited: just 15 percent of youth have received family life or sex education in school or through special programmes sponsored by the government or NGOs, ranging from less than 10 percent among the married to 17 per cent and 23 per cent among unmarried young men and women, respectively (Figure 3.4). Further analysis of Youth Study data indicates that even among those who have completed high school, just 26 per cent and 35 per cent of young men and women, respectively, had received such education.

The political backlash against the AEP further confounded its implementation. Consequently, as of September 2009, the NACO supported AEP remained suspended in 8 states, including Madhya Pradesh, Maharashtra, Kerala, Karnataka, Gujarat and Rajasthan. Moreover, just 20% of the budgetary allocation in 2009–10 has been utilised (National AIDS Control Organization, 2009). During 2009–10, the AEP was implemented in only 47,000 of over 145,000 high schools and higher secondary schools across the country (National AIDS Control Organization, 2010). The implementation of awareness raising programmes under the National Adolescent Reproductive and Sexual Health Strategy has also been poor; the 6th Joint Review Mission of the RCH Programme II observes that the majority of the states have made no concerted BCC efforts towards enhancing knowledge among young people (Ministry of Health and Family Welfare 2009a).

Third, concerns remain with regard to the quality of training imparted to the trainers and the extent to which this has succeeded in breaking down traditional inhibitions about discussing sensitive topics. The poor quality of training imparted to trainers and their inhibitions in imparting information on sexual and reproductive matters to students (Verma, Sureender, and Guruswamy, 1997) are likely to prevent many teachers from serving as a reliable source of information on these matters. Indeed, the Youth Study reports that just 10 percent of young people had received information on sexual matters from teachers (International Institute for Population Sciences and Population Council 2010). The Youth Study also show that although youth gave a generally positive assessment of the education they had received, one-fifth of young men and almost two-fifths of young women reported feeling uncomfortable or embarrassed while receiving family life or sex education, raising questions about the extent to which they were indeed able to participate freely and clarify doubts (International Institute for Population Sciences and Population Council 2010).

Finally, a number of concerns remain with regard to the content of the AEP curriculum. Recent curriculum revisions have indeed brought in a broader sexual and reproductive health focus than the earlier and narrower HIV focus, and hold promise not only to raise awareness among young people but also to enable young people to correctly understand and assess the risks they face and adopt appropriate protective actions. At the same time, although many references are made to sexual relations, what these entail is never discussed or is discussed in vague terms, such as the 'student is taught that....sex should be based on consent and respect....' or that sex is 'when male and female sex cells unite during intimate physical relationships between two people.' Likewise, discussion of contraception is extremely limited. Methods are explained in abstract and technical terms without indicating their pros and cons, how they are used or their usefulness in preventing disease. Misconceptions, such as the belief that marriage ensures safety from infection or that one cannot become pregnant at first sex, are generally not addressed. Curricula of programmes for the out-of-school are not readily available, moreover, except in the NGO sector and it is difficult to ascertain messages conveyed in these programmes. At the same time, other programmes intended to impart life skills to young people, including, for example, the KSY programme or RGSEAG (the SABLA scheme) and the University Talk AIDS programme, have great potential, but the extent to which the approaches and content of these programmes have been effective and acceptable to young people has not received much attention.

Outstanding issues in the implementation of programmes to empower girls

A number of programmes have focused on empowering adolescent girls, raising the status of the girl child, and changing gender norms.

Concerns have been raised about the implementation of these programmes. For example, conditional cash transfer programmes intended to raise the status of the girl child have been fraught with cumbersome eligibility criteria and conditions, lack of clarity, limited community involvement, and unattractive benefits (Sekher 2010). The extent to which programmes for adolescent girls, notably the KSY/SABLA programme, have resulted in significant improvements in girls' nutritional levels, acquisition of marketable skills or awareness and agency is not yet clear. In a number of these programmes, fewer girls have been reached than was anticipated, and the achievement of annual targets has been erratic. Indeed, resources allocated for various programmes for girls are severely under-utilized; for example, it observes that during the first three years of the Plan, only 31 per cent of the funds allocated for the Dhanalakshmi scheme had been utilized and that it has received no response yet from bigger states like Bihar and Uttar Pradesh (Planning Commission, 2011). Similarly, it notes that NYKS should set targets for female membership and achievement of these targets should be appropriately weighted in grading youth clubs. While orientation guides for various levels of providers do attempt to raise awareness among providers that parents and other gatekeepers may not treat girls and boys equally, training manuals do not stress gender imbalances and their health consequences, or young people's sexual and reproductive rights (Ministry of Health and Family Welfare 2006b; 2006c).

Health system limitations

A number of health system limitations have been noted that compromise young peoples' ability to attain high standards of sexual and reproductive health.

One of the key factors that inhibit young people's access to services are the attitudes of providers. Evidence from a small-scale study in Andhra Pradesh and Madhya Pradesh indicates that a major factor that might hinder health care providers' ability to provide sexual and reproductive health services to young people is their discomfort in doing so. While most stakeholders were comfortable discussing SRH matters with married young women, sizeable proportions reported discomfort in addressing young men and even unmarried young women. Male providers were less uncomfortable providing information and services to young women than were female providers about providing such services to young men (Santhya, Jejeebhoy, and Ghosh 2007). Evidence from the Youth Study reaffirms the limited reach of health care providers; just 3–7 per cent of young people had obtained information on sexual matters from a health care provider (International Institute for Population Sciences and Population Council 2010). Provider attitudes may also have influenced the skewed method mix adopted by married young women. Indeed, despite their young age, almost two in five young women in India were already sterilized, and one quarter were using traditional methods. Just two in five were using modern non-terminal methods most suited to the young. Indeed, the NFHS-3 also found that only one quarter of women seeking contraception were provided information on the range of methods appropriate for them (International Institute for Population Sciences and Macro International 2007).

Health care providers' failure to make efforts to tailor service delivery strategies to accommodate constraints faced by young people, particularly young women, also tends to limit young people's access to sexual and reproductive health services. For example, although young women's isolation is widely known, evidence from NFHS-3 shows that outreach services rarely reach them. For example, just 11 per cent of young women had received a visit at home from a health worker in the three months preceding the survey. Adolescent girls were only half as likely as young women (7 per cent versus 15 per cent), and unmarried young women were only one quarter as likely as married young women (4 per cent versus 17 per cent), to so report (International Institute for Population Sciences and Macro International 2007). Likewise, although the guidelines for ASHAs do highlight in general terms the vulnerability of young women and especially pregnant young women and although over three-quarters of the 8.3 lakh ASHAs selected have received training pertaining to adolescent issues (Ministry of Health and Family Welfare 2011), there remains a need to provide more specific information on possible strategies through which to deliver services to this group. Evidence from a recent study of some 150 ASHAs in two districts of Rajasthan indicates that their interactions with adolescent and young women remain limited; just one-third of ASHAs reported that they had counselled newly married women about contraceptives, for example

(Santhya et al. 2011b). Similarly, evaluations of the JSY indicate that women who had delivered at young ages (less than 18 years) were less likely than others to have availed of the benefits (Lim et al. 2010; Santhya et al. 2011c).

As with awareness raising programmes, uneven implementation of programmes intended to improve young people's access to sexual and reproductive health services is of concern. Adolescent health clinics are functional in many states, but are concentrated in a few (Gujarat, Madhya Pradesh, Maharashtra, Himachal Pradesh, Kerala and Punjab; Ministry of Health and Family Welfare, 2009b). Moreover, the few evaluations available suggest that the programme has neither improved access to services among youth nor quality of services they receive. Evidence from an evaluation of 21 ARSH clinics/centres in Gujarat observes that not all were functional, very few had separate OPD hours and days designated for adolescents or provided auditory and visual privacy, few young people were aware of the clinics and even fewer would use them because of lack of privacy, fear of attending clinics located in health centres and hospitals, and fear of provider attitudes (Centre for Operations Research and Training, 2009).

Although training programmes on ARSH have been imparted for various levels of providers, not all medical officers, staff nurses, ANMs, ASHAs, and other personnel have been trained, or sensitised about the unique needs of the young (Ministry of Health and Family Welfare, 2009b). Moreover, training has not always combined a focus on the content of information to be imparted with strategies for imparting the information or attention to the clarification of values. The evaluations of ARSH clinics in Gujarat and Maharashtra also raise question about the quality of provider training and the need for reorientation (CORT, 2009; IIHMR, 2010).

Finally, the poor quality of sexual and reproductive health services in the public sector has been widely observed, including such issues as lack of privacy and confidentiality. Further analysis of Youth Study data has established a link between the quality of care received on previous occasions and treatment-seeking for symptoms of infection: among married women who had experienced one or more symptoms of infection, the quality of previous contacts with health care providers was positively associated with whether or not treatment was sought, even after controlling for confounding factors (AOR 1.29, Sabarwal and Santhya 2012).

Limited attempts at engaging boys and young men

While wide gender disparities place young women at a notable disadvantage, young men are also disadvantaged in many ways. Many misuse tobacco products and alcohol, many experience unsafe premarital sex, and notable minorities even marry in adolescence. Further, their awareness of sexual and reproductive health matters is limited, many do not receive family life or sex education, and many, including the married, lack easy access, in practice, to contraceptives from a health care provider or pharmacy. Finally, many hold unequal gender norms, and power imbalances are evident within marital relations. However, programmes for adolescents and young people have not made enough effort to include boys and young men.

Insufficient attention to reach the most vulnerable and the marginalized

The evidence presented in this chapter emphasises the heterogeneity of youth not only in terms of their situation but also with regard to their needs. Also evident is the heightened vulnerability of such subgroups of young people as those growing up in poverty, belonging to socially excluded groups and who missed the chance the acquire an acceptable level of schooling. Poverty and social exclusion status have inhibited young people from achieving educational milestones and making a successful transition into work roles. Similarly, poverty, social exclusion status and lack of education pose significant obstacles to young people's attainment of good sexual and reproductive health and realization of their rights. Adverse outcomes, for example, early marriage, limited contraceptive use, early childbearing and malnutrition, were more prevalent among the poor, the socially excluded and the less educated than among other groups. Further analyses using the Youth Study data also reaffirm the vulnerability faced by young people, particularly, adolescent and young women faced with the double disadvantage of growing up in poverty and lacking education (Table 4.9). Regardless of the indicator and the sex of young people, those who face the double disadvantage of poverty and limited education were considerably less likely than their better educated counterparts from wealthy households to exercise agency and to be informed about sexual and

Table 4.9 Differences in Indicators of Young People's Agency, SRH Awareness and SRH Practices by Economic and Educational Vulnerability

Indicators of agency, awareness and practices	Men (15–24 years)		Women (15–24 years)	
	Less educated from poor households	Better educated from rich households	Less educated from poor households	Better educated from rich households
Made independent decisions on personal matters (%)	52.6	60.8	18.7	42.5
Permitted to visit a friend outside the village/neighbourhood unescorted (%)	–	–	14.9	37.8
Had comprehensive knowledge of HIV/AIDS (%)	14.6	67.6	7.4	52.6
Initiated sex before marriage by age 18 (%)	17.9	9.9	4.2	1.9
Married before age 18 (among those aged 18–24)	13.3	1.4	77.2	15.0
Among the married, became pregnant for the first time before age 18 (among those aged 18–24)	–	–	63.7	20.4

Source: Calculated from Youth Study Data.

reproductive matters, and more likely to have experienced adverse SRH outcomes, including early pre-marital sexual initiation, early marriage and early childbearing. The differences were starker for young women than young men.

Unfortunately, the reach of the programmes has been skewed towards the most advantaged, as discussed in the case of AEP in this chapter or in the case of the JSY, discussed in Chapter 3, for example.

Difficulties in breaking down patriarchal norms held by key influentials in the community

Kinship systems in India continue to be age and gender-stratified, traditional gender norms persist, and investments in girls at the family and community levels remain relatively limited. Changing deeply entrenched traditional norms and attitudes requires action on many fronts, and it is not clear that enough effort has been placed on addressing each of the key stakeholders. For example, there is evidence that the socialisation of sons and daughters continues to be gendered. Research has shown, for example, that there continues to be a gender gap in parental aspirations for and investments in the education of their sons versus daughters (Santhya and Jejeebhoy, 2012). Double standards in the socialization of sons and daughters are also evident, with daughters socialized with many more constraints than sons on mobility, freedom to develop social networks, control over money and so on—disparities that clearly influence girls' ability to exercise informed choice as they grow into adulthood (International Institute for Population Sciences and Population Council 2010). Family elders—mothers- and fathers-inlaw, for example—also play a powerful role in reinforcing gender inegalitarian norms. Likewise, teachers and health care providers are, in different ways, powerful agents of change, but it is not clear that they play a role in changing traditional gender-hierarchical norms and values. Community leaders are another group of stakeholders who are responsible for the upholding of traditional norms. None of these key stakeholder groups has been convincingly reached. Programmes intended to break down the deeply entrenched patriarchal norms held by all of these groups remain relatively rare, and there is little information available on how successful these efforts have been. While the

ARSH programme's Implementation Guide for State and District Programme Managers has included parents in the target audience, the guide contains no discussion of the specific measures to be taken to involve parents or the special messages to be imparted to them (Ministry of Health and Family Welfare 2006a). While there have been many more efforts to sensitise teachers, evaluations of their effectiveness are limited. Indeed, the discomfort experienced by teachers was a significant component of the backlash against the AEP. In-depth efforts that focus on training and building the aptitude of nodal teachers and helping them overcome their embarrassment and hesitation in discussing sexuality and reproductive health issues have traditionally been missing (UNFPA 2003) and other research has suggested that teachers are embarrassed about discussing sexual matters with adolescents, typically skip chapters relating to reproduction and at best discuss these issues in such technical terms that key areas of concern to youth remain unaddressed (Chakrabarti 2003). It is not clear that current training programmes have succeeded in changing teacher attitudes, and the recent Rajya Sabha Report highlights, moreover, the extent to which a supportive environment has not yet been created for the provision of SRH related messages even among the nation's political leadership (Rajya Sabha Committee on Petitions 2009).

Policy-related Gaps

A large number of policies formulated at the national level in the recent past have clearly articulated a commitment to meeting the sexual and reproductive health needs of adolescents and youth. However, most policies have overlooked the fact that young people are not a homogenous group. For example, the National Population Policy has neglected to discuss whether it is advocating services for all adolescents or exclusively for married adolescents. While it does not specifically indicate that unmarried adolescents are ineligible to access services, such statements as 'reproductive health services for adolescent girls and boys are especially significant in rural India, where adolescent marriage and pregnancy are widely prevalent' suggest a certain ambivalence with regard to the extent to which services will be made available to meet the sexual and reproductive health needs of the unmarried. On the other hand, the focus of the NACP 2002 is largely on unmarried young people (students in school and college) and to a certain extent, married young men.

The National Youth Policy 2003, too, remained ambiguous about the extent to which services were to be made available to the unmarried or to girls. The draft Youth Policy 2012 recognises the heterogeneity of youth, based on 'their habitat, environment in which they live, socio-economic status of the family they belong to and their own lifestyle'. It has identified several groups of youth as target groups, including students, youth in urban slums, including migrants, rural youth, tribal youth, youth at risk of substance abuse, human trafficking, working in hazardous occupations and sex workers, youth in violent conflicts, out-of-school youth, youth who suffer from social or moral stigma, and youth in institutional care. Among these target groups, three groups are considered priorities: young women, youth belonging to socially and economically disadvantaged communities and differently abled youth. The policy, however, has several limitations. Most disturbing is the exclusion of those aged 10–15 year-olds from the definition of youth, despite ample evidence that experiences in early adolescence influence the transition to adulthood and beyond. Also notable is the failure of the policy document to recognize the vulnerability of married adolescent girls and young women. Moreover, the three sub-groups of youth described in the Policy (16–21, 21–25 and 26–30 year-olds) obscure many key transitions that youth face. Additionally, beyond categorizing young people into these three sub-groups, the policy document contains no discussion of how the policy interventions will be tailored to meet the differential needs of these sub-groups. For example, the first group (ages 16–21) is described as comprising adolescents whose needs and concerns are different from those aged 22 and above; however, the policy document is completely silent about what the needs and concerns of this sub-group are and what strategies can address their needs. Similarly, the second group (ages 21–25) is described as comprising youth who are in the process of 'completing their education and getting into a career'; but fails to recognise that for the majority of young women in particular, these ages represent a period characterised by transitions to marriage and childbearing and that most have completed their education long before they are aged 21.

Similarly, although the policy document has identified a number of target groups and priority groups, strategies for meeting the needs of these groups have not been delineated in the document.

While almost all policies underscore the need to raise awareness about sexual and reproductive health issues among young people, many do not recognize young people's need for sexual and reproductive health services. For example, the NACP are notably silent about the delivery of any specially packaged services for young people. Further, policies that have recognized such needs are somewhat ambiguous about the nature of services to be made available to young people. For example, the focus of the National Population Policy 2003 and the XIth Five Year Plan is clearly on the less controversial aspects of sexual and reproductive health—counselling and dissemination of information—but not quite as clearly on the provision of services to unmarried adolescents. Likewise, the draft National Youth Policy 2012 shies away from highlighting young people's need for a wide range of sexual and reproductive health services. The emphasis seems to be tilted towards preventing HIV/AIDS and substance abuse; young people's need for such services as contraceptive counselling and supplies, safe abortion services and maternal health services is not at all mentioned.

Overall, most of the national policies discussed here are committed to addressing the gender disparities underlying the poor sexual and reproductive health situation of young people. However, most policy documents are vague about how these commitments are to be operationalized. For example, the draft National Youth Policy 2012 advocates just 'a programme of education of the community people and dialogue with leaders and elders' to prevent such harmful practices as child marriage, dowry, honour killings and so on. Likewise, while most policies indicate the need to create a safe environment for young people, the measures to be taken to do so are rarely described; at the same time, the draft National Youth Policy 2012 does not even mention the need to create a safe environment for young people. Surprisingly, the current draft has completely dropped the recommendations included in the draft National Youth Policy 2010 to engage parents and other gatekeepers to enable young people to make a healthy and safe transition to adulthood.

Gaps in existing laws and acts and their weak enforcement

India has a range of impressive laws and acts intended to promote young people's health and development. The most obvious challenge is the country's apparent inability to implement laws, the most glaring of which is the Child Marriage Restraint Act. A review of data from the National Crime Records Bureau (NCRB) indicates that very few cases of crimes against children punishable under Special and Local Laws, including the Immoral Traffic Prevention Act 1956 and the Child Marriage Restraint Act 1929, have been registered (National Crime Records Bureau, 2010). For example, crimes under the Child Marriage Restraint Act reported nationally, ranged from 58 cases in 1999 to 104 cases in 2008. Strangely, cases under the newly enacted Prohibition of Child Marriage Act 2006 have been clubbed with other crimes under Special and Local Laws. Similarly, just 89 cases were recorded in 2009 under the Indian Penal Code (IPC) 372 and 373 that deal with buying and selling of girls aged below 18 for sex work.

Lack of awareness among young people and the wider community of the provisions of laws that address young people's sexual and reproductive health constitutes another challenge. For example, awareness of the legal minimum age at marriage is not universal, even among the young: just 59 per cent and 70 per cent of young women and men, respectively, were aware of the legal minimum age at marriage for females in the country (International Institute for Population Sciences and Population Council 2010). Young people and adults, similarly, remain poorly informed about their rights under the MTP Act (International Institute for Population Sciences and Population Council, 2010; Jejeebhoy et al., 2011a; 2011b). The continuing belief among women and men, including young people, that men are justified in beating their wife in certain circumstances underscores the limited awareness of the Domestic Violence Act (International Institute for Population Sciences and Macro International 2007; International Institute for Population Sciences and Population Council 2010).

Concerns have also been raised about limitations in the provisions of several of these acts. For example, with regard to the Prohibition of Child Marriage Act, it has been argued that there is no provision in the law that stops a child bride from living with her husband and protects her from sexual and other forms of abuse. It has been argued that by not invalidating a child marriage in all circumstances, and by putting the onus of declaring such a marriage void on the child or the guardians, who would have to go through court proceedings for the same, the Act, in fact, lays the foundation for such an abuse. Moreover, the Act does not make the registration of marriages compulsory (Gonsalves 2007; Law Commission of India 2008).

Concerns have also been raised about the different definitions of 'child' in various laws (Law Commission of India 2008): for example, the Child Marriage Restraint Act defines a child as a male under 21 and a female under 18; however, according to the Immoral Traffic (Prevention) Act of 1986, a child is an individual below 16 years, and a minor is an individual aged between 16 and 18, while under the Juvenile Justice (Care and Protection of Children) Act 2000, a child is an individual below 18.

* * *

This overview has explored the major programmes related to the sexual and reproductive health of adolescents and youth in India, and assessed the extent to which these efforts have responded to young people's needs. Findings suggest that youth in India are, for the most part, unprepared to meet the needs of a globalizing world. Access to quality schooling, particularly secondary level of schooling eludes many, especially girls. Few youth are equipped with marketable skills. Also of concern is the compromised sexual and reproductive health situation of young people. Early and unsafe entry into sexual life and childbearing, exposure to the risk of unwanted pregnancy and infection, unmet need for contraception, unwanted and sometimes coercive sexual activity, and adverse reproductive health outcomes characterize the life of too many youth in India. Progress has been uneven, and gender gaps persist, with young women more likely than young men to experience adverse sexual and reproductive outcomes. The review also highlights that gaps between rural and urban youth, less and better educated youth, poor and wealthy youth and socially excluded and included youth remain. Youth residing in rural areas, with no or limited education, belonging to economically disadvantagedhouseholds and belonging to socially excluded castes, particularly scheduled tribes were more likely than others to report adverse outcomes and compromised ability and resources to take protective actions.

This review has outlined a number of barriers at the individual, family and community level as well as gaps in the policies, laws and programmes that exacerbate young people's vulnerability. At the individual level, these include their limited awareness of health promoting behaviours, limited health care seeking practices, gender power imbalances and limited agency among young women. At the family and community level, barriers include limited communication between parents and children, and lack of safe and supportive environment for young people. Several gaps remain at the programme level as well. For example, current investments in schooling and skilling of young people are yet to make a remarkable change in the situation of young people, and fall short of what is required to enable the country to harness its demographic dividend and its youth to participate in and benefit from global development. Many programmes to build awareness of sexual and reproductive health issues among young people remain poorly implemented, may not reach all groups of adolescents and youth, and little is known about their impact or quality. Delivery of and access to appropriate sexual and reproductive counselling and services falls far short of stated goals. It is clear that services are not youth-friendly; youth are inhibited from accessing services and few are approached by the health system; moreover, the limited available evidence suggests that those who do connect with the health system receive services that are no different from those received by adults, that is, services that do not recognise young people's unique service delivery needs. There is little coordination across the various sectors that implement programmes intended to foster gender equity among the young; moreover, among programmes that have attempted to address these issues, little is known about the extent to which they have stressed sexual and reproductive rights or ways of building egalitarian relations among young couples, measures that would clearly have implications for sexual and reproductive health and care-seeking.

Overriding all of these concerns is the need for greater intersectoral coordination with regard to programming for young people. Young people have multifaceted needs–for services, information and counselling, communication and negotiation skill building, programmes that foster gender equity/develop egalitarian gender norms, and access to supportive gate-keepers, for example. Many of these need and have been addressed in the programmes of several Ministries and Departments–Health and Family Welfare and the NACO, Human Resource Development and Education, Women and Child Development and Youth Affairs and Sports, in particular. While efforts have been made to establish a nodal authority to coordinate work on young people, this has not been effectively accomplished, and as a result, as apparent from this review, coordination is not always evident.

In conclusion, our review clearly shows that there is considerable recognition of the importance of young people in defining India's future, and a considerable commitment to meeting their needs, including those in the sexual and reproductive health and rights arenas. Efforts have been initiated to translate this commitment into practice. Policies and programmes –be they related to women and child development, young people, health and family welfare, or HIV/AIDS have all recognized the importance of improving sexual and reproductive health and choice among young people, and the importance of healthy, productive young women and men in shaping India's future. However, ambiguities in the policy documents (the draft National Youth Policy 2012 is a case in point, for example) and implementation challenges abound and it is not clear that activities have been implemented according to the spirit of each programme. Moreover, monitoring and evaluation has been so sporadic that it is not clear how many young people have been reached, the quality of their interactions with programmes or the extent to which programmes have indeed affected their sexual and reproductive health, awareness, and exercise of informed choices. What is needed is a commitment to ensuring that programmes do indeed reach young people, that the scope and content of programmes are expanded, and that promising lessons are assimilated and scaled up.

Appendix

Table A4.1 Percentage of 18–24 Year Old Young Men and Women Who Had Completed High School, According to State, India, 2005–06

State	Men 18–24	Women 18–24
India	**41.6**	**30.7**
North	**46.2**	**37.9**
Delhi	56.2	62.6
Haryana	59.1	45.3
Himachal Pradesh	81.6	70.1
Jammu & Kashmir	47.5	36.7
Punjab	50.0	55.2
Rajasthan	31.4	17.4
Uttarakhand	48.4	45.9
Central	**35.4**	**23.8**
Chhattisgarh	26.3	17.5
Madhya Pradesh	30.7	19.7
Uttar Pradesh	38.3	26.2
East	**35.0**	**19.3**
Bihar	41.7	18.4
Jharkhand	38.4	19.3
Odisha	34.5	22.8
West Bengal	29.3	18.5
Northeast	**29.7**	**25.0**
Arunachal Pradesh	22.0	20.6
Assam	29.7	24.2
Manipur	50.9	36.8
Meghalaya	26.8	27.6
Mizoram	28.9	31.5
Nagaland	30.3	26.4
Sikkim	27.5	28.7
Tripura	23.6	20.3
West	**46.6**	**38.5**
Goa	61.1	57.7
Gujarat	33.0	30.5

(*Continued*)

Table A4.1 *(Continued)*

State	Men 18–24	Women 18–24
Maharashtra	52.6	42.5
South	**49.9**	**41.9**
Andhra Pradesh	51.6	33.9
Karnataka	43.8	37.4
Kerala	60.8	65.0
Tamil Nadu	50.3	49.0

Source: Calculated from individual male and female respondent data from NFHS-3.

Table A4.2 WorkForce Participation Rate (Usual Status, Principal and Subsidiary) among Young People Aged 15–29 Years by Rural–Urban Residence and Sex, According to State, India, 2005–06

State	Rural		Urban	
	Males	Females	Males	Females
India	**70.5**	**33.0**	**61.0**	**15.2**
North				
Delhi	58.6	1.8	63.2	6.9
Haryana	63.4	30.2	60.6	15.1
Himachal Pradesh	57.8	50.6	51.7	19.5
Jammu & Kashmir	55.2	37.6	46.0	18.2
Punjab	64.3	24.2	63.7	9.2
Rajasthan	68.1	48.0	58.3	11.0
Uttarakhand	61.6	27.7	55.3	8.2
Central				
Chhattisgarh	75.0	60.8	60.4	16.9
Madhya Pradesh	76.7	42.3	57.6	13.1
Uttar Pradesh	68.7	17.2	56.7	8.5
East				
Bihar	68.9	16.6	47.4	5.6
Jharkhand	64.7	35.6	35.1	8.3
Odisha	74.9	34.5	54.7	14.3
West Bengal	76.6	17.9	59.4	17.5
Northeast				
Arunachal Pradesh	56.2	45.9	13.2	
Assam	67.9	19.8	52.6	10.6

State	Rural		Urban	
	Males	Females	Males	Females
Manipur	42.1	30.3	33.9	18.9
Meghalaya	67.3	46.1	46.5	21.1
Mizoram	77.4	54.5	43.4	25.6
Nagaland	62.7	59.1	27.3	17.1
Sikkim	56.5	29.5	52.5	29.5
Tripura	57.0	10.5	41.0	7.6
West				
Goa	77.8	18.8	70.2	22.1
Gujarat	81.8	44.4	74.2	15.2
Maharashtra	69.5	48.1	62.8	15.4
South				
Andhra Pradesh	76.1	56.4	63.8	21.2
Karnataka	71.3	41.7	70.2	22.5
Kerala	56.1	19.8	57.3	15.3
Tamil Nadu	67.4	37.7	64.2	24.6

Source: National Sample Survey Organization (2010).

Table A4.3 Percentage of 20–24 Year Old Women Married by Age 18, According to State, India, 2005–06

State	Women 20–24
India	47.4
North	**40.1**
Delhi	22.7
Haryana	41.2
Himachal Pradesh	12.3
Jammu & Kashmir	14.4
Punjab	19.7
Rajasthan	65.2
Uttarakhand	23.0
Central	**58.0**
Chhattisgarh	55.0
Madhya Pradesh	57.3
Uttar Pradesh	58.6

(*Continued*)

Table A4.3 *(Continued)*

State	Women 20–24
East	**57.1**
Bihar	69.0
Jharkhand	63.2
Odisha	37.2
West Bengal	54.0
Northeast	**35.5**
Arunachal Pradesh	42.0
Assam	38.6
Manipur	12.9
Meghalaya	24.6
Mizoram	20.6
Nagaland	21.4
Sikkim	30.1
Tripura	41.6
West	**38.9**
Goa	12.1
Gujarat	38.7
Maharashtra	39.4
South	**38.6**
Andhra Pradesh	54.8
Karnataka	41.8
Kerala	15.4
Tamil Nadu	22.3

Source: Calculated from individual male and female respondent data from NFHS-3.

Table A4.4 Percentage of Married Young Women Currently Using Any Contraceptive Method and a Modern Non-terminal Method, According to State, India, 2005–06

State	Any method	Any modern non-terminal method
India	**27.5**	10.5
North	**24.3**	**14.4**
Delhi	35.4	25.1

State	Any method	Any modern non-terminal method
Haryana	31.0	17.8
Himachal Pradesh	34.2	18.6
Jammu & Kashmir	22.2	13.1
Punjab	33.8	24.1
Rajasthan	17.8	9.0
Uttarakhand	23.7	15.9
Central	**22.0**	**8.7**
Chhattisgarh	17.6	6.2
Madhya Pradesh	20.3	7.6
Uttar Pradesh	23.1	9.5
East	**28.1**	**11.9**
Bihar	12.6	4.0
Jharkhand	15.5	7.0
Odisha	19.0	10.3
West Bengal	53.9	23.2
Northeast	**39.2**	**17.3**
Arunachal Pradesh	28.4	18.1
Assam	40.0	15.4
Manipur	37.9	14.3
Meghalaya	15.7	9.4
Mizoram	24.7	22.7
Nagaland	12.1	6.5
Sikkim	35.5	25.7
Tripura	55.6	34.7
West	**32.1**	**14.3**
Goa	25.6	14.2
Gujarat	34.0	14.1
Maharashtra	31.2	14.4
South	**31.1**	**4.8**
Andhra Pradesh	33.6	1.8
Karnataka	30.8	5.1
Kerala	33.0	14.9
Tamil Nadu	25.5	6.6

Source: Calculated from individual female respondent data from NFHS-3.

Table A4.5 Percentage of 20–24 Year Old Women Who Had Given Birth Before Age 18 and Married Young Women Aged 15–24 With Three or More Children, According to State

State	Given birth before age 18 (20–24)	Three or more children (15–24)
India	**21.7**	**12.9**
North	**14.6**	**12.3**
Delhi	6.3	8.2
Haryana	14.8	7.8
Himachal Pradesh	4.6	8.1
Jammu & Kashmir	7.2	13.8
Punjab	9.4	8.7
Rajasthan	22.4	15.3
Uttarakhand	9.2	11.2
Central	**24.5**	**17.4**
Chhattisgarh	24.2	15.3
Madhya Pradesh	22.7	13.8
Uttar Pradesh	25.2	19.0
East	**28.4**	**12.8**
Bihar	31.1	15.5
Jharkhand	37.0	17.4
Odisha	16.4	10.6
West Bengal	28.9	8.8
Northeast	**21.5**	**11.4**
Arunachal Pradesh	28.0	17.1
Assam	24.0	11.7
Manipur	7.2	9.8
Meghalaya	12.8	13.8
Mizoram	12.3	13.4
Nagaland	12.4	17.1
Sikkim	18.6	9.8
Tripura	21.0	6.0
West	**16.4**	**10.4**
Goa	4.4	4.4
Gujarat	13.0	11.5
Maharashtra	18.3	9.9

State	Given birth before age 18 (20–24)	Three or more children (15–24)
South	**20.0**	**9.4**
Andhra Pradesh	29.6	8.7
Karnataka	23.4	14.6
Kerala	5.6	3.2
Tamil Nadu	9.0	5.3

Source: Calculated from individual female respondent data from NFHS-3.

Table A4.6 Percentage of Births in the Five Years to Adolescent and Young Mothers That Were Unwanted, According to State, India, 2005–06

State	Women 15–24
India	**16.8**
North	**13.3**
Delhi	8.9
Haryana	10.2
Himachal Pradesh	14.9
Jammu & Kashmir	18.7
Punjab	11.2
Rajasthan	14.4
Uttarakhand	17.7
Central	**18.9**
Chhattisgarh	11.6
Madhya Pradesh	12.8
Uttar Pradesh	22.0
East	**18.5**
Bihar	13.6
Jharkhand	22.9
Odisha	13.1
West Bengal	25.5
Northeast	**17.2**
Arunachal Pradesh	19.3
Assam	12.6
Manipur	10.9

(*Continued*)

Table A4.6 (*Continued*)

State	Women 15–24
Meghalaya	42.6
Mizoram	49.1
Nagaland	20.2
Sikkim	27.3
Tripura	27.4
West	**12.9**
Goa	11.9
Gujarat	16.7
Maharashtra	10.8
South	**16.6**
Andhra Pradesh	15.9
Karnataka	19.7
Kerala	17.3
Tamil Nadu	12.9

Source: Calculated from individual male and female respondent data from NFHS-3.

Table A4.7 Percentage of Youth Who Were Moderately or Severely Anaemic, According to State, India, 2005–06

State	Men 15–24	Women 15–24
India	**11.1**	**17.5**
North	**10.4**	**16.7**
Delhi	8.1	10.6
Haryana	6.0	19.1
Himachal Pradesh	9.8	10.7
Jammu & Kashmir	9.1	15.4
Punjab	8.4	13.3
Rajasthan	13.6	19.3
Uttarakhand	13.8	15.7
Central	**11.9**	**15.7**
Chhattisgarh	11.3	19.1
Madhya Pradesh	11.7	16.6
Uttar Pradesh	12.0	14.9
East	**13.7**	**17.9**

State	Men 15–24	Women 15–24
Bihar	10.7	17.7
Jharkhand	18.5	20.0
Odisha	13.4	15.5
West Bengal	14.8	18.4
Northeast	**15.7**	**20.1**
Arunachal Pradesh	13.6	14.3
Assam	16.2	23.2
Manipur	2.7	4.6
Meghalaya	23.4	14.8
Mizoram	10.8	9.9
Nagaland	–	–
Sikkim	16.3	19.1
Tripura	15.2	15.6
West	**8.6**	**17.7**
Goa	4.6	9.7
Gujarat	10.3	20.3
Maharashtra	7.7	16.4
South	**9.0**	**19.0**
Andhra Pradesh	11.0	25.6
Karnataka	9.5	18.2
Kerala	3.6	8.3
Tamil Nadu	8.2	15.4

Source: Calculated from individual male and female respondent data from NFHS-3.

References

Acharya, R., F. Ram, S. J. Jejeebhoy, A. Singh, K.G. Santhya, U. Ram et al. 2009. *Physical and Sexual Violence within Marriage among Youth in India*: Findings from the *Youth in India, Situation and Needs Study*. Paper presented at the XXVI IUSSP International Population Conference, Marrakech, Morocco, 27 September–2 October, 2009.

Alexander, M., L. Garda, S. Kanade, S.J. Jejeebhoy, and B. Ganatra. 2007. 'Correlates of Premarital Relationships among Unmarried Youth in Pune district, Maharashtra, India', *International Family Planning Perspectives*, 33(4): 150–159.

Andrew, G. and V. Patel. 2002. *Health Needs of Adolescents: A Study of Health Needs of Adolescents in Higher Secondary Schools in Goa*, Alto-Porvorim: Resource Centre for Adolescent and Child Health.

Annual Status of Education Report (ASER). 2012. *Annual Status of Education Report (Rural) 2011, Provisional, January 16, 2012*. New Delhi: ASER Centre.

Barua, A. and K. Kurz. 2001. 'Reproductive Health-Seeking by Married Adolescent Girls in Maharashtra, India', *Reproductive Health Matters*, 9(17): 53–62.

Centre for Development and Population Activities (CEDPA). 2011. *Udaan Towards A Better Future: Improving the Lives of Young People in Jharkhand, India*. New Delhi: CEDPA.

Centre for Operations Research and Training (CORT). 2009. Assessment of Adolescent Reproductive and Sexual Health (ARSH) Centers in Gujarat. CORT: Vadodara.

Chakrabarti, V. 2003. 'Population Education in Formal and Non-Formal Sectors in India', in *Towards Adulthood: Exploring the Sexual and Reproductive Health of Adolescents in South Asia*, ed. S. Bott et al., Geneva: World Health Organisation.

Chhabra, R., S. Gupte, A. Mehta et al. 1988. 'MTP and Concurrent Contraceptive Adoption in Rural India', *Studies in Family Planning*, 19(4): 244–247.

Ganatra, B. 2000. 'Abortion Research in India: What We Know and What We Need to Know', in *Women's Reproductive Health in India*, eds. R. Ramasubban and S. Jejeebhoy. Jaipur: Rawat Publications.

Ganatra, B. and S. Hirve. 2002. 'Induced Abortions among Adolescent Women in Rural Maharashtra', *Reproductive Health Matters*, 10(19): 76–85.

Garda, L. and M. Alexander. 2009. *Parent-child Connectedness: A Pressing Need to be Addressed in Rural and Urban India*, paper presented at XXVI IUSSP International Population Conference, Marrakech, Morocco.

Gonsalves, C. 2007. *Illegal Yet Valid!* Accessed on July 21 2011 at http://www.hrln.org/admin/issue/subpdf/Illegal_yet_valid_2007.pdf.

Institute of Health Management Research (IIHMR). 2010. Evaluation Study on Adolescent Friendly Health Clinics in Maharashtra. IIHMR: Jaipur.

International Institute for Population Sciences and Macro International. 2007. *National Family Health Survey (NFHS-3), India, 2005–06*. Mumbai: IIPS.

International Institute for Population Sciences (IIPS) and Population Council. 2010. *Youth in India: Situation and Needs 2006–2007*. Mumbai: IIPS.

Jaya. 2010. *Responding to the Sexuality Education Controversy in India, Presentation Made at the International Consultation, Comprehensive Sexuality Education: Advancing Human Rights, Gender Equality and Improved Sexual and Reproductive Health, Review of Current Evidence and Experiences*. Presentation made at meeting organized by UNFPA, Bogota, Colombia in December 2010.

Jaya. and S. Yadav. 2010. *Adolescence Education Programme: Evolution, Implementation Status and Lesson Learned*. Presentation made at Second UNFPA Regional Workshop: Programming for Young People: The Framework for Action, at Kathmandu, Nepal.

Jejeebhoy, S.J. and M.P. Sebastian. 2004. 'Young People's Sexual and Reproductive Health', in *Looking Back, Looking Forward: A Profile of Sexual and Reproductive Health in India*, ed. S.J. Jejeebhoy. New Delhi: Rawat Publications.

Jejeebhoy, S.J., K.G. Santhya, and R. Acharya. 2010. Meeting the Sexual and Reproductive Health Needs of Youth: Insights from India. *Presentation made at the UNFPA and ICOMP Asia and the Pacific Regional Consultation on Family Planning in Asia and the Pacific – Dealing with the Challenges*. Bangkok.

Jejeebhoy, S.J., S. Kalyanwala, A.J. Francis Zavier, R. Kumar, and N. Jha. 2010. 'Experience Seeking Abortion among Unmarried Young Women in Bihar and Jharkhand, India: Delays and Disadvantages', *Reproductive Health Matters*, 18(35): 163–174.

Jejeebhoy, S.J. and K.G. Santhya. 2011a. *Parent-child Communication on Sexual and Reproductive Health Matters: Perspectives of Mothers and Fathers of Youth in India*. New Delhi: Population Council.

Jejeebhoy, S.J. and K.G. Santhya. 2011b. *Sexual and Reproductive Health of Young People: A Review of Policies, Laws and Programmes*. New Delhi: Population Council.

Jejeebhoy, S.J., A.J. Francis Zavier, R. Acharya et al. 2011a. *Increasing Access to Safe Abortion in Rural Maharashtra: Outcomes of a Comprehensive Abortion Care Model*. New Delhi: Population Council.

Jejeebhoy, S.J., A.J. Francis Zavier, R. Acharya et al. 2011b. *Increasing Access to Safe Abortion in Rural Rajasthan: Outcomes of a Comprehensive Abortion Care Model*. New Delhi: Population Council.

Law Commission of India. 2008. *Proposal to Amend the Prohibition of Child Marriage Act, 2006 and Other Allied Laws* (Report No. 205). New Delhi: Law Commission of India, Government of India.

Lim, S.S., L. Dandona., J.A. Hoisington, S.L. James, M.C. Hogan, and E. Gakidou. 2010. 'India's Jananki Suraksha Yojana, A Conditional Cash Transfer Programme to Increase Births in Health Facilities: An Impact Evaluation', *Lancet*, 375: 2009–23.

Mahajan, P. and N. Sharma. 2005. 'Parents' Attitude Towards Imparting Sex Education to Their Adolescent Girls', *Anthropologist*, 7(3): 197–199.

Ministry of Health and Family Welfare (MOHFW). 2006a. *Implementation Guide on RCH II: Adolescent Reproductive Sexual Health Strategy, for State and District Programme Managers*. New Delhi: MOHFW, Government of India.

Ministry of Health and Family Welfare (MOHFW). 2006b. Orientation Programme for Medical Officers to Provide Adolescent-Friendly Reproductive and Sexual Health Services: Facilitator's Guide. New Delhi: MOHFW, Government of India.

——— 2006c. Orientation on Programme for ANM/LHVs to Provide Adolescent-Friendly Reproductive and Sexual Health Services: Facilitator's Guide. New Delhi: MOHFW, Government of India.

——— 2006d. *Reading material for ASHA, Book # 3, Family planning, RTI/STIs and HIV/AIDS and ARSH*. Accessed on 4 July 2011 at http://www.mohfw.nic.in/NRHM/Documents/ASHA_Book_No_3.pdf.

——— 2006e. *Janani Suraksha Yojana: Features and Frequently Asked Questions and Answers*. Accessed on September 4 2011 at *http://mohfw.nic.in/dofwwebsite/JSY_features_FAQ_Nov_2006.htm*.

Ministry of Human Resource Development 2009a. *National Rural Health Mission, Reproductive and Child Health Program Phase 2, 6th Joint Review Mission Aide Memoire*, New Delhi: MOHFW, Government of India.

——— 2009b. *Reproductive and Sexual Health of Young People in India*, New Delhi: MOHFW, Government of India.

——— 2010. *Asha Module 6: Skills that Save Lives*, New Delhi: MOHFW, Government of India.

——— 2011. *Update on the ASHA Programme*, New Delhi: MOHFW, Government of India.

——— n.d. *School Health Programme*. Accessed on July 4 2011 at http://www.mohfw.nic.in/showfile.php.

Ministry of Human Resource Development (MOHRD). 2008. *Aide Memoire, First Joint Review Mission of Mahila Samakhya*. New Delhi: MOHRD, Government of India. Accessed on 4 July 2011 at http://education.nic.in/ms/AideMemoireJRM08.pdf.

——— 2009a. *Framework for Implementation of Rashtriya Madhyamik Shiksha Abhiyan*. New Delhi: MOHRD, Government of India. Accessed on 4 July 2011 at http://education.nic.in/secedu/Framework_Final_RMSA.pdf.

——— 2009b. *Saakshar Bharat*. New Delhi: MOHRD, Government of India. Accessed on 4 July 2011 at http://education.nic.in/Elementary/SaaksharBharat.pdf.

Ministry of Human Resource Development (MOHRD). 2011. *Working Group Report on Secondary and Vocational Education 12th Five Year Plan 2012–2017*. New Delhi: Department of School Education and Literacy, MOHRD, Government of India.

Ministry of Labour. 2009. *National Policy on Skill Development*. New Delhi: Ministry of Labour, Government of India. Accessed on July 4 2001 at http://www.labour.nic.in/policy/NationalSkillDevelopmentPolicyMar09.pdf.

Ministry of Labour and Employment. 2011. *Report of the Working Group on Skill Development and Training For XII Five Year Plan 2012–1017*. New Delhi: Ministry of Labour and Employment, Government of India.

Ministry of Women and Child Development (MOWCD). 2010. *Implementation Plan of Rajiv Gandhi Scheme for Empowerment of Adolescent Girls [RGSEAG] SABLA*. Agenda No. 3. New Delhi: MOWCD, Government of India. Accessed on 21 June 2010 at www.wcd.nic.in/agenda16062010/agenda_16062010_item3.pdf.

Ministry of Youth Affairs and Sports (MOYAS). n.d. National Programme for Youth and Adolescent Development: Scheme Guidelines. Accessed on July 4 2011 at http://www.yas.nic.in/writereaddata/linkimages/5349309212.pdf.

Narayan, G. and Jaya. 2011. *Strategy for Reaching Adolescents in out-of-school Settings Through Nehru Yuva Kendra Sangathan (NYKS) in collaboration with Ministry of Youth Affairs and Sports (MOYAS)*. Presentation made to the Joint Secretary, Ministry of Youth Affairs and Sports, New Delhi.

National AIDS Control Organization (NACO). 2004. *Annual Report 2002–2004*. New Delhi: NACO.

———. 2006. *National AIDS Control Programme, Phase III (2006–2011), Strategy and Implementation Plan*, New Delhi: NACO.

———. 2008a. *Adolescence Education Programme, Life Skills Development*. Accessed on 10 March 2011 at http://www.nacoonline.org/upload/NACOinActiion/AEP-TeachersWorkbook.pdf.

———. 2008b. *Adolescence Education Programme, Life Skills Development: Facilitators' Guide*. Accessed on 10 March 2011 at http://www.nacoonline.org/upload/NACOinActiion/FacilitatorsGuide.pdf.

———. 2009. *Project Directors' Review Meeting, 1 September, 2009*. Accessed on 10 March 2011 at http://www.nacoonline.org/upload/Meetings_conferences_Workshops/PDreview.

———. 2010. *Annual Report 2009–10*, New Delhi: NACO.

———. n.d. *Adolescence Education Programme*. Accessed on 10 March 2011 at http://nacoonline.org/Quick_Links/Youth/School_Age_Education_Program_SAEP.

National Council of Educational Research and Training (NCERT). 2011. *Training and Resource Materials under the Adolescence Education Programme*. Accessed on 4 July 2011 at http://www.ncert.nic.in/programmes/aep/aep.html

National Crime Records Bureau (NCRB). 2010. *Crime in India 2009*. New Delhi: NCRB, Government of India.

National Institute of Medical Statistics and National AIDS Control Organization. 2008. *National Behavioural Surveillance Survey (BSS), 2006, Youth (15–24 Years)*. New Delhi: NACO, Ministry of Health and Family Welfare, Government of India. Accessed on 5 January 2012 at http://www.nacoonline.org/Quick_Links/Publication/ME_and_Research_Surveillance/Reports_and_Surveys/National_BSS_20062.

National Sample Survey Organisation (NSSO). 2006. *Employment and Unemployment Situation in India 2004–05, Part I, NSS 61*st *Round*. New Delhi: NSSO, Government of India.

——— 2010. *Employment and Unemployment Situation in India 2007–08, NSS 64th Round*. New Delhi: NSSO, Government of India.

Office of the Registrar General, India. 2009. *Special Bulletin on Maternal Mortality in India 2004–06*. New Delhi: Office of Registrar General, India.

Office of the Registrar General and Census Commissioner India. 2006. *Population Projections for India and States 2001–2026 (Revised December 2006)*. New Delhi: Office of the Registrar General and Census Commissioner.

Parasuraman, S., S. Kishor, S.K. Singh and Y. Vaidehi. 2009. A Profile of Youth in India, National Family Health Survey (NFHS-3), India, 2006–06, Mumbai: IIPS.

Planning Commission. 2011. *Mid-Term Appraisal Eleventh Five Year Plan 2007–2012*. New Delhi: Oxford University Press.

Prasad, J.H., S. Abraham, V. George, M.K. Lalitha, R. John, M.N. Jayapaul, et al. 2005. 'Reproductive Tract Infections Among Young Married Women in Tamil Nadu, India,' *International Family Planning Perspectives*, 31(2): 73–8.

Pratham Resource Centre. 2011. *Annual Status of Education Report (Rural) 2010*, Mumbai: Pratham Resource Centre.

Rajya Sabha Committee on Petitions. 2009. *Hundred and Thirty-Fifth Report on Petition Praying for National Debate and evolving Consensus on the Implementation of the Policy for the Introduction of Sex Education in the Schools and Holding Back its Introduction Until Then*. Accessed on 3 June 2009 at <http://164.100.47.5:8080/committeereports/reports.aspx>.

Rani, M. and S. Bonu. 2003. 'Rural Indian Women's Care-Seeking Behavior and Choice of Provider for Gynaecological Symptoms,' *Studies in Family Planning*, 34(3): 173–185.

Sabarwal, S. and K.G. Santhya. 2012. 'Treatment-seeking for Symptoms of Reproductive Tract Infection Among Married and Unmarried Young Women in India,' *International Perspectives on Sexual and Reproductive Health,* 38(2): 90–98.

Santhya, K.G, N. Haberland, E. McGrory, A. Joshi, A. Mehta, and A. Das. 2003. 'Supporting Married Adolescent Girls: Encouraging Positive Partner Involvement'. Paper presented at the meeting *Reaching Men to Improve Reproductive Health for All*, Washington, September 15–18.

Santhya, K.G., S. Ghosh, and S.J. Jejeebhoy 2007. *Addressing the Sexual and Reproductive Health Needs of Young People: Perspectives and Experiences of Stakeholders from the Health and Non-Health Sectors*. New Delhi: Population Council.

Santhya, K.G. and S.J. Jejeebhoy. 2007. Young People's Sexual and Reproductive Health in India: Policies, Programmes and Realities. *South and East Asia Regional Working Paper No. 19*. New Delhi: Population Council.

Santhya, K.G., R. Acharya, and S.J. Jejeebhoy. 2011a. 'Condom Use Before Marriage and Its Correlates: Evidence from India', *International Perspectives on Sexual and Reproductive Health*, 37(4): 170–180.

Santhya, K.G., S.J. Jejeebhoy, and A.J. Francis Zavier. 2011b. *Implementing the Janani Suraksha Yojana: Perspectives and Experiences of Accredited Social Health Activists in Rajasthan*. New Delhi: Population Council.

Santhya, K.G., S.J. Jejeebhoy, R. Acharya, and A.J.F. Zavier. 2011c. *Effects of the Janani Suraksha Yojana on Maternal and Newborn Care Practices: Women's Experience in Rajasthan*. New Delhi: Population Council.

Santhya, K.G., R. Acharya, S.J. Jejeebhoy, and U. Ram. 2011d. Timing of First Sex Before Marriage And Its Correlates: Evidence from India, *Culture, Health and Sexuality*, 13(3): 327–341.

Santhya, K.G. and S.J. Jejeebhoy. 2012. *Gender Differences in Educational Attainment Among Youth in India: An Exploratory Study of Parental Aspirations about and Investment in Young People's Schooling*. unpublished report.

Sekher, T.V. 2010. *Special Financial Incentive Schemes for the Girl Child in India: A Review of Select Schemes*, Mumbai: IIPS.

Shetty, P., S. Kowli, and V. Patil. n.d. Attitude of Mothers Towards Sex Education of Adolescent Girls, *Regional Health Forum WHO South-East Asia Region* (Volume 3). Accessed on 29 March 2011 at http://www.searo.who.int/en/Section1243/Section1310/Section1343/Section1344/Section1351/Section1686_7197.htm

Solapurkar, M.L and R.N. Sangam. 1985. 'Has the MTP Act in India Proved Beneficial?', *Journal of Family Welfare,* 31(3): 46–52.

Soletti, A.B., V. Guilamo-Ramos, D. Burnette, S. Sharma, and A. Bouris. 2009. 'India-US Collaboration to Prevent Adolescent HIV Infection: The Feasibility of a Family-Based HIV-prevention Intervention for Rural Indian Youth', *Journal of the International AIDS Society,* 12: 35.

Sujay, Rachna. 2009. Premarital Sexual Behaviour Amongst Unmarried College Students Of Gujarat, India, *Health and Population Innovation Fellowship Programme Working Paper, No. 9*. New Delhi: Population Council.

Verma R.K., S. Sureender, and M. Guruswamy. 1997. 'What Do School Children and Teachers in Rural Maharashtra Think of Aids and Sex?', *Health Transition Review, 37(Suppl.)*: 481–86.

Verma R.K., J. Pulerwitz, V. Mahendra S. Khandekar, G. Barker, P. Fulpagare, et al. 2006. 'Challenging and Changing gender Attitudes Among Young Men in Mumbai, India,' *Reproductive Health Matters,* 14(28): 135–143.

United Nations Population Fund (UNFPA). 2003. *UNFPA-Supported Project for Adolescents during the UNFPA Fifth Country Programme (1997–2002): A Compendium*. New Delhi: UNFPA.

5

Women's Empowerment and Gender Equity

Shireen J. Jejeebhoy
K.G. Santhya

The principle of gender equality is enshrined in the Indian Constitution. India has, moreover, made many commitments to empowering women. It ratified the Convention on the Elimination of All Forms of Discrimination against Women (CEDAW) in 1993, and is a signatory to the Millennium Development Goals (2000), of which Goal 3 refers specifically to promoting gender equality and empowering women. Over the past two decades, moreover, there has been an explicit recognition of the extent to which the prevailing inequalities and women's lack of empowerment have impeded national development and violated women's rights. A number of policies as well as programmes initiated by government and civil society organizations have therefore focused on empowering women and enhancing gender equality and equity, and strides have been made in reducing gaps between men and women, and in enabling women to realize their rights. Policies and laws relating to empowering women and narrowing gender gaps have been described in Chapter 1.

Notwithstanding these policies and commitments, gender inequities and violations of women's rights persist, as noted by many, including the Working Group on Women's Agency and Empowerment constituted to inform the XIIth Five Year Plan (Ministry of Women and Child Development, 2011). This chapter describes key programmes, summarizes the situation with regard to gender disparities and women's empowerment, and where possible, the changes in this situation over time, and highlights the challenges in and opportunities for meeting the commitments outlined in India's policies and programmes.

Key Programmes Relating to Women's Empowerment and Gender

Several programmes that aim to enhance women's ability to exercise informed choices and promote gender equality and equity exist. While public sector programmes intended to redress gender inequities and promote women's empowerment fall under the responsibilities of many sectors (Human Resource Development, Health and Family Welfare, Youth Affairs, Women and Child Development for example), most programmes in this area are implemented by the Ministry of Women and Child Development (Ministry of Women and Child Development, 2010). Key among its programmes to empower women is the National Mission for the Empowerment of Women. This mission was launched in 2010 with the goal of achieving inter-sectoral convergence of all pro-women programmes: focus areas include economic empowerment, elimination of violence against women, social empowerment, notably in the areas of health and education, gender mainstreaming of programmes and policies, and awareness generation and advocacy to enable women to demand schemes and programmes for which they are entitled. Accomplishments to date have not been documented.

Specific schemes that address women's limited access to health care have also been promoted. Notable among these is the recently launched Indira Gandhi Matritva Sahyog Yojana (IGMSY). This scheme provides conditional cash transfers to pregnant and lactating women that complements similar transfers provided by the *Janani Suraksha Yojana* (JSY) implemented by the Ministry of Health and Family Welfare, and is implemented using the Integrated Child

Development Services (ICDS) platform, initially on a pilot basis in 52 districts of the country (for more information, see Chapter 3).

Other schemes have focused on raising the status of adolescent girls. For example, the Rajiv Gandhi Scheme for the Empowerment of Adolescent Girls (RGSEAG) (SABLA) and the *Kishori Shakti Yojana* (KSY) are intended to provide nutritional supplementation and life skills education to girls aged 11–18 (for more information, see Chapter 4). Schemes have also been instituted that focus on providing cash transfers for daughters, as a means of reversing the acute problem of a declining child sex ratio. The Dhanalakshmi project was launched in 2008 that provides a set of staggered cash transfers (totalling some Rs 13,500) to the family, preferably the mother, of a girl on the fulfilment of certain conditions, including birth registration, immunization, enrolment and continuation in school, and delayed marriage (18 or later). The scheme was introduced on a pilot basis in 11 blocks across seven states (Andhra Pradesh, Bihar, Chhattisgarh, Odisha, Jharkhand, Punjab, and Uttar Pradesh) (Ministry of Women and Child Development 2010). The *apni beti apna dhan*, and the *ladli* schemes are similar conditional cash transfer programmes for girls that act upon both girls' wellbeing as well as attitudes towards them (Department of Women and Child Development 2005).

There have also been special programmes to encourage girls' education. The National Programme for Education of Girls at Elementary Level provides additional support for elementary education of underprivileged or disadvantaged girls. Kasturba Gandhi Balika Vidyalayas, residential schools for girls belonging predominantly to socially excluded groups, have been established in educationally backward blocks. Moreover, a cash transfer scheme has been initiated that provides incentives to girls to encourage secondary education attendance; under this scheme, primarily for girls belonging to socially excluded groups, a sum of Rs. 3,000 is deposited into an account in the name of girls who have completed Class 8 and are enrolled in secondary school, and may be withdrawn when the girl reaches age 18 (Ministry of Human Resource Development n.d.). Other schemes, including the provision of bicycles, free uniforms, and free textbooks have been implemented by several state governments to promote girls' education.

Several schemes have been initiated that address the economic empowerment of women, including encouraging group formation, providing credit and financial autonomy for women, and raising women's awareness of their rights. For example, the *Mahila Samakhya*, implemented in selected states, seeks to enable women to gain better access to education and health services, open up economic options for women and enhance their role in local government. The Support to Training and Employment Programme (STEP) for Women has been ongoing for 25 years and is intended to build skills and awareness and improve access to credit among asset-less women in ten traditional sectors (agriculture, handloom, handicraft, etc). The scheme has recently been revised to include training based on market needs. The *Priyadarshini* programme for women's empowerment and livelihood in six districts of Uttar Pradesh and Bihar supports self-help groups for women, and aims to both build women's livelihood opportunities and equip them with the skills to exercise rights; support is provided, moreover, for the establishment of small and medium sized enterprises. *Swayamsiddha* is an integrated scheme for women's empowerment through Self Help Group (SHGs). It seeks to achieve holistic empowerment of women through awareness generation, economic empowerment and convergence of various schemes. Finally, the *Rashtriya Mahila Kosh* (National Credit Fund for Women), launched in 1993, aims to meet the credit needs of poor women in the informal sector. The programme has implemented a number of measures to raise awareness of micro-financing, thrift and credit, formation and stabilization of SHGs and enterprise development. Through intermediary micro-financing organisations, credit is disbursed to poor women without collateral, for livelihood activities, housing, micro-enterprises, etc.

Programmes for skill development for women have also been articulated. The XIth Plan recognizes the constraints women have faced in securing employment and suggests the need to work towards mainstreaming women in new and emerging areas of the economy through necessary skill training, vocational training and technology education, and advocates social policies that mitigate the adverse impact of globalization on women. It calls for public-private partnerships and use of corporate social responsibility programmes for advancing training and capacity building of women, while at the same time, discusses the need to recognize traditional skills and market women's products (eg. weaving, food processing). It also discusses the need to ensure that NREGA does not discriminate against women. The National Skill Development Initiative has also recognised the need to ensure equitable access to skill development opportunities to all, in particular women (Planning Commission 2011).

Other schemes have addressed the needs of special groups of vulnerable women. The Swadhar scheme has been ongoing for 10 years and is intended to provide food and shelter, vocational skill building, and legal and/or health related services for women in difficult circumstances, including deserted widows, trafficked women, the mentally challenged and those with HIV/AIDS. The Ujjawala scheme, launched in 2007, is intended to support trafficked women and girls, and addresses not only rescue and rehabilitation needs but also prevention.

Notwithstanding this range of programmes and schemes, and notwithstanding the steps outlined in the XIth Plan, the achievement of targets set out in the XIth Plan were, by the Ministry's own reckoning, no more than partially achieved (Ministry of Women and Child Development 2011). The Working Group on Women's Agency and Empowerment highlights a roadmap to strengthen efforts toward empowering women over the course of the XIIth Plan. In the economic arena, it advocates, for example, increasing women's workforce participation, notably in secondary and tertiary sectors, ensuring decent work for women, financial inclusion, including access to credit, increasing women's asset base, and creating skill building opportunities for women and girls. Focus is also placed on ensuring women's right to reproductive health services and eradicating malnutrition and anaemia among them. It argues for greater access to secondary and tertiary education for girls, and a gender-sensitive and girl-friendly educational system. It calls for efforts to eliminate violence against women as a 'non-negotiable deliverable' of the XIIth Plan: strengthening existing legislation, ensuring effective enforcement of laws and policies, ensuring prompt action through fast track courts, support for victims of violence, and expansion of activities to ensure wide dissemination of the legal rights of women. Finally, it recognies that while women's political representation in local governance has increased, the extent and quality of their participation remains compromised as a result of prevailing gender inequities: the thrust of the XIIth Plan is to promote alliances of female Panchayati Raj Institutions (PRIs), pre-election preparation of candidates and training, and capacity building of elected women representatives.

Women's Empowerment and Gender Equity: The Situation

In this section, we explore the situation of women and prevailing gender gaps in terms of education, health, economic activity, and political participation, and explore the extent to which these have changed over time.

Educational Status: Trends and Differentials

Literacy and educational attainment levels among women have clearly been increasing. The 2011 census reveals literacy rates of 65 per cent among females, compared to 81 per cent among males. Even so, as Figure 5.1 suggests, the female literacy rate in 2011 has just equalled that attained by males twenty years earlier. Statewise data, presented in Table A5.1 confirm huge statewise variation in female literacy rates. While the female literacy rate is 73 per cent in Tamil Nadu and 92 per cent in Kerala, it region ranges from 52 per cent to 59 per cent in such states as Bihar, Jharkhand, Madhya Pradesh, Rajasthan, and Uttar Pradesh.

Figure 5.1 and Table A5.1 also show that the gender gap has narrowed, from a 25 point difference in 1991 to a 16 point difference by 2011, suggesting that the pace of increase in literacy has been more impressive, over this last decade, among females than males. However, the male–female gap in literacy persists in almost every state except Kerala. Meghalaya and Mizoram (where it is 3 to 4 percentage points), as seen in Table A5.1. Indeed, the difference is 20 percentage points or more in several states: Jammu and Kashmir and Rajasthan in the north, all three central states (Chhattisgarh, Madhya Pradesh, and Uttar Pradesh), and Bihar and Jharkhand in the east.

There is evidence that the gender gap in school attendance has also narrowed (Table 5.1). As of 2005–06, more than three-quarters of girls aged 6–14 were in school, compared to 83 per cent of boys; the gender difference in school attendance rates declined from 17 points in

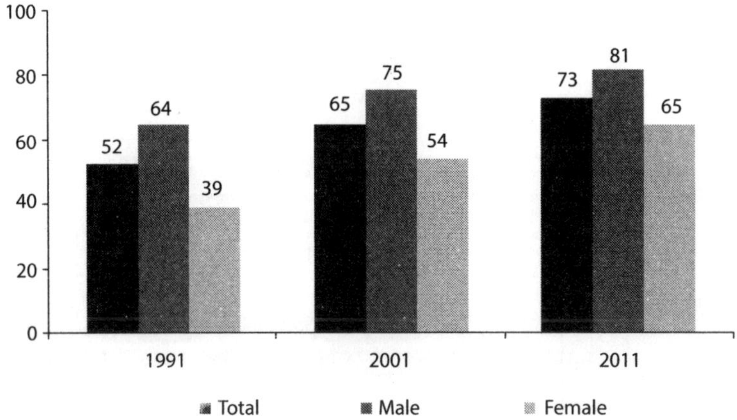

Figure 5.1 Literacy Rates 1991–2011: Trends and Gender Disparities
Source: Office of the Registrar General and Census Commissioner, India (2013).

1992–93 to 9 points in 1998–99 and 6 points in 2005–06 (International Institute for Population Sciences and Macro International 2007).

School attendance, moreover, differs considerably by such socio-demographic factors as age, rural-urban residence, religion, caste, and economic status (Figure 5.2). For example, school attendance among those aged 6–14 ranged from 64 per cent among girls from scheduled tribes to 83 per cent among those from general castes, a 19 percentage point difference, and from 58 per cent among girls from the poorest households to 95 per cent among those in the wealthiest ones; corresponding differences are somewhat narrower among boys

Table 5.1 Percentage of Children Aged 6–14 years Attending School by Sex, 1992–93 to 2005-06, India*

Year	Males	Females	M–F gap in school attendance
1992–93	75.5	58.9	16.6
1998–99	83.1	73.7	9.4
2005–06	82.6	76.4	6.2

Note: **de facto* household population
Source: International Institute for Population Studies (1995); International Institute for Population Studies and ORC Macro (2000) and International Institute for Population Sciences and Macro International (2007).

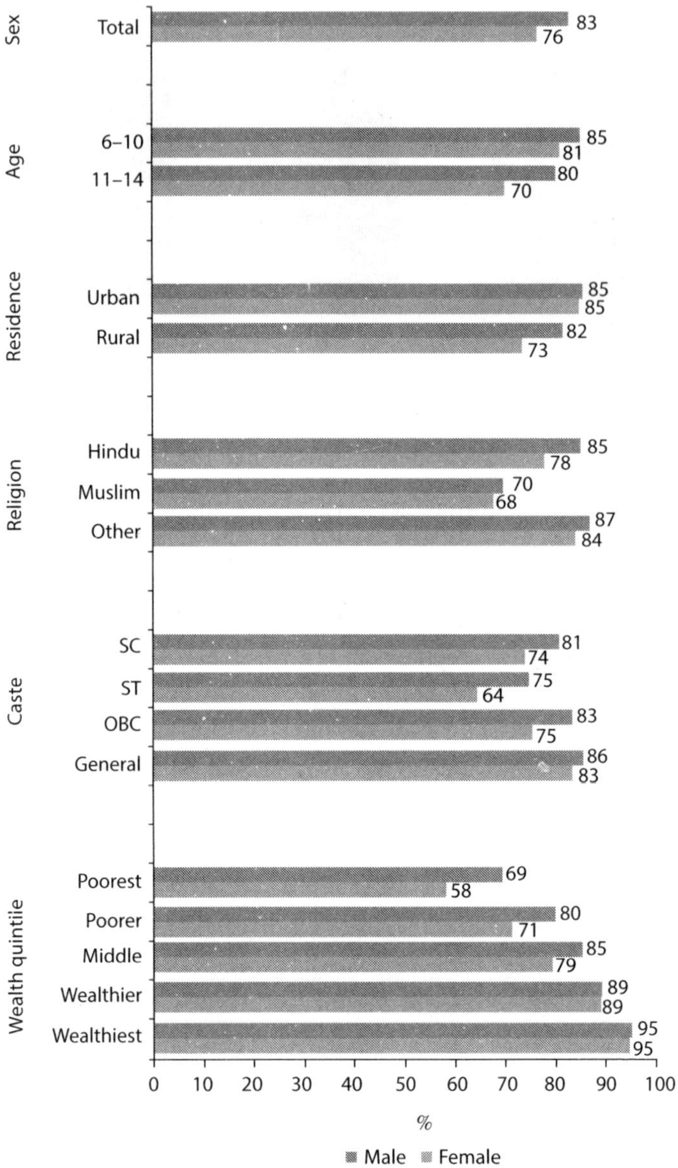

Figure 5.2 School Attendance, Boys and Girls Aged 6–14, by Selected Background Characteristics, India, 2005–06

Source: Calculated from NFHS 2005–06 household data; *De facto household population age 6–14.

(75 per cent and 86 per cent, respectively in the case of caste, and 69 per cent and 95 per cent in the case of economic status).

The gender gap in school attendance also differs considerably by socio-demographic and economic characteristics (Figure 5.2). The difference in the percentage of boys and girls attending school in 2005–06 was just 4 points (85 per cent versus 81 per cent) among those aged 6–10 years, it increased to 10 points (80 per cent versus 70 per cent) among those aged 11–14. While no gender gap was observed in urban areas, a gap of some 8 points was apparent in rural areas. A 7–10 point gender gap persisted among those belonging to scheduled castes, scheduled tribes and other backward castes, while it was almost negligible among those belonging to the general castes (2 points). Data also highlight that the gender gap in school attendance narrowed steadily with household economic status, from 11 points among those belonging to the poorest households to less than one point among those belonging to the richest households. In most states (Appendix 5.2), the gender gap in school attendance was narrow; it exceeded 10 points in such states as Jharkhand (11 points), Bihar (12 points) and Rajasthan (18 points).

Educational attainment levels continue to be low in general, and particularly for females (International Institute for Population Sciences and Macro International 2007). As of 2005–06, just 21per cent of women aged 20–49 had completed a high school education (Class 10) compared to 34 per cent of men. Further analysis of NFHS-3 data, presented in Figure 5.3, highlights that marked improvements have taken place over progressively younger cohorts in terms of secondary school completion, and gender gaps, while persisting, have narrowed. For example, a comparison of the cohorts aged 20–24 and 30–39 suggests that 30 per cent of young women aged 20–24 had completed high school, compared to 18 per cent of their older counterparts; the corresponding increase was much milder among men (41 per cent versus 34 per cent, an 11 point difference). The gender gap narrowed from 16 percentage points among those aged 30–39 to 11 points among those aged 20–24.

High school completion, like school attendance, suggests huge variation by socio-demographic status as well (Figure 5.3). For example, just 8per cent of females and 16 per cent of males from scheduled tribes had completed secondary school, compared to 35

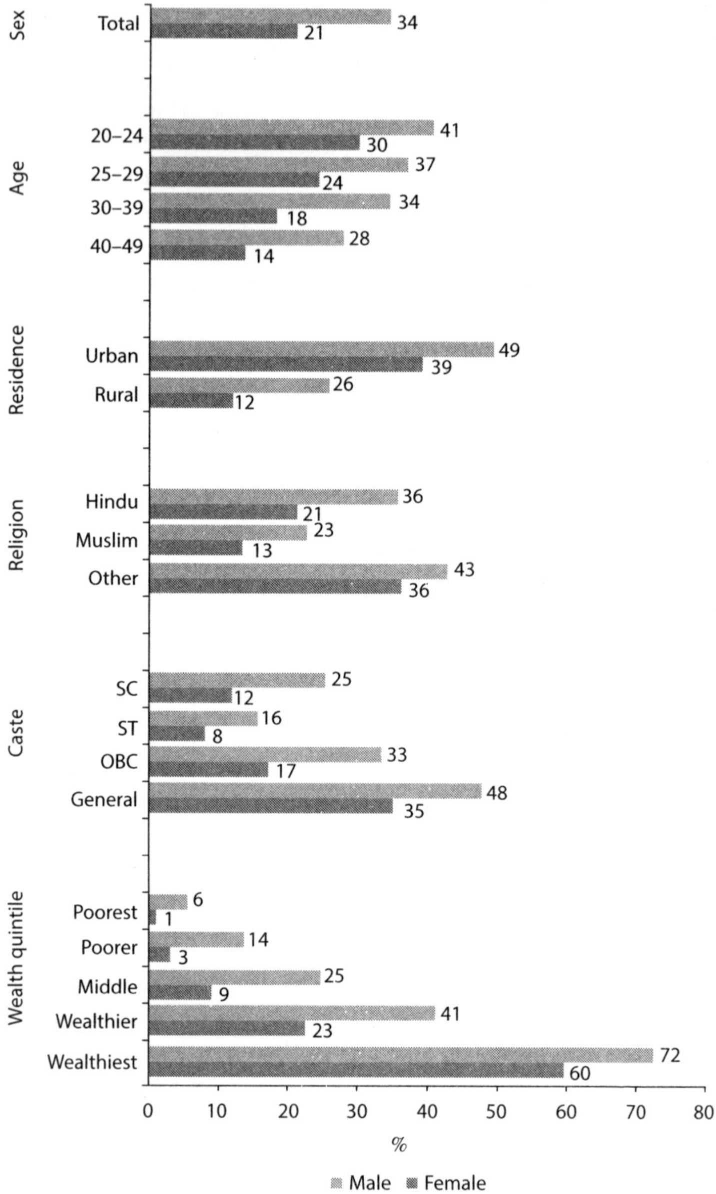

Figure 5.3 Percent of Men and Women aged 20–49 Who Completed High School Education by Selected Background Characteristics, India, 2005–06

Source: Calculated from NFHS (2005–06) individual data.

per cent and 48 per cent of their counterparts from general castes. Differences by wealth status are particularly wide, ranging from 1 per cent among females from the poorest households to 60 per cent of those from the wealthiest households, and from 6 per cent to 72 per cent, respectively, among males. What is also notable is the persistence of gender differences even when socio-demographic levels are identical and the fact that gender differences are narrower among the poor than they are among the better off. For example, whereas there is a 5 percentage point difference in secondary school completion rates of males and females from the poorest households, the difference increases to 12 points among those from economically better off households.

State-wise differences were also apparent. Fewer than 15 per cent of women aged 20–49 had completed high school in Rajasthan, Chhattisgarh, Madhya Pradesh, Bihar, Jharkhand compared to more than 40 per cent of those in Delhi, Goa, Himachal Pradesh, and Kerala. Moreover, the gender gap in high school completion was in the range of 15–24 points in 9 out of the 29 states (see Table A5.2).

Work Participation

While almost all women contribute hugely to the labour force, including in the home, the family farm or the family business, their participation in wage work, an important source of empowerment, is relatively limited. Moreover, gender disparities in employment remain wide.

Gender differences persist in terms of the extent of the work force participation rate, as evident from data drawn from progressive rounds of NSSO surveys. Data, presented in Table 5.2, show that in 2007–08, 55 per cent of males and 25 per cent of females were employed (principal and subsidiary). Also notable is the finding that rates for both males and females, and those in both rural and urban areas, have remained basically unchanged between 1993–94 and 2007–08, and the gender gap has remained on the order of 26–30 percentage points; the difference was much narrower—in the range of 22–26 percentage points—in rural areas than in urban areas, in which it was as wide as 37–42 percentage points.

Table 5.2 Work Force Participation Rate (usual status, principal and subsidiary) by Sex and Rural-Urban Residence, India, 1993–94 to 2007–08

Year	Total			Rural			Urban		
	Males	Females	M–F gap	Males	Females	M–F gap	Males	Females	M–F gap
1993–94	54.5	28.6	25.9	55.3	32.8	22.5	52.1	15.5	36.6
1999–00	52.7	25.9	26.8	53.1	29.9	23.2	51.8	13.9	37.9
2004–05	54.7	28.7	26.0	54.6	32.7	21.9	54.9	16.6	38.3
2007–08	55.0	25.0	30.0	54.8	28.9	25.9	55.4	13.8	41.6

Source: National Sample Survey Organisation (2006, 2010).

State-wise differences were also evident (Table A5.3). For example, among the large states, just 15 per cent of rural women in Bihar and West Bengal were employed, compared to almost half in Andhra Pradesh, Chhattisgarh, and Himachal Pradesh. Likewise, among the urban population, work force participation rates ranged from 7 per cent among women in Bihar to 20 per cent or more in Himachal Pradesh and Tamil Nadu. In almost every state, the gender gap was wider among the urban as compared to the rural population. Moreover, of the 29 states, the gender gap was of the order of 30 percentage points or more in the rural areas of 9 states and in the urban areas of 26 states (National Sample Survey Organisation 2010).

Notable socio-demographic differentials were observed. Among women, employment increased with age from 33 per cent among those aged 15–29 to 54 per cent among those aged 30–59 in rural areas; the corresponding percentages were 15 and 24 in urban areas. Percentages employed fell steadily from among those with no education (36 per cent and 16 per cent in rural and urban areas, respectively) to those with 12 years of schooling (20 per cent and 11per cent, respectively), and increased thereafter among those with post graduate degrees or more (53 and 39 per cent, respectively) (National Sample Survey Organisation 2010).

Gender disparities in patterns of work further highlight disparities between men and women. For example, in rural areas, while 84 per cent of employed women were engaged in agricultural activities, 67 per cent of men were so engaged (National Sample Survey Organisation 2010). Data from NFHS-3 show that men were far less likely than women to report that their work was not remunerated: 6 per cent versus 22 per cent (International Institute for Population Sciences and Macro International 2007). Data from the NSSO reiterate gender disparities in average wages earned. For example, in 2007–08, a male regular wage earner earned nearly 1.6 times that of a female in rural areas (Rs 175 versus Rs 108) and about 1.3 times that of a female in urban areas (Rs 276 versus Rs 213). Disparities in wage rates were apparent even among those who had completed a graduate degree or more (Rs 298 versus Rs 214 in rural areas and Rs 511 versus Rs 381 in urban areas) (National Sample Survey Organisation 2010).

In short, findings suggest that women continue to be hugely disadvantaged: they are far less likely than men to work, and among those employed, far less likely to have worked continuously or to have been engaged in activities for which they were remunerated. Among those remunerated, moreover, wage disparities were evident. Women are far more likely to work in the informal sector than men, where they are not protected by labour laws, have no control over the terms and conditions of their employment and do not have access to regular work.

Women's Participation in Political Spheres

Concerted efforts have been made to ensure that women are engaged in political life. The most notable of these are the 73rd and 74th constitutional amendments that reserve one third of seats for women in PRIs. Evidence suggests the actual representation of women in PRIs has now crossed the one-third mark: as of 2008, women constituted 37 per cent each of elected representatives of village, intermediate and district panchayats (Ministry of Panchayati Raj 2011).

As mentioned earlier, the Women's Reservation Bill has not yet been passed by the Lok Sabha. The representation of women at national level remains low and increases in the percentage of women representatives have been mild. For example, women constituted just 11 per cent of the 15th Lok Sabha constituted in 2009 (60 of 543 sitting members), and 11 per cent of the Rajya Sabha (26 of 242 sitting members) (Lok Sabha 2009).

Agency

Agency has been defined as the capacity to make choices through the acquisition of a sense of self and a sense of personal competence (National Research Council and Institute of Medicine, 2005); the ability to make strategic life choices (Kabeer, 2001) and to affect well-being and to exert influence over life matters (Mensch, 2006). What is available, moreover, from the literature on empowerment among women suggests that central elements of the capacity to make choices include decision-making capacity, freedom of movement, a sense of self-worth and access to resources (Malhotra, Schuler, and Boender, 2002). In the gender-stratified and patriarchal social system prevailing in India, women have limited agency. While data on trends in women's agency are not available, evidence from a number of recent surveys including the NFHS and the Youth in India surveys (International Institute for Population Sciences and Macro International, 2007; International Institute for Population Sciences and Population Council, 2010) confirms that women have limited control over economic resources, freedom of movement and decision-making authority.

Control over economic resources, for example, was measured in the NFHS-3 in terms of whether women had access to money of their own that they could decide how to use. As evident from Figure 5.4, in total, just 45 per cent of women aged 15–49 reported such access. At the same time, just 15 per cent of all women had a bank account of their own. As Figure 5.4 shows, control over economic resources, measured by way of both of these indicators—increases quite sharply by age, educational status and wealth status. While women belonging to general castes are just moderately more likely to report access to money than those belonging to scheduled castes and tribes, they are far more likely to report ownership of bank accounts.

Freedom of movement and decision-making authority are also severely constrained for large proportions of women. Indeed, Figure 5.5 shows that one-third of currently married women aged 15–49 were permitted to go alone to the market, the health centre, and outside their community, and just 37 per cent participated in decisions relating to their own health care, purchases for daily needs, purchases of large household good and visits to the natal family (International Institute for Population Sciences and Macro International 2007). Figure 5.5 also establishes the links between a number of sociodemographic factors and these indicators of women's agency. As in the case of control over economic resources, age relaxes constraints on decision making authority and freedom of movement on women; young women's agency in these respects is particularly constrained. Household economic status is also consistently and positively associated with these indicators of agency. Patterns by educational attainment levels were not as clearly inverted; however, women with 12 or more years of education were far more likely to report agency on both of these indicators than uneducated women or those with some education. Differences by caste were narrower, but suggest that those from general castes were mildly more likely than those from

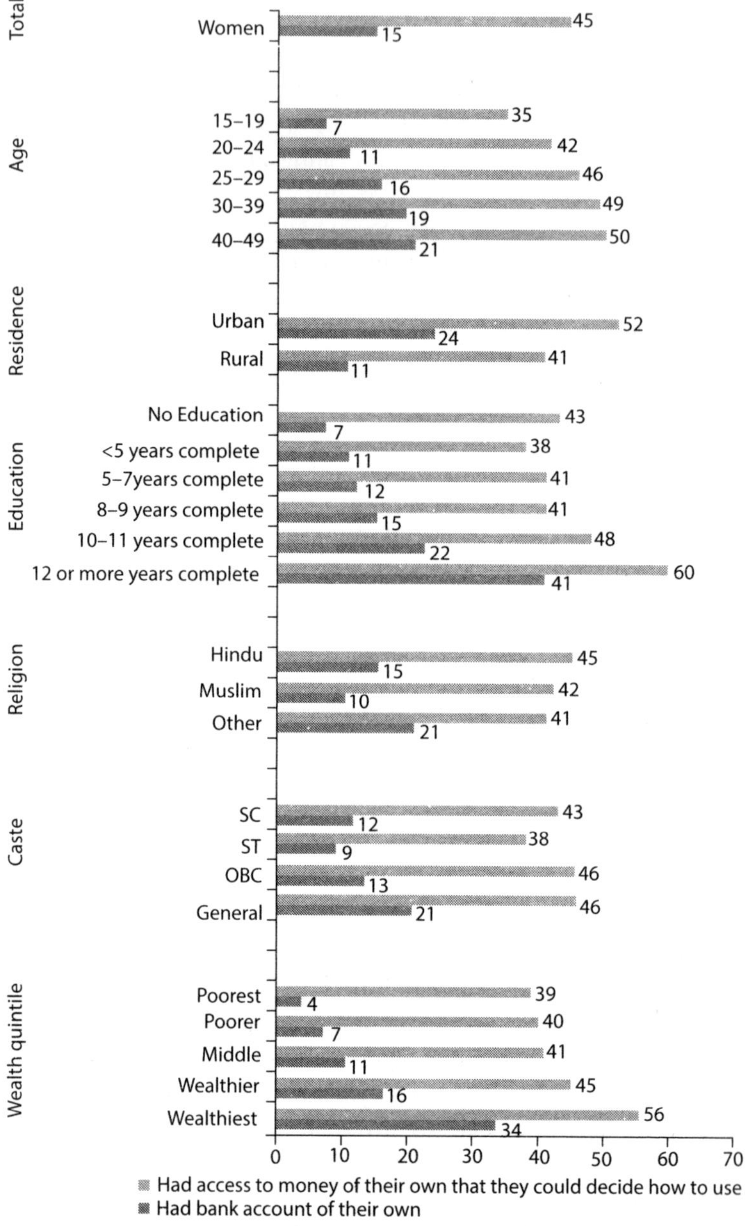

Figure 5.4 Access to and Control Over Financial Resources among Women Aged 15–49 by Selected Background Characteristics, India, 2005–06

Source: International Institute for Population Sciences and Macro International (2007).

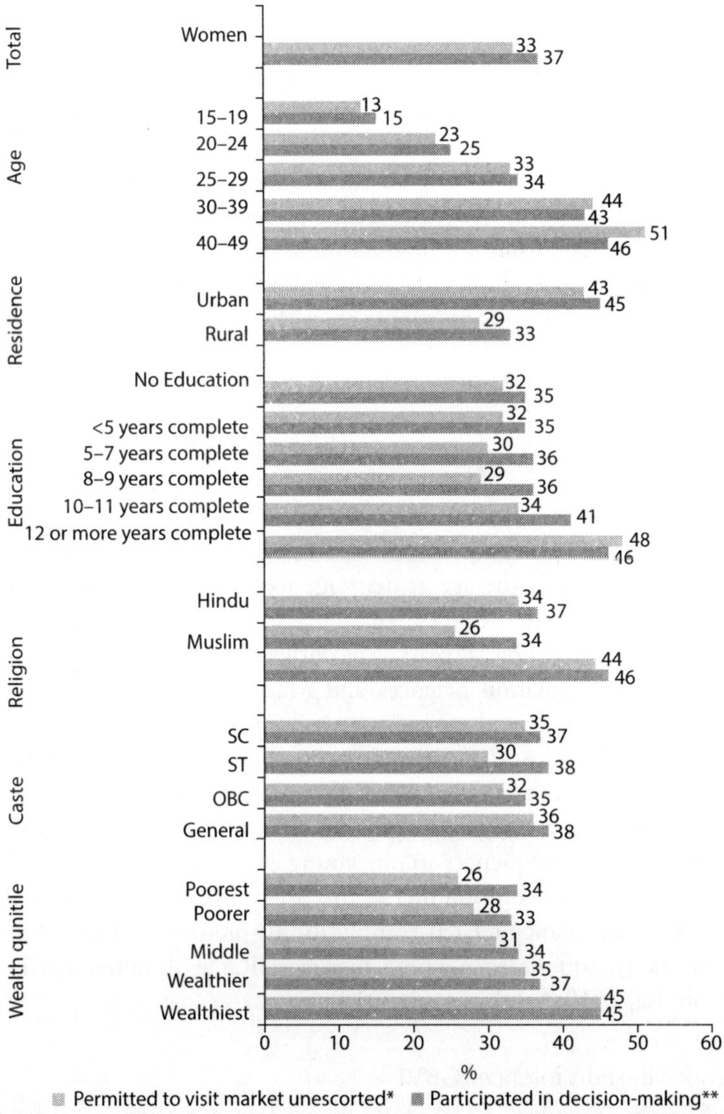

Figure 5.5 Decision-making Authority and Freedom of Movement Exercised by Women Aged 15–49 by Selected Background Characteristics, India, 2005–06

*To visit market, a health centre and places outside the village/community, all women.

** Participated in decision regarding their own health care, purchases for daily needs, visits to the natal family and purchase of large household goods, currently married women.

Source: International Institute for Population Sciences and Macro International (2007).

scheduled tribes to exercise agency. Differences by religion show that Muslim women are less likely than their Hindu counterparts to report decision-making authority and freedom of movement, but both are far less likely than those from other religions to report such freedom.

While evidence from men on these three dimensions of agency is not available from NFHS, evidence presented in Chapter 4 has shown, using data from the *Youth in India* survey, that gender differences in control over money, decision making authority and freedom of movement among young people are wide.

Child Marriage

Despite the enactment of laws, several harmful practices that compromise women's exercise of informed choices in life, violate their rights and undermine their sexual and reproductive health persist in India. Key among these is the persistence of child marriage. As described in Chapter 4, while the age at marriage for women has undergone a secular increase, the reality is that almost half of all women aged 20–24 were married by 18 years as recently as in 2006 (International Institute for Population Sciences and Macro International 2007). Trend data show that the percentage of women marrying as children declined by just 7 percentage points between 1992 and 2006 (Ministry of Health and Family Welfare 2009). Recent studies in India highlight that early marriage is clearly correlated with a range of adverse health consequences among young women and their children even after a host of confounding factors are controlled—unintended pregnancy, pregnancy-related complications, pre-term delivery, foetal mortality, and violence within marriage (Raj et al. 2009, 2010a, 2010b; Raj 2010, Santhya et al. 2010).

Gender Based Violence (GBV)

Despite a plethora of laws intended to protect women from violence within the home, in the workplace, and in society more generally, the practice continues in India. Violence within marriage is commonly experienced, and trafficking of women and children, violence in the workplace, sexual harassment, and other crimes against women, show no signs of abating.

Violence within marriage

Marital violence is pervasive in India. Nationally, NFHS-3 found that about two in five (39 per cent) of all currently married women aged 15–49 had experienced physical, sexual or emotional violence in their married life, and more than one-quarter (27 per cent) had so experienced in the year prior to the interview. The leading form of violence was physical, with 35 per cent and 21 per cent having experienced this form of violence ever in their married life and in the last year, respectively (International Institute for Population Sciences and Macro International 2007). As evident from Table A5.4, percentages of women who had ever experienced marital violence varied widely by state: from 20 per cent or less in such states as Delhi, Goa, Himachal Pradesh, Jammu and Kashmir, Kerala, Meghalaya and Sikkim to 61 per cent in Bihar, and from 31 per cent in the southern states to 48 per cent in the eastern states.

A synthesis of studies of marital violence in India corroborates the finding of pervasive marital violence. It found that between one-tenth and half of women had experienced physical violence, and between one in twenty and one in three women had experienced sexual violence perpetrated by their husband. Sizeable proportions had experienced physical and/or sexual violence even when they were pregnant– between one in eight and one in two in the case of physical violence and between one in twenty and one in three in the case of sexual violence. Evidence available from men on the perpetration of violence also reflects the pervasiveness of marital violence, including among young men, with almost one-quarter of men reporting the perpetration of physical violence, and between one-sixth and almost one-third reporting the perpetration of sexual violence against their wife (Jejeebhoy, Santhya, and Acharya 2010). Moreover, data from the National Crime Records Bureau (NCRB) indicate that torture (cruelty by husband and other relatives) constituted the leading crime against women– accounting for more than 40 per cent of the 0.2 million incidents of crime against women registered in both 2009 and 2010 (National Crime Records Bureau 2010; 2011).

Marital violence is evident from an early age. For example, NFHS-3 data show that 23 per cent of all ever married women—or 62 per cent of ever married women who had ever experienced physical or sexual violence perpetrated by their husband—had experienced such violence for the first time in the first two years of marriage (International Institute for Population Sciences and Macro International, 2007). Likewise, the review of available studies cited earlier showed that considerable proportions of married young women—those aged 15–24—had also experienced spousal violence: between one in five and three in five had experienced physical violence, and between one in ten and three in five had experienced sexual violence within marriage (Jejeebhoy, Santhya, and Acharya, 2010).

As far as the correlates of marital violence are concerned, findings from NFHS-3 suggest that factors protecting women from ever experiencing spousal violence included education and household economic status, urban residence, and belonging to general castes (Figure 5.6). Further analysis of NFHS-3 data also show that factors associated with the recent experience (12 months preceding the interview) of sexual or physical violence included, aside from education and wealth status, the husband's non-consumption of alcohol and not witnessing of parental violence; early marriage and number of surviving children were significant correlates of physical but not sexual violence (Kishor and Gupta, 2009). Additionally, an emerging body of evidence shows that women's agency tends to reduce women's risk of experiencing physical and sexual violence in marriage. For example, evidence from a prospective study indicates that financial autonomy and freedom of movement considerably reduced women's risk of experiencing physical violence within marriage (Sabarwal, Santhya, and Jejeebhoy 2013). Another study, using cross-sectional data, reports that women's agency, as measured by a summary measure that took into consideration decision-making autonomy, freedom of movement and control over resources, was inversely correlated with women's experience of sexual violence within marriage (Acharya, Sabarwal and Jejeebhoy 2012). Yet another study that explored these associations among young women reports that those who made decisions were significantly less likely than those who did not to have experienced physical or sexual violence, and those who reported self-efficacy were considerably less likely than others to experience violence (Acharya et al. 2009).

Evidence from various studies also reiterates the adverse health and social consequences of marital violence among women in general, and young women in particular, even after a host of socio-demographic

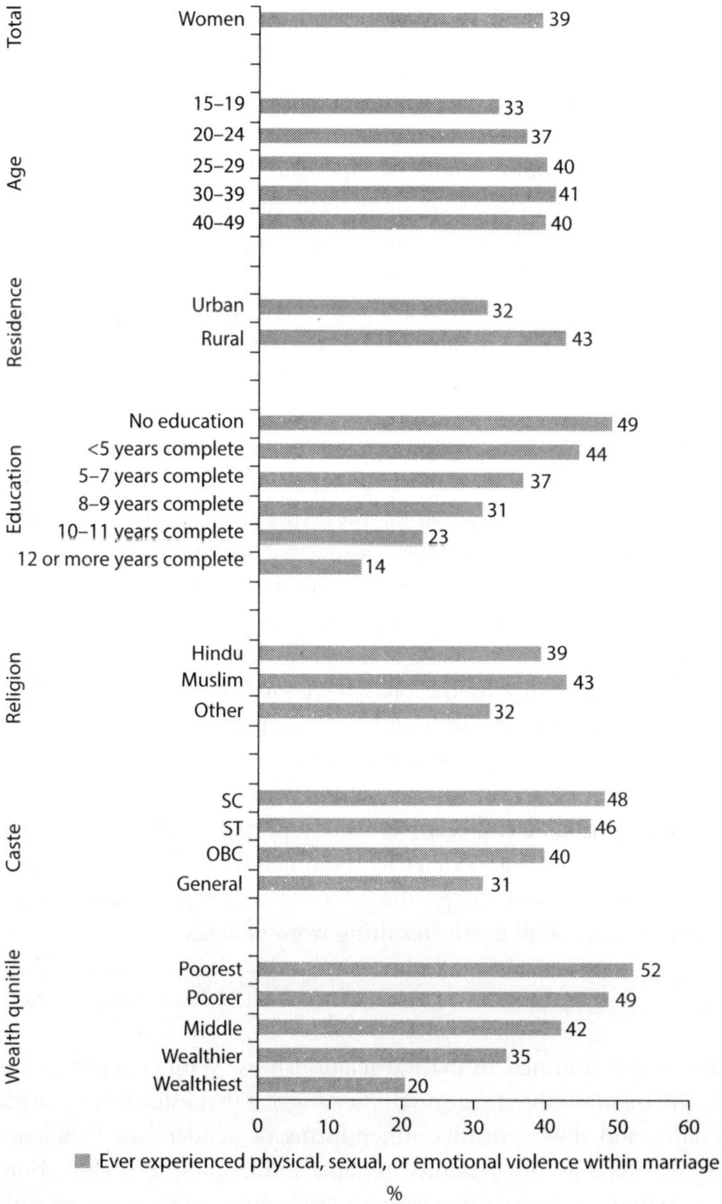

Figure 5.6 Currently Married Women's Experience of Violence within Marriage by Selected Background Characteristics, India, 2005–06
Source: Calculated from NFHS-3 (2005–06) individual data.

factors are controlled (for a review, see Jejeebhoy, Santhya, and Acharya 2010). Among sexual, reproductive and child health outcomes, women who had experienced physical and/or sexual violence were more likely than others to report unwanted pregnancy; this association was observed even when young women were considered. Similarly, women–all and young–who had experienced physical and/or sexual violence within marriage were more likely than others to have experienced symptoms of RTI/STI, and, in one study, to be HIV+. Finally, in many studies and settings, women who had experienced physical and/or sexual violence within marriage were significantly more likely than other women to have experienced pregnancy-related complications, and foetal, infant and child mortality. Findings from studies among young women show, moreover, that many of these associations are observed early in marriage, suggesting that women are at risk of ill-health for much of their married life. Aside from sexual, reproductive and child health outcomes, the experience of physical and/or sexual violence within marriage is associated with poor mental health outcomes. These effects are observed in almost all studies, covering women of all ages, and also young women in particular.

Data on domestic violence and deaths due to domestic violence are regularly reported by the NCRB. A total of 6,787 dowry death cases were reported in 2005 and this number increased by 27 per cent to 8618 by 2011; in both years, these deaths comprised 4 per cent of all crimes against women. Likewise, a total of 58,319 cases of cruelty by husband and relatives were reported in 2005, increasing by 70 per cent to 99,135 by 2011 (National Crime Records Bureau, 2012). It is difficult to assess the extent to which these numbers are underestimates of all deaths resulting from violence.

Other forms of GBV

GBV is not confined to marital relationships. While data from the NCRB are undoubtedly limited, they suggest that aside from marital violence and dowry deaths, other forms of gender based violence are considerable. Such crimes as rape, kidnapping and abduction, molestation, and sexual harassment are perpetrated against sizeable number of women. For the year 2011, the NCRB recorded a total of 228,650 crimes against women, an increase of 23 per cent over the preceding five years. Of all crimes against women recorded in 2011, 11 per cent were rape cases (24,206), 19 per cent were molestation cases (42,968), 16 per cent were kidnapping and abduction cases (35,565), and 4per cent were sexual harassment cases (8,570) (National Crime Records Bureau 2012).

Sexual harassment in the workplace is also considerable. A qualitative study of sexual harassment in the health sector reports that of the 135 women interviewed, 77 reported having experienced some form of sexual harassment in their current or previous workplace; the forms of sexual harassment included psychological harassment (45), verbal harassment (41), unwanted touch (27) and sexual gestures and exhibitionism (16) (Chaudhuri, 2006). Another study, conducted among 600 women working in both the organized and unorganised sectors in four regions of Maharashtra, reports that 37 per cent of women had experienced sexual harassment in their workplace (Yugantar Education Society, n.d., accessed at ncw.nic.in).

Finally, trafficking of women and children persists. While the magnitude of trafficking is not correctly known, a study commissioned by the Ministry of Women and Child Development estimated that about 2.8 million women are victims of trafficking, of whom more than one-third are children (Ministry of Women and Child Development, 2011). A study on trafficking in women and children in 13 states and union territories reports that one-quarter of the survivors of trafficking (that is, trafficked into commercial sexual exploitation and then rescued) and almost one-tenth of victims of trafficking (that is, trafficked into commercial sexual exploitation and not rescued) interviewed in the study were indeed victims of re-trafficking (NHRC, UNIFEM, and ISS 2004).

Son Preference and Gender Imbalance in the Child Sex Ratio

Perhaps the most fundamental expression of gender inequality in India is the preference for sons over daughters. Survey after survey have underscored the persistence of son preference, and, as seen in earlier chapters, son preference, which had manifested itself in gendered health care and feeding practices of children, has increasingly manifested itself in the practice of sex selection and termination of pregnancies carrying a female foetus.

Successive NFHS surveys have highlighted the strength of the desire for a son. As Table 5.3 shows, ideal family size has fallen by about half a child between 1992–93 and 2005–06, and the percentage of women desiring more sons than daughters has declined from 42 per cent to 26 per cent over the same period. Statewise variation in son preference is considerable (Table A5.5). While about two-fifths of all women (38–42 per cent) in such states as Bihar, Chhattisgarh, Rajasthan and Uttar Pradesh continued to desire more sons than daughters, just 10–12 per cent in the southern states of Andhra Pradesh, Kerala and Tamil Nadu so desired (International Institute for Population Sciences and Macro International, 2007).

Findings suggest, moreover, that strong son preference falls systematically with education and wealth status and was much lower among urban than rural women, and among women from general as opposed to other castes. The preference for sons has declined just marginally among younger cohorts: for example, while 29 per cent of women aged 40–49 wanted more sons than daughters, 23–25 per cent of those aged 15–24 expressed this preference (Figure 5.7).

Notwithstanding declining family size preferences and desires for at least one son, sex ratios at birth and of the child population have actually worsened, as observed in Table 5.3 using data from successive NFHS surveys. Indeed, the sex ratio at birth is estimated to have fallen from 941 to 919, and the child sex ratio

Table 5.3 Ideal Family Size, Son Preference, and Children Sex Ratio, 1992–93 to 2005–06, India

Year	Ideal family size and son preference, currently married women		Sex ratios	
	Mean ideal number of children[1]	% who want more sons than daughters[1]	Child sex ratio[2]	Sex ratio at birth[2]
1992–93	2.9	41.5	934	941
1998–99	2.7	33.4	926	938
2005–06	2.4	25.5	918	919

Source: [1]Calculated from different rounds of NFHS; [2]Kishor and Gupta (2009).

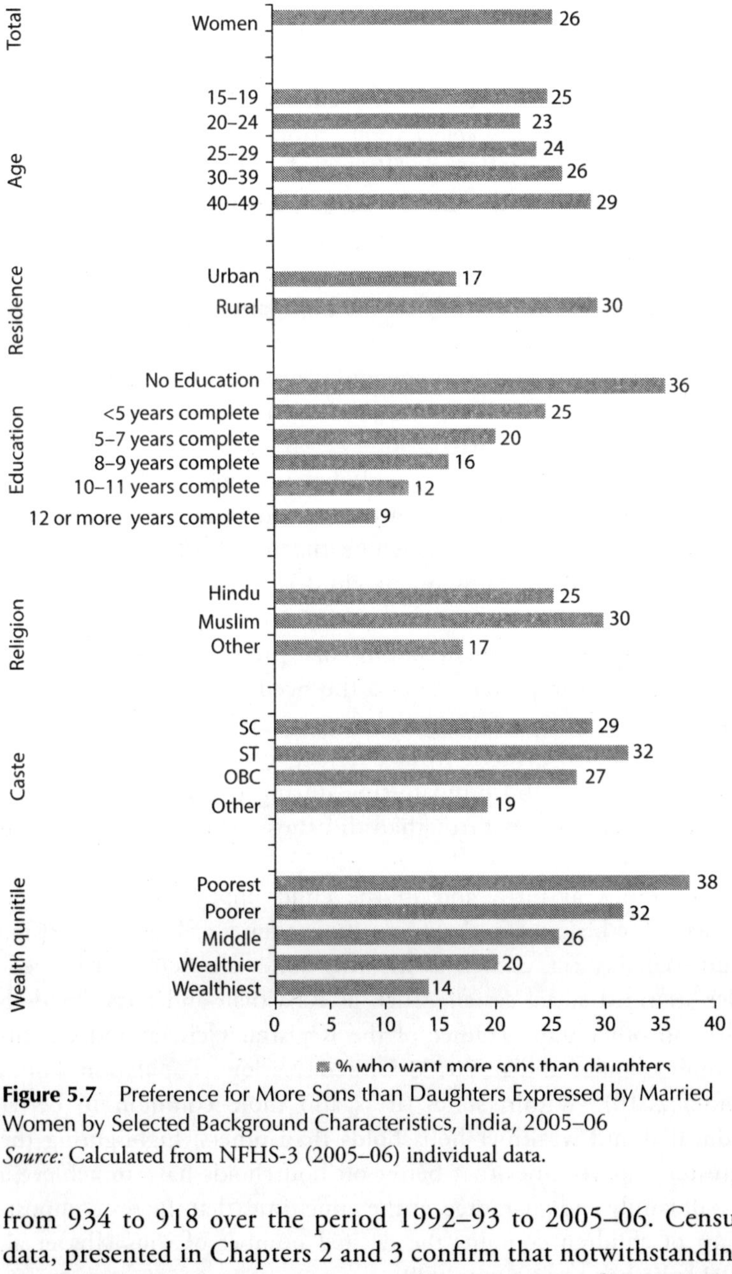

Figure 5.7 Preference for More Sons than Daughters Expressed by Married Women by Selected Background Characteristics, India, 2005–06
Source: Calculated from NFHS-3 (2005–06) individual data.

from 934 to 918 over the period 1992–93 to 2005–06. Census data, presented in Chapters 2 and 3 confirm that notwithstanding the PCPNDT Act, sex selection and termination of pregnancies carrying a female foetus is pervasive: as of 2011, the child sex ratio had plummeted to 919, from an already dismal 927 in 2001, and 945 in 1991(Office of the Registrar General and Census Commissioner, India, 2013). Indeed, recent studies have noted that as a result of sex selective abortion, about 0.5–0.6 million girls are missing each year (Jha et al., 2006; United Nations Population Fund, India, 2010). Large parts of India may have an excess of young men by up to 20 percent by 2030 (Hesketh et al., 2011). Indeed, the proportion of India's population residing in states in which the sex ratio of the population aged 0–6 is below 920 girls per 1,000 boys increased from 11 in 1991 to 43 in 2001 (Office of the Registrar General and Census Commissioner, India, 2004) to 51 in 2011 (Office of the Registrar General and Census Commissioner India 2013).

Analysis of NFHS data highlights that where the first born child is female, the sex ratio of the second child is highly skewed towards males; in contrast, where the first born child is male, the sex ratio of the subsequent child is not affected. Sex ratios at birth were most distorted at parity 2 (as low as 762), clearly, the consequence of small family size preferences accompanied by persisting son preference and the need to ensure that at least one child is a boy (Kishor and Gupta, 2009). The link to sex-selection is also evident from data suggesting that women who had undergone ultrasound testing during pregnancy reported a far lower sex ratio at birth than did those who had not done so (851 versus 941).

Sex ratios at birth and in the child populations have been observed to be lower in the more affluent states of Punjab, Haryana and Maharashtra, as well as in other states characterized by gender stratified social systems such as Rajasthan and Uttar Pradesh than in other states (Office of the Registrar General and Census Commissioner, India, 2013; United Nations Population Fund, India 2010). Within states, it is also more common in better educated and wealthier households than others, highlighting the greater opportunities that better off households have to achieve a small family and guarantee, at the same time, that the sex composition of children contains the desired number of sons (Jha et al. 2011; Kishor and Gupta 2009).

Obstacles to Women's Empowerment and Gender Equity

India's performance in achieving gender equality and equity, and in enhancing the situation of women has been, for the most part, disappointing. There has, of course, been improvement on several fronts: for example, there has been an impressive narrowing of the gender gap in educational attainment levels. However, many disturbing trends persist: the child sex ratio has worsened considerably, women's agency remains constrained, and violence against women is widespread. A number of obstacles are evident that must be overcome.

Difficulties in Reversing Traditional Norms of Masculinity and Femininity

Clearly, difficulties in breaking down patriarchal norms and men's sense of entitlement lie at the heart of the slow pace of change in empowering women and promoting gender equality and equity. Kinship systems in India continue to be age- and gender-stratified, traditional gender norms persist, and investments in girls and women at family and community level remain relatively limited. For example, there is evidence that the socialization of sons and daughters continues to be gendered. Research has shown, for example, that there continues to be a gender gap in parental aspirations for and investments in the education of their sons versus daughters (Santhya and Jejeebhoy 2012). Double standards in the socialization of sons and daughters are also evident, with daughters socialized with many more constraints than sons on mobility, freedom to develop social networks, control over money and so on—disparities that clearly influence girls' ability to exercise informed choice as they grow into adulthood (International Institute for Population Sciences and Population Council 2010).

Traditional notions of masculinity and entitlement persist among men. For example, findings from the *Youth Study* show that 70 per cent of young men and somewhat smaller percentages of young women (64 per cent) believe that a woman must take her husband's permission for most things (International Institute for Population Sciences and Population Council 2010). National, sub-national and local studies note that men, including young men, condone marital violence in at least one situation; a study of men in Mumbai found

31 per cent believed that a woman deserves to be beaten at times, and 36 per cent believed that a woman should tolerate violence to keep her family together. Moreover, considerable proportions of young men in this study maintained that a man should dominate a woman in sexual and reproductive matters: for example, 42 per cent believed that it is a man who decides about sex, and 29 per cent believed that a man needs other women even if his relationship with his wife is good (Verma et al. 2006). Gender double standards are also evident: for example, while 64 per cent of young men in the *Youth Study* believed that a young man's future would be ruined if he had sex before marriage, many more—82 per cent—believed that a young woman's future would be ruined if she had premarital sex (International Institute for Population Sciences and Population Council, 2010). The NFHS-3 found that some 11 per cent of men believed that women have no right to refuse sex or insist on condom use if the husband has an STI; the poor and uneducated were considerably more likely than the better off to so report (for example, 25 per cent of the uneducated versus 2 per cent of those with 12 or more years of education agreed that women had no right to refuse sex or ask their partner to use a condom if infected (International Institute for Population Sciences and Macro International 2007).

Family elders—mothers and fathers-in-law for example—also play a powerful role in reinforcing gender in-egalitarian norms. Likewise, teachers and health care providers, although in a position to change traditional gender hierarchical norms and values, tend to promote gender stereotypes (Santhya, Zavier, and Jejeebhoy 2012). Community leaders are another group of stakeholders who are responsible for the upholding of traditional norms.

Failure of the Media to Play a Proactive Role in Promoting Gender Equitable Norms

Although the media can powerfully shape and transmit new ideas and attitudes, the popular media in India have tended to uphold and reinforce—rather than question—traditional notions of masculinity, a limitation also noted in the midterm review of the Eleventh Plan (Planning Commission 2011). Opportunities to promote new role models have therefore been lost. Indeed, efforts to change norms and build new role models by exploiting both the traditional media and new information technologies, including mobile phones and the internet, have been extremely limited.

Programme Challenges in Promoting Women's Empowerment and Narrowing Gender Disparities

Although many programmatic innovations have been implemented to empower women and promote gender equality and equity, gaps remain.

Gaps in Programme Implementation

While an impressive set of programmes exist that address women's empowerment and that work towards narrowing gaps in marketable skills, access to credit, and employment opportunities, their implementation has been weak. A number of concerns have been expressed that must be addressed.

First, fewer women have been reached than was anticipated in a number of programmes, and the achievement of targets among women's empowerment programmes have been somewhat erratic and unsuccessful. For example, the STEP programme's annual targets rose from 40,000 in 2007–08 to 70,000 in 2008–09 and fell again to 30,000 in 2009–2010, raising questions about how targets are established. This becomes even more pertinent when we find that the programme has not reached its targeted number of beneficiaries in recent years. For example, while it achieved its target in 2007–08, of the 70,000 women targeted in 2008–09, it succeeded in reaching just 46 per cent; and of the 30,000 targeted for 2009–10, it reached, in 10 months, just 13,986 (47 per cent of the full year's target) (Ministry of Women and Child Development 2010).

Second, as far as skill building programmes are concerned, their focus on training women in skills relevant to traditional sectors has limited the extent to which women trained under such programmes as STEP did indeed obtain a marketable skill. We note that in 2007 this scheme was revised to encompass a broader range of skills relevant for market demand, however the extent to which women have been trained in marketable skills is not available (Planning Commission 2011).

Third, there is a need to review programme content and assess the extent to which they address the social isolation and lack of support that many women face. Opportunities to establish social networks and provide safe spaces to women to meet and build solidarity have not been emphasised thus far in available programmes. NGO and SHG examples may exist and their operation and effects need to be better understood.

Fourth, while efforts to narrow the gender gap have indeed been implemented at national and state levels, in government and civil society programmes, promising actions, including conditional and unconditional cash transfers, have not been well evaluated or upscaled. Few of these have been assessed for their effectiveness in changing gender norms or in empowering women and girls.

Fifth, programmes to support women who experience harmful practices—early marriage and violence for example—are lacking, despite the evidence that early marriage and violence against women continue to be experienced by large numbers of women. Alongside programmes intended to prevent these practice, efforts are needed that identify or screen, and support women who experience violence. For one, programmes are needed that support and empower girls married as children, breaking down their social isolation, building their negotiation skills and informing them about rights and services to which they are entitled. Equal effort is needed within the health sector to integrate violence screening and referral into other services for women, for example, family planning, ICTC and other HIV-related services, as well as the ICDS; at the same time, effective strategies that address the needs of women for legal support, shelter and financial assistance must be devised, and linkages between the health and other sectors to provide these services must be established.

Finally, resources allocated for various programmes for women are severely under-utilized. The Rashtriya Mahila Kosh (Ministry of Women and Child Development, 2010) has extended its intermediary micro-finance organisations to all states, and reports impressive recovery rates (over 90 per cent). Overall, however, it has disbursed loans amounting to Rs 235 crores, benefitting 6.6 lakh women, and in the 9 months from April to December 2009, loans amounting to just Rs 4.1 crores were disbursed, benefitting only 3,431 women. The midterm review of the XIth Plan noted, moreover, that while the Rashtriya Mahila Kosh lends to intermediate microfinance organizations at an interest rate of eight percent, onward lending results in women borrowers paying a considerably higher interest rates, perhaps resulting in the smaller than targeted number of beneficiaries (Planning Commission 2011). Likewise, the Dhanalakshmi programme, initiated on a pilot basis in a few blocks and intended to enhance the status of daughters and redress the adverse child sex ratio has been both poorly conceptualised and implemented. For example, cash transfers are made on the achievement of a large number of 17 conditions, but the total amount disbursed is just Rs 13,500, an amount hardly likely to change deep rooted under investment in girls; at the same time, the scheme has been under-utilised, with just 31per cent of funds used by 2010 (Planning Commission 2011). Indeed, the Report of the XIIth Plan's Working Group on Women's Agency and Empowerment (Ministry of Women and Child Development 2011) has acknowledged that the targets set out in the XIth Plan have only been partially achieved.

Multipronged programmes and upscaling of promising approaches that address issues of gender equity and harmful practices are needed. A number of civil society groups have piloted programmes that provide an opportunity to document lessons and challenges, as well as potential for scaling up and these opportunities need to be supported. At the same time, there is no escaping the fact that the maximum reach can be obtained only through government action.

Limited Attention to Raising Awareness About Available Laws and Programmes

While laws and programmes for women exist, efforts to promote awareness of these have been limited. Consequently, for the most part, neither women nor the wider community are aware of women's rights and the programmes to which they are entitled. For example, efforts to raise awareness of the legal minimum age at marriage have been half-hearted and awareness is limited, even among the young: just 59 per cent and 70 per cent of young women and men were aware of the legal minimum age at marriage for females in the country (International Institute for Population Sciences and Population Council 2010). Attention to informing women about their rights under the MTP Act has been limited, and few women are correctly aware about their rights (Jejeebhoy et al. 2011a; 2011b). With regard to domestic violence, the midterm review of the XIth Plan, for example) highlights that awareness of the Domestic Violence Act is limited; indeed, the Act has not even been translated into regional languages, and IEC efforts have not been undertaken at community level or among the police or in courts to inform communities about their rights. As such, it is no surprise that vast numbers of women and men continue to maintain that men are justified in beating their wife in some circumstances (International Institute for Population Sciences and Macro International 2007). With regard to various programmes and schemes for women, likewise, awareness remains limited among potential beneficiaries. For example, awareness of empowerment schemes—for example, the STEP programme—is limited and this lack of awareness may have effectively compromised poor and socially excluded women's access to programmes for which they are eligible (Planning Commission 2011). Similarly, hardly any recently delivered women who had availed of JSY benefits knew that women delivering in an accredited private facility are entitled to receive cash benefits, and few were aware of the full range of services to which they were entitled (Santhya et al. 2011). Programmes have not recognised, moreover, that women with limited agency may need support in accessing available programmes, schemes, and services to which they are entitled.

Neglect of Men and Other Key Stakeholders in Efforts to Promote Gender Equity and Equality

Changing deeply entrenched traditional norms and attitudes require action on many fronts, and it is not clear that enough effort has been placed on addressing each of the key stakeholders. For example, men remain relatively neglected in efforts to change norms, notwithstanding their role in inhibiting women's empowerment. There is, however, evidence that interventions intended to reverse traditional notions of masculinity and entitlement have succeeded in promoting gender equitable attitudes and behaviours among men, for example, reducing marital violence, increasing condom use and reducing reported symptoms of infection among men (Verma et al.

2008). Efforts to expand and upscale such promising interventions among men, and, at the same time, initiate programmes intended to change norms from an early age, have been limited. Life skills education programmes have, for the most part, excluded boys, and the school and health systems, which are most likely to interact with boys and young men, have not used this opportunity to build teacher and health care provider—particularly males—skills in engaging boys and young men. Similarly, programmes intended to break down the deeply entrenched patriarchal norms held by key stakeholder groups, including parents, teachers, health care providers and community leaders remain relatively rare; even when efforts have been made to engage many of these groups, there is little information available on their reach and content, or on how successful they have been.

Lack of Multi-sectoral Coordination

India has a range of well-conceptualized policies and programmes intended to promote gender equity and equality and enhance women's empowerment. Unfortunately, implementation of programmes and policies, and political commitment, have not kept up with the promises made.

Achieving gender equity and equality and empowering women requires the commitment and coordination of many sectors. It is with this in mind that the Women and Child Development Ministry was established. The extent to which inter-sectoral coordination has been achieved is, however, unclear. In some instances, parallel schemes are introduced by different sectors: for example, the conditional cash transfer scheme to enhance institutional delivery, the flagship programme of the Ministry of Health and Family Welfare ongoing since 2006, was supplemented in 2010 by the IGMSY of the Ministry of Women and Child Development. The rationale for and the efficiency implied in the implementation of two similar schemes is unclear. Likewise, while the Ministry of Women and Child Development implements a programme for out-of-school girls (SABLA), its programmes do not extend to efforts to reduce school discontinuation or provide livelihood training to those in school.

Gaps in Policies and Laws

Weak Enforcement of Laws and Acts

India has a range of impressive laws and Acts intended to promote gender justice and counter prevailing gender inequities, such as, for example, laws prohibiting child marriage, protecting women from domestic violence and sexual harassment, and ensuring that pre-natal sex selection does not take place. It is discouraging to note that these laws and Acts have been systematically violated, and that neither the state nor communities have taken concerted steps to enforce or abide by them. There is little evidence of prosecution of those who have violated these laws. At the same time, while there have been several NGO efforts to inform communities about laws and available services, change attitudes about child marriage, domestic violence and sex selection, these efforts have been typically small, their effects have not been well documented, and few have been taken to scale. Indeed, the Midterm Appraisal of the XIth Plan (Planning Commission 2011) has noted that procedures for implementation of the Domestic Violence Act have not even been put in place. Likewise, the Working Group on Women's Agency and Empowerment has highlighted that conviction rates relating to crimes against women remain low, reflecting the gaps in prosecution processes (Ministry of Women and Child Development 2011). Particularly in cases of gender based violence, evidence suggests that procedures are far from woman or girl-friendly. Invasive police investigations and medical examinations, repeated questioning and requirements of statements to various authorities, and lack of medical attention and counselling, pose significant obstacles to women's and children's readiness to institute criminal procedures in cases of violence (Ministry of Women and Child Development 2011).

Lack of Political Will

At the same time, political will to work for gender equity has largely been weak. The Women's Reservation Bill has been pending for 15 years. It was first introduced in parliament in 1996 and thereafter several more times under different governments, but failed to obtain the necessary consensus. It was finally passed by the Rajya

Sabha in 2010, but remains to be passed by the Lok Sabha even in 2011. Clearly, obtaining commitment from politicians and law makers remains a huge challenge to women's political empowerment. Lack of political will is evident also from the resources allocated to women's programmes in the XIth Plan. Indeed, the midterm review of the XIth Plan has noted that 86 per cent of the total plan outlay on women's agency was allocated for ICDS alone, leaving just the remaining 14 per cent (Rs 4,345 crores) for schemes focusing on women. The report notes that most of the schemes relating to women have unrealistic cost norms (Planning Commission 2011).

Efforts to better understand the implementation challenges faced by each programme, to build accountability among programme implementers, and strengthen advocacy measures to engage the political leadership are essential in order that promises made can be realised.

* * *

This chapter has described a range of programmes intended to empower women and enhance gender equity and equality, has explored the situation in terms of women's agency and gender disparities, and has outlined the socio-cultural, programmatic, and policy level factors that pose challenges to the attainment of stated goals. Clearly, a number of commitments have been made toward empowering women and ensuring gender equality and equity, nevertheless, the pace of change has been slow, and in many dimensions, there is little evidence of empowerment or a reduction in gender disparities.

In the area of education, while gender inequities have certainly narrowed, yet, literacy rates attained by females in 2011 have only just reached those attained by males twenty years earlier. Likewise, while school attendance and completion rates have also increased among women and gender disparities have narrowed, just one in five of those aged 20–49 have attained a high school education, compared to one in three men. In terms of economic activity, while almost all women contribute hugely to the labour force, their participation in wage work remains relatively limited and the gender gap—of the order of 26–30 points–has shown no signs of narrowing over the past two decades. Women's work remains concentrated in agriculture and the unorganized sector, wage disparities persist, and women's access to marketable skills remains limited. In the political arena, although women's participation in political life at panchayat level has increased notably, the representation of women at national level remains dismal: they constitute just 11per cent of the 15th Lok Sabha constituted in 2009, and 11per cent of the Rajya Sabha.

In the gender-stratified and patriarchal social system prevailing in India, women have limited agency, defined as the ability to make strategic life choices. Women have limited access to money and control over economic resources, few women own a bank account. Freedom of movement and decision-making authority remain hugely curtailed, and despite the enactment of laws, gender-based violence persists, within marriage and relationships, in the workplace, and in terms of other crimes against women, including torture, rape, dowry deaths, and trafficking. One of the most fundamental expressions of gender inequality in India is the preference for sons over daughters. It has manifested itself in gendered health care and feeding practices of children, and, in the practice of sex selection and termination of pregnancies carrying a female foetus that has reached such proportions that the sex ratio of the child population is hugely distorted.

This review has outlined a number of barriers that have compromised the nation's commitments to empower women and build gender equity and equality. At the individual, family and community levels, these have included difficulties in breaking down patriarchal norms and failure of the media to break down these norms. Several gaps remain at programme and policy levels as well. Awareness of entitlements, by way of services, programmes and schemes remain limited among women, yet few efforts have been made to raise such awareness or connect women to claim their rights. Programmes have had limited success in meeting targets and resources allocated for various programmes are severely under-utilized; skill building efforts have had limited success in building marketable skills among women; programmes have faced considerable difficulty in breaking down women's social isolation; promising actions, including conditional and unconditional cash transfers have not been well-evaluated or scaled up; programmes have neglected men; and programmes intended to prevent early marriage, gender based violence and other crimes against women remain poorly implemented. Laws and acts remain poorly enforced, political will to work for gender equity has largely been weak, and notwithstanding a range of well conceptualized policies and programmes intended to promote gender equity and equality, there is little coordination across the various sectors that implement programmes intended to foster gender equity.

Evidence presented in this chapter concurs with the conclusions of the midterm appraisal of the XIth Plan that improvements in gender issues have been uneven (Planning Commission, 2011), and that the challenges impeding progress in terms of gender equality, equity and women's empowerment are multi-faceted and require multi-sectoral action. While many of the gaps outlined above fall outside of the health sector per se—for example those that focus on political participation, economic empowerment or reducing gender gaps in education—improvements in these domains will clearly have implications for sexual and reproductive health and exercise of reproductive rights.

Appendix

Table A5.1 Literacy Rates by State, India, 2011

	Literacy rate (%)			
	Person	Male	Female	M–F gap
India	**73.0**	**80.9**	**64.6**	**16.3**
North	**72.9**	**82.2**	**62.7**	**19.4**
Delhi	86.2	90.9	80.8	10.2
Haryana	75.6	84.1	65.9	18.1
Himachal Pradesh	82.8	89.5	75.9	13.6
Jammu & Kashmir	67.2	76.8	56.4	20.3
Punjab	75.8	80.4	70.7	9.7
Rajasthan	66.1	79.2	52.1	27.1
Uttarakhand	78.8	87.4	70.0	17.3
Chandigarh	86.0	90.0	81.2	8.8
Central	**68.3**	**77.9**	**58.0**	**19.9**
Chhattisgarh	70.3	80.3	60.2	20.0

(Continued)

Table A5.1 (*Continued*)

	Literacy rate (%)			
	Person	Male	Female	M–F gap
Madhya Pradesh	69.3	78.7	59.2	19.5
Uttar Pradesh	67.7	77.3	57.2	20.1
East	**69.2**	**77.2**	**60.8**	**16.4**
Bihar	61.8	71.2	51.5	19.7
Jharkhand	66.4	76.8	55.4	21.4
Odisha	72.9	81.6	64.0	17.6
West Bengal	76.3	81.7	70.5	11.2
Andaman & Nicobar Islands	86.6	90.3	82.4	7.8
Northeast	**74.7**	**79.9**	**69.3**	**10.6**
Arunachal Pradesh	65.4	72.6	57.7	14.9
Assam	72.2	77.8	66.3	11.6
Manipur	79.2	86.1	72.4	13.7
Meghalaya	74.4	76.0	72.9	3.1
Mizoram	91.3	93.3	89.3	4.1
Nagaland	79.6	82.8	76.1	6.6
Sikkim	81.4	86.6	75.6	10.9
Tripura	87.2	91.5	82.7	8.8
West	**80.9**	**87.5**	**73.8**	**13.7**
Goa	88.7	92.6	84.7	8.0
Gujarat	78.0	85.8	69.7	16.1
Maharashtra	82.3	88.4	75.9	12.5
Dadra Nagar Haveli	76.2	85.2	64.3	20.9
Daman & Diu	87.1	91.5	79.5	12.0
South	**76.5**	**82.9**	**70.0**	**12.9**
Andhra Pradesh	67.0	74.9	59.1	15.7
Karnataka	75.4	82.5	68.1	14.4
Kerala	94.0	96.1	92.1	4.0
Tamil Nadu	80.1	86.8	73.4	13.3
Lakshadweep	91.8	95.6	87.9	7.6
Puducherry	85.8	91.3	80.7	10.6

Source: Office of the Registrar General and Census Commissioner, India (2013).

Table A5.2 Percentage of the *De Facto* Household Population Aged 6–14 Years Attending School, Population Aged 20–49 Years Who Had Completed High School Education, by State, India, 2005–06

	De facto household (population aged 6–14 years attending school) (%)[1]			High school completion (population aged 20–49) (%)[2]		
	Male	Female	M–F gap	Male	Female	M–F gap
India	**82.6**	**76.4**	**6.2**	**34.4**	**21.0**	**13.4**
North	**86.3**	**76.0**	**10.3**	**39.0**	**26.2**	**12.8**
Delhi	86.7	87.0	–0.3	60.9	53.9	7.0
Haryana	86.5	81.2	5.3	43.5	26.4	17.1
Himachal Pradesh	97.1	95.2	1.9	59.4	41.6	17.8
Jammu and Kashmir	89.7	85.7	4.0	35.9	26.1	9.8
Punjab	85.9	84.7	1.2	42.2	37.5	4.7
Rajasthan	84.2	65.9	18.3	26.4	11.3	15.1
Uttarakhand	92.4	88.1	4.3	46.1	32.8	13.3
Central	**80.5**	**74.8**	**5.7**	**30.6**	**15.0**	**15.6**
Chhattisgarh	84.6	77.6	7.0	27.5	12.2	15.3
Madhya Pradesh	80.1	76.9	3.2	27.8	13.2	14.6
Uttar Pradesh	80.2	73.8	6.4	32.3	16.1	16.2
East	**74.8**	**67.7**	**7.1**	**30.1**	**14.7**	**15.4**
Bihar	68.3	56.2	12.1	36.5	12.8	23.7
Jharkhand	77.2	66.1	11.1	29.5	14.3	15.2
Odisha	80.3	74.7	5.6	25.8	15.5	10.3
West Bengal	79.4	80.1	–0.7	27.7	16.1	11.6
Northeast	**83.0**	**82.3**	**0.7**	**31.3**	**21.0**	**10.3**
Arunachal Pradesh	75.8	69.0	6.8	25.0	16.7	8.3
Assam	85.1	83.6	1.5	31.2	19.7	11.5
Manipur	85.9	84.2	1.7	54.7	37.1	17.6
Meghalaya	64.3	68.6	–4.3	28.1	25.4	2.7
Mizoram	91.5	88.3	3.2	31.7	28.9	2.8
Nagaland	74.9	78.1	–3.2	31.4	22.7	8.7
Sikkim	81.8	82.7	–0.9	31.7	24.0	7.7

(*Continued*)

Table A5.2 *(Continued)*

	De facto household (population aged 6–14 years attending school) (%)[1]			High school completion (population aged 20–49) (%)[2]		
	Male	Female	M–F gap	Male	Female	M–F gap
Tripura	86.5	88.6	–2.1	23.2	16.3	6.9
West	**88.2**	**83.3**	**4.9**	**39.6**	**27.5**	**12.1**
Goa	95.0	92.0	3.0	47.6	47.6	0.0
Gujarat	87.0	78.5	8.5	31.1	23.1	8.0
Maharashtra	88.7	85.5	3.2	43.8	29.5	14.3
South	**88.9**	**84.8**	**4.1**	**36.5**	**25.6**	**10.9**
Andhra Pradesh	84.6	78.1	6.5	33.4	17.4	16.0
Karnataka	85.9	82.0	3.9	36.4	24.6	11.8
Kerala	97.6	97.7	–0.1	45.5	44.4	1.1
Tamil Nadu	95.1	92.6	2.5	36.8	27.9	8.9

Source: [1]Calculated from NFHS 2005–06 household data; [2]Calculated from NFHS 2005–06 individual data.

Table A5.3 Workforce Participation Rate According to Usual Status (PS+SS), by State, India, 2007–08

	Workforce participation rate (%)					
	Rural			Urban		
	Male	Female	M–F gap	Male	Female	M–F gap
India	**54.8**	**28.9**	**25.9**	**55.4**	**13.8**	**41.6**
North						
Delhi	51.4	2.9	**48.5**	55.4	5.2	**50.2**
Haryana	49.8	27.8	**22.0**	53.1	14.9	**38.2**
Himachal Pradesh	56.0	46.4	**9.6**	55.9	21.3	**34.6**
Jammu and Kashmir	54.0	30.3	**23.7**	53.1	14.0	**39.1**
Punjab	54.9	23.8	**31.1**	59.4	10.5	**48.9**
Rajasthan	50.1	37.0	**13.1**	52.3	11.4	**40.9**
Uttarakhand	53.0	29.4	**23.6**	50.9	8.9	**42.0**
Chandigarh	73.2	6.6	**66.6**	47.9	13.1	**34.8**

	Workforce participation rate (%)					
	Rural			Urban		
	Male	Female	M–F gap	Male	Female	M–F gap
Central						
Chhattisgarh	56.2	47.1	**9.1**	51.2	16.9	**34.3**
Madhya Pradesh	55.2	32.0	**23.2**	52.1	12.9	**39.2**
Uttar Pradesh	49.3	19.0	**30.3**	50.4	8.1	**42.3**
East						
Bihar	47.8	14.9	**32.9**	46.6	6.7	**39.9**
Jharkhand	50.6	28.7	**21.9**	46.2	8.9	**37.3**
Odisha	58.8	29.3	**29.5**	54.1	13.2	**40.9**
West Bengal	59.0	14.6	**44.4**	59.4	14.2	**45.2**
Andaman & Nicobar Islands	57.9	19.3	**38.6**	61.0	10.5	**50.5**
Northeast						
Arunachal Pradesh	52.3	35.2	**17.1**	46.4	14.0	**32.4**
Assam	56.4	15.3	**41.1**	54.1	8.7	**45.4**
Manipur	50.5	25.0	**25.5**	48.2	16.7	**31.5**
Meghalaya	52.6	35.4	**17.2**	46.6	20.3	**26.3**
Mizoram	59.9	37.1	**22.8**	48.7	27.2	**21.5**
Nagaland	58.2	48.3	**9.9**	45.1	18.1	**27.0**
Sikkim	53.4	28.5	**24.9**	57.1	24.6	**32.5**
Tripura	55.6	11.0	**44.6**	55.2	13.6	**41.6**
West						
Goa	62.6	13.6	**49.0**	61.1	15.3	**45.8**
Gujarat	60.2	35.9	**24.3**	59.3	13.1	**46.2**
Maharashtra	59.2	43.6	**15.6**	56.7	14.2	**42.5**
Dadra and Nagar Haveli	57.0	5.9	**51.1**	59.3	8.7	**50.6**
Daman & Diu	64.0	18.0	**46.0**	53.6	13.7	**39.9**
South						
Andhra Pradesh	62.0	47.1	**14.9**	56.6	18.9	**37.7**
Karnataka	60.4	39.2	**21.2**	59.7	17.8	**41.9**
Kerala	55.6	22.1	**33.5**	57.7	17.7	**40.0**

(*Continued*)

Table A5.3 (*Continued*)

	Workforce participation rate (%)					
	Rural			Urban		
	Male	Female	M–F gap	Male	Female	M–F gap
Tamil Nadu	59.8	38.9	**20.9**	59.8	21.6	**38.2**
Lakshadweep	48.9	10.8	**38.1**	47.4	13.3	**34.1**
Puducherry	53.6	26.7	**26.9**	51.1	11.5	**39.6**

Source: National Sample Survey Organisation (2010).

Table A5.4 Marital Violence Experienced by Married Women Aged 15–49 by State, India, 2005–06

	Ever experienced physical, sexual, or emotional violence (%)
India	**39.2**
North	**34.3**
Delhi	16.7
Haryana	28.0
Himachal Pradesh	6.4
Jammu and Kashmir	14.6
Punjab	26.0
Rajasthan	49.8
Uttarakhand	29.6
Central	**44.8**
Chhattisgarh	31.0
Madhya Pradesh	48.5
Uttar Pradesh	45.2
East	**48.1**
Bihar	61.2
Jharkhand	40.7
Odisha	40.8
West Bengal	40.9
Northeast	**38.8**
Arunachal Pradesh	43.3

	Ever experienced physical, sexual, or emotional violence (%)
Assam	40.9
Manipur	44.9
Meghalaya	14.0
Mizoram	22.3
Nagaland	20.6
Sikkim	17.5
Tripura	44.6
West	**32.7**
Goa	18.1
Gujarat	33.4
Maharashtra	32.6
South	**30.9**
Andhra Pradesh	35.6
Karnataka	20.1
Kerala	18.1
Tamil Nadu	42.4

Source: Calculated from NFHS-3 (2005–06) individual data.

Table A5.5 Currently Married Women by Mean Ideal Family Size, Percentage Wanting More Sons Than Daughters and Percentage Wanting At Least One Son by State, India, 2005–06

	Mean ideal number of children	Wants more sons than daughters (%)	Wants at least one son (%)
India	**2.4**	**25.5**	**81.0**
North	**2.4**	**29.0**	**83.8**
Delhi	2.2	14.1	65.7
Haryana	2.3	25.2	86.6
Himachal Pradesh	2.0	13.4	80.0
Jammu and Kashmir	2.4	29.3	83.8
Punjab	2.0	20.6	77.7
Rajasthan	2.8	38.7	90.2

(*Continued*)

Table A5.5 *(Continued)*

	Mean ideal number of children	Wants more sons than daughters (%)	Wants at least one son (%)
Uttarakhand	2.3	25.5	77.6
Central	**2.7**	**37.2**	**86.9**
Chhattisgarh	2.8	37.8	87.0
Madhya Pradesh	2.6	34.6	90.2
Uttar Pradesh	2.7	38.1	85.6
East	**2.4**	**29.7**	**85.0**
Bihar	2.7	42.3	90.5
Jharkhand	2.7	31.6	82.1
Odisha	2.4	28.9	87.5
West Bengal	2.1	17.3	79.4
Northeast	**2.5**	**26.1**	**82.0**
Arunachal Pradesh	3.1	31.1	89.3
Assam	2.3	27.6	80.8
Manipur	3.1	31.2	96.6
Meghalaya	3.6	14.3	89.9
Mizoram	4.0	29.8	98.2
Nagaland	3.5	23.0	84.4
Sikkim	1.9	17.1	76.8
Tripura	2.1	19.1	74.7
West	**2.2**	**19.7**	**78.1**
Goa	2.1	10.7	63.8
Gujarat	2.2	26.1	74.9
Maharashtra	2.1	16.7	79.9
South	**2.2**	**10.4**	**70.3**
Andhra Pradesh	2.2	10.4	71.6
Karnataka	2.1	13.5	73.5
Kerala	2.4	11.7	67.8
Tamil Nadu	2.0	6.4	66.3

Source: Calculated from NFHS-3 (2005–06) individual data.

References

Acharya, R., F. Ram, S.J. Jejeebhoy, A. Singh, K.G. Santhya, U. Ram, et al. 2009. 'Physical and Sexual Violence Within Marriage among Youth in India: The Youth in India, Situation and Needs Study'. Paper presented at the XXVI IUSSP International Population Conference, Marrakech, Morocco, 27 September–2 October, 2009.

Acharya, R, Sabarwal, S, and Jejeebhoy S.J., 2011. 'Women's Empowerment and Forced Sex within Marriage in Rural India,' *Economic and Political Weekly*, 47(2): 65–69.

Chaudhuri, P. 2006. 'Sexual Harassment in the Workplace: Experiences of Women in the Health Sector'. *Health and Population Innovation Fellowship Programme, Working Paper No. 1*. New Delhi: Population Council.

Department of Women and Child Development. 2005. *LADLI: The New Scheme for the Girl Child*. Haryana: Department of Women and Child Development, Government of Haryana. Accessed on 1 June 2011 at *http://www.wcdhry.gov.in/new_schemes_F.htm*.

Hesketh, Therese, L. Lu, and Zhu Wei Xing. 2011. 'The Consequences of Son Preference and Sex-Selective Abortion in China and Other Asian countries', *Canadian Medical Association Journal* (March 15).

International Institute for Population Studies (IIPS). 1995. *National Family Health Survey (NFHS), India, 1992–93*. Mumbai: IIPS.

International Institute for Population Studies (IIPS) and ORC Macro. 2000. *National Family Health Survey (NFHS-2), India, 1998–99*. Mumbai: IIPS.

International Institute for Population Sciences (IIPS) and Macro International. 2007. *National Family Health Survey (NFHS-3), India, 2005–06*. Mumbai: IIPS.

International Institute for Population Sciences (IIPS) and Population Council. 2010. *Youth in India: Situation and Needs 2006–2007*. Mumbai: IIPS.

Jejeebhoy, S.J., K.G. Santhya, and R. Acharya. 2010. *Health and Social Consequences of Marital Violence: A Synthesis of Evidence from India*. New Delhi: Population Council.

Jejeebhoy, S.J., A.J. Francis Zavier, R. Acharya, and S. Kalyanwala. 2011a. *Increasing Access to Safe Abortion in Rural Maharashtra: Outcomes of a Comprehensive Abortion Care Model*. New Delhi: Population Council.

Jejeebhoy, S.J., A.J. Francis Zavier, R. Acharya, and S. Kalyanwala. 2011b. *Increasing Access to Safe Abortion in Rural Rajasthan: Outcomes of a Comprehensive Abortion Care Model*. New Delhi: Population Council.

Jha, P., R. Kumar, P. Vasa, D. Thiruchelvam, and R. Moineddin. 2006. 'Low Male-to-Female Sex Ratio of Children Born in India: National Survey of 1.1 Million Households', *The Lancet*, 367(9056): 211–218.

Jha, P., M.A. Kesler., R. Kumar, F. Ram, U. Ram, L Aleksandrowicz, et al. 2011. 'Trends in Selective Abortions of Girls in India: Analysis of Nationally Representative Birth Histories from 1990 to 2005 and Census Data from 1991 to 2011', *The Lancet*, published online DOI: 10.1016/S0140–6736(11): 60649–1.

Kabeer, N. 2001. 'Resources, Agency, Achievements: Reflections on the Measurement of Women's Empowerment', in *Discussing Women's Empowerment—Theory and Practice*, Sida Studies No 3, NovumGrafiska AB, Stockholm.

Kishor, S. and K. Gupta. 2009. *Gender Equality and Women's Empowerment in India*. National Family Health Survey (NFHS-3), India, 2005–06. Mumbai: International Institute for Population Sciences; Calverton, Maryland, USA: ICF Macro.

Lok Sabha. 2009. *Fifteenth Lok Sabha (18/5/2009): Women Members*. Accessed on 5 June 2011 at www.parliamentofindia.nic.in.

Malhotra, A., S. Schuler, and C. Boender. 2002. *Measuring Women's Empowerment as a Variable in International Development on Women*. Paper commissioned by the Gender and Development Group of the World Bank and by the World Bank's Social Development Group.

Mensch, B. 2006. 'Issues in Defining, Measuring and Evaluating Interventions to Enhance Agency among Young Women', Presentation made at the meeting Programming for Young People: New Evidence on Young People's Situation and Needs. New Delhi: Population Council.

Ministry of Health and Family Welfare (MOHFW). 2009. *Reproductive and Sexual Health of Young People in India*. New Delhi: MOHFW, Government of India.

Ministry of Panchayati Raj. 2011. *Annual Report 2007–2008*. New Delhi: Ministry of Panchayati Raj, Government of India. Accessed on www.panchayat.nic.in.

——— 2010. *Annual Report 2010–11*. New Delhi: Ministry of Women and Child Development, MOWCD, Government of India.

Ministry of Women and Child Development (MOWCD). 2011. *XII Five Year Plan Report of the Working Group on Women's Agency and Empowerment*. New Delhi: Ministry of Women and Child Development, MOWCD, Government of India.

National Crime Records Bureau (NCRB). 2010. *Crime in India 2010*. New Delhi: Ministry of Home Affairs, Government of India.

——— 2012. *Crime in India: 2011 Compendium*. New Delhi: Ministry of Home Affairs, Government of India.

National Research Council and Institute of Medicine. 2005. *Growing Up Global: The Changing Transition to Adulthood in Developing Countries.* Washington, DC: National Academies Press.

National Sample Survey Organisation (NSSO). 2006. *Employment and Unemployment Situation in India 2004–05, Part I, NSS 61*st *Round.* New Delhi: NSSO, Government of India.

——— 2010. *Employment and Unemployment Situation in India 2007–08, NSS 64*th *Round.* New Delhi: NSSO, Government of India.

NHRC, UNIFEM, and ISS. 2004. A Report on Trafficking in Women and Children in India, 2002–2003. Accessed on 5 June 2011 at http://nhrc.nic.in/Documents/ReportonTrafficking.pdf.

Office of the Registrar General and Census Commissioner, India. 2004. Primary Census Abstract: Total Population Table, A–5 Series 1, New Delhi: Office of the Registrar General and Census Commissioner.

——— 2013. *Census of India 2011: Primary Census Abstract: Data Highlights, India, Series 1.* New Delhi: Office of the Registrar General.

Planning Commission. 2011. *Mid-Term Appraisal Eleventh Five Year Plan 2007–2012.* New Delhi: Oxford University Press.

Raj A, N. Saggurti, D. Balaiah, and J.G. Silverman. 2009. 'Prevalence of Child Marriage and Its Effect on Fertility and Fertility-Control Outcomes of Young Women in India: A Cross-Sectional, Observational Study'. *The Lancet,* 373: 1883–1889.

Raj A. 2010. 'When the Mother is a Child: The Impact of Child Marriage on the Health and Human Rights of Girls', *Archives of Disease in Childhood* 95: 931–935.

Raj A., N. Saggurti, D. Lawrence, D. Balaiah, and JG Silverman. 2010a. 'Association Between Adolescent Marriage and Marital' Violence among Young Adult Women in India', *International Journal of Gynecology and Obstetrics* 110: 35–39.

Raj A., N. Saggurti, M, Winter A. Labonte, M.R. Decker, D. Balaiah et al. 2010b. 'The Effect of Maternal Child Marriage on Morbidity and Mortality of Children Under 5 in India: Cross-sectional Study of a Nationally Representative Sample', *British Medical Journal,* 340: b4258.

Registrar General of India. 2011. *Sample Registration System Bulletin, Volume 45 No. 1.* New Delhi: Office of the Registrar General.

Santhya, K.G., U. Ram., R. Acharya, S.J. Jejeebhoy, F. Ram, and A. Singh. 2010. 'Associations Between Early Marriage and Young Women's Marital and Reproductive Health Outcomes: Evidence from India', *International Perspectives on Sexual and Reproductive Health,* 36(3): 132–139.

Sabarwal, S., K.G. Santhya and S.J. Jejeebhoy. 2013. 'Women's Autonomy and Experience of Physical Violence Within Marriage in Rural India:

Evidence from a Prospective Study' *Journal of Interpersonal Violence*. Doi: 10.1177/0886260513505144.

Santhya, K.G. and S.J. Jejeebhoy 2012. *Gender Differences in Educational Attainment among Youth in India: An Exploratory Study of Parental Aspirations about and Investment in Young People's Schooling* (unpublished report).

Santhya, K.G., S.J. Jejeebhoy., R. Acharya, and A.J.F. Zavier. 2011. *Effects of the Janani Suraksha Yojana on Maternal and Newborn Care Practices: Women's Experience in Rajasthan*. New Delhi: Population Council.

Santhya, K.G, A.J.F. Zavier, and S.J. Jejeebhoy. 2012. *Associations Between Secondary School Quality and Outcomes for Adolescents: Evidence from Bihar, India* (unpublished report).

United Nations Population Fund, India (UNFPA). 2010. *Trends in Sex Ratio at Birth and Estimates of Girls Missing at Birth in India*. UNFPA: New Delhi.

Verma, R.K., J. Pulerwitz, V. Mahendra S. Khandekar, G. Barker, P. Fulpagare et al. 2006. 'Challenging and Changing Gender Attitudes among Young Men in Mumbai, India', *Reproductive Health Matters* 14(28): 135–143.

Verma, R.K., J. Pulerwitz, V.S. Mahendra S. Khandekar, A.K. Singh. S.S. Das et al. 2008. Promoting Gender Equity As a Strategy to Reduce HIV Risk and Gender-Based Violence Among Young Men in India. *Horizons Final Report*: New Delhi: Population Council.

Yugantar Education Society. n.d. A Research Study on the Nature, Incidence, Extent and Impact of Sexual Harassment of Women at Workplace in the State of Maharashtra. Accessed on 5 June 2011 at http://ncw.nic.in/pdfReports/sexualpercent20harassment%20in%20Maharashtra-report.pdf.

6

Role of Partners

Firoza Mehrotra

India, one of the fastest growing economies of the world, is now categorized as a middle-income country and has become one of the emerging economies in Asia. On the other hand however, a large part of the population appears to have been left out of this growth curve. Home to one third of the world's poor, India is still grappling with adverse social indicators, aggravated by poor governance and corruption. Two main challenges confront India's development–how can social, economic, and political development be made more inclusive and all encompassing so that it reaches the most marginalised populations and those residing in the remotest areas, and how best to bring about structural reforms that result in good governance, a conducive environment for growth, increased productivity, and a life of dignity for all.

Description of Partners

Partners can broadly be divided into four categories: governments, bilaterals, multilaterals, and civil society.

India's growth story has a large unfinished agenda, which can only be achieved if strategic partnerships are forged and nurtured. Successful and appropriate partnerships are crucial, because even if a single partner can fulfill a number of roles, it is not clear that such an arrangement would be advisable or an optimal use of its resources (human, financial and time). Most partners participate in one or more of a variety of activities such as (1) policy advocacy and formulation; (2) planning and designing programmes; (3) research, reviews, assessments and analyses; (4) capacity building and training; (5) service delivery; (6) developing and testing pilots and innovations; (7) awareness building and behavioural/attitudinal change communication; and (8) monitoring and evaluation. Most development partners specialise in one or more of these activities, in particular geographical locations. While identifying partnerships, besides technical competency/skills and reach, one should also take into account the networks the partner may have or are able to build, capacity to influence policies/programmes, capacity to leverage other partners' resources, and long term sustainability.

Governments

Governments include those at the central and state levels and their affiliated organisations and institutions. As in any country, the Government in India is the primary partner as it plays multiple roles: in policy formulation as well as in advocacy, planning, service delivery, research, monitoring and evaluation, capacity building, and rolling out plans and schemes. It also has the unique role of convening interactions along with multilateral and bilateral organizations.

Table 6.1 outlines the outlays for health, family welfare and health research from the Third Plan period to the Eleventh Plan, both for the Centre and the States and Union Territories (UTs).

Table 6.1 indicates that there has been a steeper growth of outlays for Family Welfare, from Rs 24.9 crores in the Third Plan to Rs 90,558 crores in the Eleventh Plan, compared to the growth in the Health sector from Rs 225.9 crores in the Third Plan to Rs 41,092.9 crores in the Eleventh Plan. Even if we look at the percentage share of health and family welfare in the total plan, it ranges from .67 to 2.6 per cent for health and between 0.3 to 2.48 per cent for family

Table 6.1 Plan Outlay on Health & Family Welfare in Different Plan Periods for Centre, States and UTs

(Rs. in crores)

Period	Health	Family Welfare	Health Research	Sub-total	Total Plan	% of Health to Total	% of Family Welfare to Total
Third Plan (1961–66)	225.9	24.9		250.8	8,576.5	2.6	0.3
Annual Plan (1966–69)	140.2	70.4		210.6	6,625.4	2.1	1.1
Fourth Plan (1969–74)	335.5	278.0		613.5	15,778.8	2.1	1.8
Fifth Plan (1974–79)	760.8	491.8		1,252.6	39,426.2	1.9	1.2
Annual Plan (1979–80)	223.1	118.5		341.6	12,176.5	1.8	1.0
Sixth Plan (1980–85)	1,821.0	1,010.0		2,831.0	97,500.0	1.9	1.0
Seventh Plan (1985–90)	3,392.9	3,256.3		6,649.2	180,000.0	1.9	1.8

(*Continued*)

Table 6.1 *(Continued)*

Period	Health	Family Welfare	Health Research	Sub-total	Total Plan	% of Health to Total	% of Family Welfare to Total
Annual Plans							
1990–91	960.9	784.9		1,745.8	61,518.1	1.6	1.3
1991–92	1,042.3	856.6		1,898.9	65,855.8	1.6	1.3
Eigth Plan (1992–97)	7,575.9	6,500.0		14,075.9	434,100.0	1.7	1.5
Ninth Plan (1997–2002)	12,073.0	14,170.0*		4,463.7	859,200.0	1.4	1.6
Tenth Plan (2002–2007)	10,252.0	26,126.0		36,378.0	1,525,639	.67	1.71
Eleventh Plan (2007–2012)	41,092.92	90,558.00	4,496.08	136,147.00	3,644,718	1.25 (including health research)	2.48

Note: *Figure excludes arrears.

Source: Planning Commission, quoted in Government of India (2009); 'Family Welfare Statistics in India 2009', Ministry of Health and Family Welfare, 2009. New Delhi-Accessed in March 2011 at https://nrhm-mis.nic.in/familywelfare2009.html.

welfare, during the Third to Eleventh plans. Mindful of the fact that these are outlays and not actual expenditures, a comparison of the 10th Plan outlay against expenditure revealed that against an outlay of Rs 26,126 crores, there was an expenditure of Rs 26,350 crores. Further analysis has been constrained by the lack of data. The above table however is a good indicator of the trends in outlays of the Government for the health sector.

Bilateral External Assistance

The changing aid scenario in the country has brought in a paradigm shift in the role of development partners in India. The Indian economy today is no longer reliant on external assistance for the financing of its plan outlays or for gross capital formation. The early reliance on food aid has been done away with and the country moved away from the compulsions of accepting tied aid from February 2003. External assistance today plays more of a supportive role in financing major infrastructure projects, social sector activities, and in building institutional capacities.

The present policy on external assistance, which was recast in January 2006, emphasizes the reform orientation in India's economic policy. While bilateral aid is accepted only from G-8 countries, namely USA, UK, Japan, Germany, France, Italy, Canada and the Russian Federation, as well as from the European Commission, tied aid is not accepted at all. All other countries (as well as the above) can provide bilateral development assistance either through multilateral organizations to promote greater aid harmonization, or directly to autonomous institutions, universities, Non-government Organizations (NGOs), etc through a simplified procedure. It was felt that directing smaller amounts of external assistance towards the non government sector would help this sector to remain a development partner and strengthen civil society.

Bilateral assistance is encouraged if it is in the form of technical assistance that aims to enhance the knowledge/skills of Indian nationals. Only a limited component is permitted for the provision of equipment/hardware.

There has also been a shift in the focus sectors, from a focus on basic infrastructure sectors such as power and railways in the mid

1990s to the social sectors, such as health and education. This shift is largely in consonance with national commitments to fulfil the Millennium Development Goals (MDGs).

Trends in external assistance have been captured in Table 6.2. The biggest grant donor is the UK. Although Japan has provided more assistance than any other country, its assistance is almost entirely (98 per cent) in the form of loans rather than grants. Likewise, assistance from Russia is also entirely in the form of loans.

Among bilateral partners, the three most prominent players in India in the population and health sector at present are the Department for International Development (DFID), the US Agency for International Development (USAID) and the European Union (EU).

Department for International Development (DFID) The Government of UK has been providing Bilateral Assistance to India since 1958. At present, the UK is the largest external bilateral development partner providing grants in India (www.dfid.gov.uk). UK assistance is channelled through the DFID. The priority areas of UK assistance are Health & Family Welfare, Rural Development, Environment, Slum Development, Education, Urban Services, and programmes relating to expediting the achievement of MDGs. The priority states for UK assistance are Andhra Pradesh, Madhya Pradesh, Odisha, and West Bengal.

The agency's top priorities are presently to ensure that the poorest girls and women get quality schooling, health care and nutrition, and to support the private sector to deliver jobs, products, infrastructure and basic services in key areas. This new approach focuses on India's poorest states and poorest people and seeks to share expertise, support innovation, and build skills to help India's public and private resources go further.

DFID spends 48 per cent of its aid on the health sector. They endeavour to spend an average of £280 million per year in India, and will do so until 2015. The Reproductive and Child Health (RCH) programme is one of the biggest programmes of DFID in India, amounting to £139,030,100 from 1-5-2005 to 31-3-2012. DFID discontinued their pooling of funds support to RCH II, though they continue to provide technical assistance to the programme.

Table 6.2 Trends in Bilateral Disbursements by Major Donors, 2000–01 to 2006–07

(Rupees in crores)

Donor	2000–01	2001–02	2002–03	2003–04	2004–05	2005–06	2006–07
Japan	2,729.78	3,728.95	3,328.88	3,277.64	2,971.18	2,710.36	2,097.62
	(99.4/0.6)	(100/0)	(99.7/0.3)	(99.84/0.16)	(98/2)	(97.92/2.08)	(98.28/1.72)
UK	307.30	808.37	778.73	1,279.94	1,506.93	1,371.94	1,310.32
	(0/100)	(0/100)	(0/100)	(0/100)	(0/100)	(0/100)	(0/100)
Germany	386.69	444.66	381.16	333.41	121.18	188.24	278.32
	(82.5/17.5)	(65.9/34.1)	(50.83/49.17)	(59.21/40.79)	(14.87/85.12)	(18.25/81.75)	(36.48/63.52)
EEC	36.28	181.89	326.03	147.54	426.31	820.51	397.88
	(0/100)	(0/100)	(0/100)	(0/100)	(0/100)	(0/100)	(0/100)
USA	81.11	66.18	49.86	110.56	80.17	52.66	44.56
	(0/100)	(0/100)	(0/100)	(0/100)	(0/100)	(0/100)	(0/100)
Russian	130.09	23.03	316.06	771.71	1,194.82	1,106.83	1,404.41
Federation	(100/0)	(100/0)	(100/0)	(100/0)	(100/0)	(100/0)	(100/0)
Total Bilateral	**3,866.18**	**5,624.77**	**5,399.46**	**6,218.05**	**6,446.38**	**6,309.14**	**5,531.26**
Assistance	**(83.5/16.5)**	**(72.4/27.6)**	**(71.94/28.06)**	**(68.97/31.03)**	**(64.84/35.05)**	**(60.52/39.48)**	**(64.60/35.40)**

Note: The loan/grant mix is given in brackets.

The above figures indicate donor-wise total disbursement in respect of governmental as well as non-governmental projects.

Data Source: Department of Economic Affairs, Government of India.

US Agency for International Development's (USAID) US bilateral development assistance to India started in 1951. This assistance mainly comprises development assistance, agricultural commodities and technical assistance. US assistance, presently entirely in the form of grants, is mainly administered through the USAID.

USAID's strategy to address health in India includes support to increase access to family health care, provide nutrition for mothers and children, fight infectious diseases, and prevent HIV/AIDS (www.usaid.gov/in). Health activities focus on increasing the use of reproductive health and family planning services through initiatives targeted in the north of India. To improve the effectiveness of child survival interventions, USAID helps to develop urban health plans in various cities, and supports child health research activities as well as polio eradication efforts. USAID also helps promote proven health and diagnostic products through private sector markets. The focus of USAID's support is shifting from a disease-specific approach to a health systems approach, under the Health Partnership Program. The objective is to strengthen health systems to address the health needs of vulnerable populations. USAID works together with the government to achieve a broad set of intermediate results which contribute to the GOI's national health programs, including, but not limited to, the RCH programme and the National AIDS Control Programme. Though USAID did not join RCH II as a pooling partner, it provides valuable technical assistance to RCH II.

The European Union (EU) The EU's Country Strategy Paper for India 2007–2013 (€470 million) focuses on health, education, and the implementation of the Joint Action Plan. The Joint Action Plan, revised in 2008, aims to promote peace and security, sustainable development, research and technology, people-to-people contacts, and cultural exchanges (European Commission 2007). The EU is adopting a two-pronged approach. First, it focuses on assisting India in meeting the MDGs by providing budget support to the social sector (health/education), encouraging the inclusion of best practice models in good governance, focusing on decentralised decision-making and development, including innovative methods for improved service delivery to address poverty, gender issues, institutional reforms and public sector management. Second, it focuses on implementing the ambitious EU-India Action Plan with a view to supporting India's pro-poor sector reform policies, promote dialogue in areas of mutual interest, and enhance economic co-operation.

The EU did not join RCH II as a pooling partner initially. However, it recently showed interest in joining the pool, and was advised by the GOI to contribute budgetary support to the health sector instead of becoming a pooling partner.

Multilateral Agencies

There are a host of multilateral agencies operating in India, but the ones directly or indirectly connected with the population sector are UNFPA, UNICEF, the World Bank, WHO, and UNDP.

The United Nations Population Fund (UNFPA) UNFPA is the main UN agency concerned with issues of population and reproductive health. It promotes the right of every woman, man and child to enjoy a life of health and equal opportunity. UNFPA supports countries to use population data for policies and programmes intended to reduce poverty and to ensure that every pregnancy is wanted, every birth is safe, every young person is free of HIV/AIDS, and every girl and woman is treated with dignity and respect. UNFPA has played a critical role in assisting India to redirect its population efforts away from family planning targets and quotas and focusing instead on providing high-quality services within a comprehensive reproductive health care system. UNFPA is helping India in supporting the strategy endorsed by the 1994 International Conference on Population and Development (ICPD), which emphasised population and development, and focused on meeting individuals' needs rather than demographic targets (www.unfpa.org.in).

UNICEF The RCH Programme contributes to the reduction of infant and maternal mortality by increasing the percentage of children fully immunized, improving quality and access to the health system, improving home-based practices including the management of childhood illness in selected districts, and promoting care practices for pregnant and lactating women and newborns (www.unicef.org/india).

The World Health Organization (WHO) is the international agency within the United Nations system responsible for health. WHO's objective, as set out in its constitution, is the attainment by all peoples of the highest possible standard of health. Health is defined in WHO's constitution as a state of complete physical, mental and social well-being and not merely the absence of disease or infirmity. Its broad areas of work are communicable diseases, non-communicable diseases, mental health, family and community health, and health systems strengthening.

United Nations Development Programme (UNDP) UNDP is the largest source of Development Cooperation in the UN System. The overall mission of UNDP is sustainable human development, and as such it allocates high priority to poverty alleviation, gender equity and women's empowerment, and environmental protection.

The World Bank IDA, the soft loan affiliate of the Bank began in June 1961 and has been an important component of external assistance in various sectors (www.worldbank.org.in).

The World Bank's Country Strategy (CAS) for India for 2009–2012 focuses on helping the country to fast-track the development of much-needed infrastructure and to support the seven poorest states (Bihar, Chhattisgarh, Jharkhand, Madhya Pradesh, Odisha, Rajasthan, and Uttar Pradesh) to achieve higher standards of living for their people. Preparations are underway to provide lending to support: (i) health system development in Uttar Pradesh, and (ii) programs to improve childhood nutrition nationwide.

The Bank's new strategy focuses on an interlocking set of measures to alter processes, incentives, and accountabilities to improve coverage, quality, effectiveness, and efficiency of service delivery and public health interventions, or, in short, make services work for the poor.

Reproductive and Child Health (RCH) programme This is the Government's flagship programme for population and reproductive health and is a 'sector wide approach programme' (SWAP). The World Bank was the only non-governmental pooling partner in RCH-I. The RCH-II programme, which ended on March 2012, was funded by the GOI to the extent of 92 per cent, and by three donors to the extent of

8 per cent. Of the donor pool, DFID contributed 52 per cent, World Bank 42 per cent and UNFPA 6 per cent. In the initial days of SWAP, there was a differentiation between 'core' partners who contributed to the pool and 'expanded' partners (such as UNICEF and USAID) that contributed only technical assistance. Later, however, the distinction disappeared and a 'Development Partners' Forum' came into existence, where all development partners have a more or less equal say in the implementation and monitoring of the RCH programme.

After the formal culmination of RCH-II, the Government decided not to continue with the programme as a pooling programme. The RCH programme is an integral part of the National Rural Health Mission (NRHM) but as it is no longer a sector wide pooling programme. There is no donor support from 1 April 2012.

Civil society organizations

This category is perhaps the most varied and vibrant. The civil society organisations group can further be categorized as below. Each of these sub-categories has its own niche and comparative advantages. It would be advisable to keep these in view while designing and implementing initiatives at the field level.

a. Private philanthropic foundations and trusts – Bill and Melinda Gates Foundation, Ford Foundation etc.
b. Education/training institutions – Schools, Medical colleges, etc
c. Research institutions – Indian Council of Medical Research, International Institute for Population Studies, Indian Institute of Health Management Research
d. Professional bodies – Indian Medical Association, Federation of Obstetric and Gynecological Societies of India, National Commission for Women
e. Network organizations – Voluntary Health Association of India, National Alliance of Women, Voluntary Action Network India, HEALTH WATCH
f. Private service providers – private doctors, paramedics, birth attendants, clinics, nursing – homes, hospitals, diagnostic facilities etc

g. NGOs & Trusts
h. Communication & Advertising agencies
i. Media & entertainment agencies and industry
j. International NGOs
k. Peoples' representatives – Members of Parliament, Members of Legislative Assemblies, local body representatives
l. Private sector Industry – Corporate social responsibility cells
m. Opinion leaders – Religious/spiritual leaders, teachers, parents, elderly
n. Formal and informal associations/bodies – self help groups, Youth bodies, National Service Schemes, Nehru Yuvak Kendras
o. Trade unions, staff associations, and Cooperative societies
p. Regulatory Bodies – Medical Council of India

Recommendations

The changing partner environment calls for new partnerships and more of a focus on ensuring the sustainability and institutionalization of successful initiatives. Besides making recommendations, this section also highlights emerging issues.

Strengthening Existing and Forging New Partnerships in the Public Sector

Depending on the nature and scope of interventions to be undertaken, new partnerships with different ministries/departments of government are needed. More specifically, the Ministry of Social Justice and Empowerment at the level of the central government, and Departments of Social Welfare in state governments may be mobilized for addressing issues of the elderly. Partnerships with the National Skill Development Mission may enable access to groups of youth who could be exposed to life skills programme as well as population and development issues. The Ministry of Urban Development (at the central government level) or Departments of Urban Affairs/Town and Country Planning (at state levels), and urban local bodies including their representatives, may be useful partners for issues relating to urban health.

Strengthening Existing and Forging New Partnerships in the Private Sector

Private foundations and trusts, both national and international, are another very attractive partnership for the government to explore. They are often very receptive and have flexible modalities.

At the same time, considering the role played by private medical service providers, there is huge potential to build partnerships with this sector, build their capacities, including regarding the use of new technologies, and include them more actively in the provision of health services for family planning, safe abortion, and adolescent reproductive and sexual health.

The growing private industrial sector in India has tremendous scope for partnerships. As part of corporate social responsibility, many in this sector are obliged to invest in development, but are unclear about where to invest their resources. Partnering with them has the advantage of obtaining access to resources, as well as concentrating action in a clearly defined geographical area, and often some physical infrastructure as well.

An essential component of work regarding population, reproductive health and gender justice involves change in attitudes and behaviours. The media, entertainment industry and opinion makers like spiritual and religious personalities, can play a key role in behaviour change communication. Partnerships with them should be encouraged.

Redefining the Role of Government

Today there are many more players in the development sector than even two decades ago, when the government was the primary and often the only player and provider of services. Without abdicating its responsibility of providing basic health services, the government should consider playing more of a regulatory role-setting standards, laying down protocols, enforcement etc. Policy and systemic issues and structural reforms should engage government more. The government may also consider buying services from the private sector/NGOs in certain areas, but making sure of quality. This may generate healthy competition between government service providers and private providers.

Ensuring the Sustainability and Institutionalization of Successful Initiatives

As often happens with donor funding, once the funding stops, the initiatives also cease. This is definitely not desirable. Exit strategies must be built into projects at the design stage itself. This is especially important when NGOs are supported or pilots tested. It is equally important to ensure that systemic changes are made and components integrated into regular training/education systems, after having been tested and evaluated. Realistic time frames must be provided for this to happen.

Leveraging Partnerships and Working in Synergy

It is not uncommon for stakeholders and development partners to work in isolation of each other, often doing the same or similar things, reinventing the wheel and sometimes creating unhealthy competition. It is recommended that mechanisms be put in place, like the 'Development Partners' Forum', so that stakeholders may share information with each other, leverage each other's work, build on it or around it, and work in harmony and synergy.

References

Department of Economic Affairs, Government of India. Accessed on 10 July 2013 at http://finmin.nic.in/the-ministry/dept_eco_affairs/aids_accounts_audit/aid_index1.asp.

Department for International Development (DFID). *DFID India Operational Plan 2011–2015*. Accessed on 10 July 2013 at http://www.gov.uk/government/uploads/system/uploads/attachment_data/file/67379/india-2011.pdf

European Commission. *India Country Strategy Paper 2007–2013*. Accessed on 10 March 2013 at http://eeas.europa.eu/india/csp/07_13_en.pdf.

———. 2013. *Mid-Term Review of Country* HYPERLINK "http://eeas.europa.eu/india/csp/07_13_en.pdf" \o "Country Strategy Paper for India 2007-2013" *Strategy Paper 2007-2013*. Accessed on 10 March 2013 at http://eeas.europa.eu/india/csp/11_13_mtr_en.pdf.

Ministry of Finance. 2008. *Position Paper on External Assistance Received by India*. New Delhi: Ministry of Finance, Department of Economic Affairs,

Project Monitoring Unit. Accessed on 10 July, 2013 at http://finmin.nic/the_ministry/dept_eco_affairs/pmu/PositionPaper_ExtAssist.pdf.

Ministry of Health and Family Welfare. 2009. *Family Welfare Statistics in India 2009*. New Delhi: Ministry of Health and Family Welfare, Government of India. Accessed on 10 July, 2013 at http://nrhm-mis.nic/familywelfare2009.html.

Planning Commision. 2011. *Mid-Term Appraisal Eleventh Five Year Plan 2007–2012*. New Delhi: Planning Commission.

UNICEF. n.d. *Official Website for India*. Accessed on 10 July, 2013 at www.unicef.org/india/

UNFPA. n.d. *Overview and Programmes from Official Website*. Accessed on 10 March, 2011 at http://india.unfpa.org/

USAID. n.d. *Overview and Programs from Official Website*. Accessed on 10 March, 2011 at http://www.usaid.gov/india.

World Bank. n.d *Reproductive and Child Health Overview and Programs*. Accessed on 10 March, 2011 at http://www.worldbank.org/en/country/india.

———. *India Country Strategy (CAS) 2009–2012*. Accessed on 10 March, 2011 at http://www.worldbank.org/en/news/feature/2010/04/06/india-coutry-strategy

7

Moving Forward

Shireen J. Jejeebhoy

K.G. Santhya

P.M. Kulkarni

Firoza Mehrotra

India has expressed its commitment to improving the quality of its population, including its sexual and reproductive health, through a large number of policies and programmes. Additionally, legislative measures in the area of sexual and reproductive health, youth, and gender issues underscore the nation's commitment to addressing reproductive rights of women, men and young people. The evidence compiled in this book suggests that remarkable achievements have been made in meeting the health and development needs of the nation's 1.21 billion people. Almost all of its children are in school, life expectancy has increased, gender disparities in schooling and life expectancy have narrowed, maternal and infant mortality have declined, more and more couples have exercised their right to bear only the children they want, and HIV rates have fallen. Apprehensions about population explosion and the disastrous situation it portended have been unfounded. Over the last decade, the population growth rate has slowed down and projections suggest that the population will increase modestly and reach replacement levels by the middle of this century. Projections place India's population between 1.5 and 1.8 billion at the middle of the century. An impressive set of laws and Acts exist that are intended to promote gender justice and counter prevailing gender inequities, such as laws prohibiting child marriage, protecting women from domestic violence and sexual harassment, and ensuring that pre-natal sex selection does not take place.

At the same time, there remain many areas in which progress has been uneven, and which, if not addressed soon, will affect people's wellbeing and violate their rights. There is a huge schism between the articulation of commitment to improving the quality of India's population and its operationalization at the community and grassroots level. This volume is replete with instances of India's record of making and breaking goals and targets set in policies, plans and international agreements. Political will to stand up for gender equity, sexual and reproductive health, and young people's health and development, has been indifferent, and this lack of political will may underlie India's poor record in both enforcing laws and meeting goals. The rights-based approach articulated in several policies has not yet filtered down to communities and women. The exercise of reproductive rights and informed sexual and reproductive choice continues to elude the most vulnerable. Neither health sector reforms nor the service environments can be said to have fully implemented the rights-based approach.

While there are obvious overlaps, we provide below our recommendations in four specific areas: sexual and reproductive health, young people's health and development, women's empowerment and gender equity, and emerging issues in population and sexual and reproductive health arenas. Cutting across these four areas is the need for a greater commitment to enforcing laws, meeting goals and targets set in policies and programmes, and strengthening inter-sectoral linkages and public-private partnerships. There is an urgent need to strengthen the implementation of laws, and work with agencies, both governmental and non-governmental, to make examples of those violating the laws. Likewise, there is clearly a need to set achievable targets on the one hand, and ensure that these are met, on the other. Efforts to better understand the implementation challenges faced by each programme, to build accountability among programme implementers, and strengthen advocacy measures to engage the political leadership, are essential in order to ensure that promises made can be realized.

We also note that meeting the wide range of population and sexual and reproductive health needs described in this book cannot be satisfied by a single sector. For example, the population, women's empowerment and sexual and reproductive health agenda require the active engagement of Ministries of Health and Family Welfare, Women and Child Development, Human Resource Development, and notably Education and Social Welfare, Youth Affairs and Sports, Urban Development, Social Justice and Empowerment, and Panchayati Raj. Linkages between various ministries need to be more clearly drawn at both decision-making and ground levels.

Other partnerships must also be forged. India has a thriving civil society network engaged in addressing population and sexual and reproductive health needs, and successful models implemented by this sector need to be reviewed and up-scaled. The time has come to explore synergies and develop partnerships, including by way of financial commitments, with multi and bilateral agencies, private foundations/trusts, corporate bodies, media, the commercial advertising and entertainment industries, and the civil society. Moreover, with regard to the health system, successful models of public-private partnerships exist and must be exploited so that inequities in access to health and social sector services can be addressed.

Meeting Commitments to Improve Sexual and Reproductive health

In order to meet commitments to improve sexual and reproductive health, action is required on multiple fronts, ranging from the individual to the systemic, from awareness building to service delivery, and from increasing access to improving quality and respect for rights.

Accelerate Efforts to Reduce Maternal and Newborn Mortality

Although India has taken significant steps to increase skilled attendance at delivery and reduce maternal mortality, it appears that the country is likely to hold the world from realising MDG 5 (WHO, 2012). While institutional delivery has increased impressively since the introduction of the *Janani Suraksha Yojana* (JSY), complete antenatal care, postpartum care and newborn care have not kept pace. Quality of care is uneven, harmful pregnancy related practices, including unmonitored intrapartum oxytocin use continue to be observed, access to emergency obstetric care has not increased as rapidly as expected, and the volume of complications addressed within the public health system remains sub-optimal. Efforts made under the National Rural Health Mission (NRHM) and its flagship JSY and Accredited Social Health Activist (ASHA) programmes need to be accelerated to ensure that the poorest and socially excluded women are reached with maternal and newborn health services, that all pregnant women are identified as soon as possible and followed up until their newborn has passed the neonatal stages, and that the quality of services is acceptable. Findings indicating young women's limited access to maternal health services, even at the time of the first, and often the most risky, pregnancy, highlight the need for reproductive and child health programmes in the country to build a demand for, as well as improve the availability of, such services among young people.

Accelerate Efforts to Reduce Unmet Need for Contraception, and Meet Fertility Goals

Failure to meet fertility goals and persisting unmet need for contraception in several segments of the population and notably among the young calls for greater efforts to ensure that women in need of contraception are reached in ways that are respectful of their reproductive rights. Moreover, although the programme is said to provide a cafeteria of contraceptive methods, choices offered are, in practice, limited, and efforts to encourage a wider method mix and expand non-terminal method use have not, thus far, been very successful. There is a need to ensure that services are client centred, and respect client choices. At the same time, non-terminal method options must be encouraged: new methods, injectables for example, should be considered for inclusion in the basket of contraceptive choices available, given the increasing evidence of its acceptability among women seeking contraception.

Efforts must be made to ensure the regular and wide availability of popular non-terminal methods and emergency contraceptives.

Counselling must be strengthened that encourages non-terminal method use, postpartum and post-abortion contraceptive practice. The condom must be repositioned as a suitable method of family planning, especially for the young, and efforts must be made that enable young couples to postpone the first pregnancy. In this connection, there is a need to address the lack of provider motivation, particularly inadequate attention to postpartum contraception, and limited emphasis placed on counselling, especially for postpartum and post-abortion contraception and follow up. There is a need to emphasise the importance of involving women in the selection of contraceptive methods, and providing them information that could help them arrive at a decision for themselves, including about how the method works, what the likely side effects are, and how these side-effects can be managed.

Efforts are needed that reduce the distance between communities and contraceptive supplies: community-based family planning services, including counselling, distribution of contraceptives and referral services through ASHAs, VHNDs and VHSCs need to be operationalised (Ministry of Health and Family Welfare 2010). At the same time, public private partnerships for the delivery of family planning services must be effectively forged (Ministry of Health and Family Welfare 2009). Equally, the quality of contraceptive service provision must be reviewed and much more attention paid to respect the clients' right to make contraceptive choices.

Raise Awareness of Health Promoting Practices and Available Services

Previous chapters have highlighted limited awareness of health promoting practices, rights and entitlements, and available services and the location of these services. There is clearly a need to fill this gap, to recognise that the medium and message need to be tailored to meet the needs of different sub-groups, notably, women, men and young people, and inform them about their rights, as well as about various programmes and schemes that relate to population and sexual and reproductive health.

Given the gender-stratified family systems prevailing in much of rural India, and the limited education and agency experienced by women, the mainstay of IEC and BCC efforts for rural women will continue to be interpersonal contacts. ASHAs, ANMs and AWWs are credible and locally available and are expected, in different ways, to raise community awareness. More attention needs to be paid, however, to sensitise and train these providers about key messages to be conveyed, to tailor messages to suit the needs of individual women (for example, special messages for newlyweds, first time pregnant women, women with one child/daughter and so on), and to make special efforts to communicate with the most vulnerable (for example, the young, those from scheduled castes and tribes, the poorest, etc) and those least likely to visit a health centre on their own. For example, these providers must be trained and charged with the responsibility of reaching married young women and men, including those who have not yet experienced pregnancy, with information regarding contraception and other reproductive health matters as well as contraceptive supplies. Many married young women lack the freedom of movement to seek health care, underscoring the need for health workers to reach these women, particularly those newly married and first time pregnant, in their homes. ASHAs, ANMs and AWWs also need to raise women's awareness about their eligibility for health services and the location of these services, and play the role of an intermediary who can connect poor women with available programmes.

Efforts are needed, moreover, that raise awareness at individual, community and stakeholder levels about women's rights, laws protecting women, and action that can be taken if rights are violated. These efforts need to change attitudes among women themselves as well as stakeholders and gatekeepers (police, teachers, health care providers, community leaders) about intervening to prevent violations of women's rights.

Our findings also underscore the need for a strong commitment to ensuring that educational programmes that are ongoing and aim to impart information on sexual and reproductive matters to young people do indeed reach young people, both those in school and out-of-school, married and unmarried, and rural and urban. It is important that such programmes are revived in states in which they have been stalled. These programmes should be age-appropriate. While the recent revisions of the Adolescence Education Programme (AEP) curriculum have brought in a broader sexual and reproductive health focus than the earlier and narrower HIV focus, it is important that these programmes should be designed not only to raise awareness among the youth, but to also enable young people to correctly understand and assess the risks they face and to adopt appropriate protective actions. In addition, special attention needs to be paid to the training of trainers. It is important that teachers, health care providers and other experts who provide life skill education undergo training that enables them to overcome their reluctance to communicate with the youth on sensitive sexual and reproductive matters, dispels their misconceptions on these matters, and enhances both their communication skills and their technical knowledge of these issues. Moreover, it is time to consider age-appropriate education that is initiated from a much earlier age.

Although men have also been observed to be poorly informed about both reproductive health matters, and the rights and needs of women and young people, programmes to enhance awareness among them have been limited. Community-based efforts through which to reach populations more broadly also need to be explored. For example, the NRHM has empowered communities and panchayats to play a role in reproductive health matters and it would be important to involve panchayat members and community leaders in conveying information at the community level to both women and men.

Address Health System Limitations in Infrastructure and Shortcomings in Provider Capacity

In the area of sexual and reproductive health, many remarkable advances have been made: the JSY and ASHA schemes hold huge promise for changing the reproductive health landscape of India. Nevertheless, health system weaknesses abound and their role in thwarting the achievement of good sexual and reproductive health have been highlighted throughout the book. A number of recommendations arise. Efforts must be made to meet the norms set by the NRHM in improving the health infrastructure, all FRUs must be made fully functional with comprehensive EmOC services including blood storage/blood bank, at least half of all primary health centres (PHCs) must be equipped to provide round the clock services and must be easily accessible. Stocks of supplies such as gloves, syringes, and drugs need to rectified. At the same time, in order to overcome concerns about limited access to services, promising experiences of public-private partnerships need to be reviewed and their scale expanded.

Likewise, more investment in provider training and mentoring is essential for the effective functioning of the health system. There is a need to review pre- and in-service training curricula for various categories of providers, revise materials as necessary, and ensure that all providers are fully trained prior to the rollout of programmes. For example, shortfalls in the number of ASHAs trained in all the modules relating to their activities need to be met. Moreover, where new tasks are added to providers' activities, such as, requiring ANMs and MOs to provide reproductive and sexual health information and services to adolescents, including the unmarried, it is essential that training covers not only the content of the information to be imparted, but also strategies for imparting the information in ways that resonate with the target audience. All providers need opportunities to clarify values and address discomfort about imparting information and services relating to sexual and reproductive life, and need to be sensitised about gender issues, respect for reproductive rights, and the importance of providing respectful services. In short, training of health care cadres needs to be far more systematic, comprehensive and regular, and supportive supervision of frontline workers must be far better implemented.

Considering the role played by private medical service providers and the precedent set by various programmes described in our volume, there is huge potential for building capacities of private medical service providers and involving them more actively in the provision of health services. Indeed, involving the private sector in the provision of services relating to maternal health, family planning, safe abortion and adolescent reproductive and sexual health would go a long way in increasing access to services.

Improve the Quality of Reproductive Health Services

The poor quality of sexual and reproductive health services in the public sector has been widely observed, and such issues as lack of cleanliness, long waiting times, shortages of drugs, demands for unauthorised payments, lack of visual and auditory privacy during consultations, and absence of respectful treatment documented. Moreover, findings have reiterated that the full range of services is not always available to women. Several aspects of reproductive health, such as treatment of gynaecological morbidities, preventing unsafe abortion, addressing the fertility desires of the infertile and those with HIV, addressing the sexual health needs of the young, and addressing the needs of older women, have been relatively neglected.

Attention must be paid to improving the quality of services, including with regard to providing counselling and referral services, ensuring privacy for clients, and addressing clients' needs in a more holistic way. Training must emphasise the need to provide good quality services as much as it focuses on developing technical skills. Providers must appreciate and act upon the possibility that women seeking care for one reproductive health matter may need services or screening for other needs as well. At the same time, although there is a clear preference for private sector services, the private sector's role is poorly understood and quite unregulated, and efforts are needed to better understand the quality of care provided in the private sector, including in terms of fees and charges for services rendered.

Improving the quality of services implies greater attention to mainstreaming gender in RCH programming at multiple levels. Integrating gender concerns into the formulation, implementation and monitoring of the programme must take place. It calls for increasing the availability and skills of frontline workers, including ANMs at sub-centre level, training and orienting managers and service providers about gender and equity, and the inclusion of parameters reflecting responsiveness to gender issues in quality assurance checklists (e.g. screens/partitions to ensure privacy), and measures to prevent sexual harassment in the work place.

Overcome Obstacles in Meeting Women's Need for Safe Abortion Services

Abortion accounts for eight percent of all maternal deaths, and the overwhelming majority of women who undergo abortion do so in potentially unsafe conditions. Our review argues for bold steps to increase women's access to safe abortion. To make safe abortion more accessible, a key recommendation is to increase the number of safe abortion providers. To do so, there is a need to make procedures for certification of providers and registration of facilities less cumbersome, and ensure that norms regarding the provision of abortion services at PHC/FRU level are operationalised. At the same time, there is a need to enable task shifting so as to expand the provider base for the provision of first trimester abortions to include nurses and AYUSH physicians; these providers have been found to be as safe, effective and acceptable as doctors (Jejeebhoy et al. 2011, 2012). Amendments to the MTP Act have been formulated so as to enable nurses and AYUSH physicians to provide MA and MVA; these amendments need to be approved expeditiously (Ministry of Health and Family Welfare, Expert Group on Amendments to the MTP Act 2010). A second potentially promising way of increasing access to safe abortion is to build upon successful public-private partnerships observed in the case of institutional delivery on the one hand, and the pilot implemented in Bihar to increase access to safe abortion on the other. Third, there is a need to review and reduce cumbersome and perhaps unnecessary procedures for obtaining medical abortion, explore ways of enabling chemists to provide information, supplies and referrals to women seeking medical abortion, and raise awareness more generally among women about the use of medical abortion. Finally, efforts are needed at community and facility levels that increase awareness of the Act and provider responsibilities at facility level, and assure better functioning of district level MTP committees.

Invest in Young People's Health and Development

We note that the demographic dividend provides India with a window, available only for the next 3–4 decades, of demographic opportunity. While some dividend will accrue naturally because of changes in the age structure and the dependency burden, India will not be able to reap the full impact of this demographic opportunity without an educated, productive, skilled and healthy population. Investment is urgently needed in ensuring the wellbeing of India's youth. At the same time, there must be a greater commitment to close gaps between young women and men, and between socially excluded and included youth, so that all youth and not simply young men and the more advantaged may support efforts to reap the demographic dividend.

Ensure a Well Educated, Skilled, and Healthy Youth Population

Evidence synthesized in this book shows that notwithstanding the many national programmes that aim to address the needs of the young, Indian youth are, for the most part, unprepared to meet the needs of a globalizing world. Too few young people complete high school, the quality of education received by many is poor, many lack livelihood skills and employment opportunities, and the health of many is compromised by early and unsafe entry into sexual life and childbearing, exposure to the risk of unwanted pregnancy and infection, unmet need for contraception, widespread anaemia, and worrying levels of mental health problems. Progress has been uneven, and gender gaps and gaps between the socially excluded and included persist.

The road ahead is obvious and requires multi-sectoral action. A major thrust area is to increase investments in addressing obstacles to universal school enrolment and secondary school completion, access to skill building and employment opportunities among young people. The government has articulated its commitment to improving the schooling situation in the country in several policies and acts including most recently, the Right to Education Act. What is needed is a strong commitment to ensuring that these programmes are effectively implemented, and that these do indeed reach the most disadvantaged groups. A number of central and state-sponsored programmes are ongoing that aim to reduce the cost of education and it is important to ensure that these ongoing government programmes do indeed reach the most disadvantaged groups. Additional inputs by way of conditional grants that encourage school completion among disadvantaged groups also need to be considered. At the same time, activities directed at parents are needed that promote positive attitudes towards education and school completion, raise their aspirations about their children's education, and encourage greater parental involvement in their children's education. Activities must also address school-level barriers, notably, poor infrastructure, quality of education and academic failure, particularly among young women.

There is a need to incorporate livelihood skill building models within the school setting that will not only raise young people's aspirations regarding their education and careers, but also provide them opportunities to gain market-driven job skills. There is also a need to focus on providing better training and ensuring accountability for teachers, investments that are likely to improve the quality of schooling experiences for the youth.

A second thrust area is to create greater opportunities for vocational skill acquisition by young people and link skilled youth with market opportunities. The proposed National Skills Development Mission and the Skill Development Initiative Scheme (Planning Commission 2011) is a step in the right direction and it is important that this initiative is implemented without any delay. At the same time, efforts are needed to promote self-employment and entrepreneurship through various livelihood schemes, for example, providing soft loans to youth to enable them to set up their own business enterprises. The significant constraints on young women's education and access to wage work call, moreover, for programmes specially targeted towards young women.

There must be a focus on improving mental, sexual and reproductive health, the major causes of the burden of disease among the youth, and build the skills, the supportive environment and youth-friendly health services that together will enable young people to make informed and healthy life choices. In the sexual and reproductive health arena, efforts are needed that strengthen life skills and sexuality education for those in school and out of school, that make the health system less threatening and health care providers less judgemental of young people with sexual health concerns. An increasing number of intervention models to build agency and promote egalitarian gender role attitudes among young people have been tested in India. These models should be reviewed and replicated or scaled up as appropriate.

Eliminate Child Marriage but Meet the Special Needs of Married Girls

Early marriage and early childbearing persist, in violation of a girl's rights and in violation of the law, and compromise the health and development of millions of girls. There is a need for a multi-pronged approach to eliminate the practice of early marriage. Strategies are needed that mobilise communities to help parents resist pressures that foster the practice of early marriage. Moreover, strategies are needed that establish new norms and practices, that actively engage influential persons in the community, including religious and political leaders, as well as those that initiate campaigns highlighting the adverse consequences of early marriage and the extent to which it is a violation of the rights of a child. Efforts to delay marriage also require providing girls with viable alternatives to marriage in the form of accessible and quality schooling and opportunities to build and use livelihood skills.

Equally important is to ensure greater commitment on the part of law enforcement agencies to enforce existing laws on the minimum age of marriage and the registration of marriages, and to levy penalties on violators. Allowing anonymous reporting, making law enforcement agencies and others aware that the practice of early marriage is not a minor violation, and making the guidelines for penalties clear to enforcement agencies and the wider community, are possible steps in this direction.

Given the slow pace of decline in the practice of child marriage, the needs of child brides cannot be ignored. They are the most vulnerable, the most secluded, and the most at risk of adverse pregnancy related outcomes, and the least likely to be informed about health promoting practices, and need programmes that address their unique needs.

Engage Parents to Provide Young People a Safe and Supportive Environment

Young people in general lack a safe and supportive environment, a shortcoming that is likely to pose major obstacles to their achievement of good sexual and reproductive health and the realisation of their rights. While evidence on models that are effective in bridging the distance between parents and children or that enable parents to adopt more gender-egalitarian socialisation practices is not currently available, programmes must be implemented that address parental inhibitions about discussing sexual matters with their children, and encourage greater openness and interaction between parents and children. Programmes that aim to encourage universal education or eliminate child marriage must, likewise, address parental concerns about the potential consequences of keeping daughters in school or delaying their marriage.

Make Youth-Friendly Health Services a Reality

Although there are a host of policies and programmes that seek to improve young people's access to sexual and reproductive health services, many young people lack access, in practice, to such services. Programmes intended to improve young people's access to sexual and reproductive health services have not been successful for many reasons. For example, functional adolescent health clinics are unevenly located across states (Gujarat, Maharashtra, Madhya Pradesh, Himachal Pradesh, Kerala and Punjab; MOHFW 2009), awareness of programmes for young people tends to be limited, provider attitudes continue to be judgemental, and the quality of provider-youth client interaction is frequently described as threatening.

Attention is required on many fronts. For one, evidence presented earlier suggests that efforts to smoothen the implementation of the ARSH strategy and adolescent friendly health clinics nationwide are much needed. Secondly, efforts are needed that raise community level awareness of these programmes, notably adolescent friendly clinics in all states. Thirdly, notwithstanding efforts to sensitise various categories of health care providers to the needs of adolescents, the quality and content of provider-training needs far more attention. Sensitisation and values-clarification of providers serving young people's sexual and reproductive health needs far more attention than is currently the case. Fourthly, far more cognizance must be taken of the obstacles that young people face in accessing services through adolescent clinics, notably the lack of confidentiality and privacy, and threatening provider attitudes. It is important that the working of existing adolescent clinics is reviewed, and lessons are derived from these for the modification and expansion of adolescent clinics. Different strategies should be attempted, for example, projecting the adolescent clinic as a facility reserved for adolescent health needs in general, rather than for specific, and perhaps stigmatised, sexual and reproductive health problems. At the same time, the feasibility of implementing various financing strategies needs to be addressed, for example, health insurance, competitive voucher schemes and community financing schemes, which will allow the youth to have a wider choice of providers and enhance the possibility of obtaining quality care.

Empower Women and Promote Gender Equity and Equality

India has articulated, in many policies and programmes, a commitment to women's rights and empowerment and gender equality. Yet a number of gaps remain that call for redoubling efforts to realise commitments made toward empowering women and establishing gender equity and equality.

Arrest the Declining Child Sex Ratio and Sex Selection Practices

The alarming decline in the child (0–6) sex ratio to 919 females per 1,000 males as of 2011, as against a goal of 935 by 2012, highlights the unchecked and widespread use of selective abortion to terminate pregnancies carrying a female foetus. This disturbing trend must be arrested swiftly and with multipronged measures. The PCPNDT Act must be enforced and violations on the part of ultrasound facilities and all those facilitating prenatal sex detection must be identified and punished to the full extent of the law, and such actions must be widely publicised so as to deter others. Even more important are efforts to address the root cause of sex selective abortions, that is, patriarchal norms and strong son-preference. Programmes that address gender inequities from an early age and that empower girls and women using multiple mechanisms, including providing cash transfers, skill building and employment opportunities, and access to financial products, need to be strengthened and implemented vigorously. Sustained community level campaigns and BCC activities, and creative media messaging, must be a priority.

Maintain the Rights and Gender Focus, Strengthen Efforts to Empower Women and Girls

Notwithstanding the policy and programme commitments to building women's agency, our findings have suggested that change has been unacceptably slow, that gender in-egalitarian norms persist, and that gender inequities remain. Far more attention must be paid on implementing programme and meeting policy commitments to women and girls, whether in the education, labour, skill development or health arenas. Investments in programmes intended to redress gender inequities and limited female agency must be expanded, and must be initiated among girls as well as adult women, and among females as well as the males and others who act as their gatekeepers.

Empowering women starts with a focus on equity in the access to and the quality of education of girls, Best practices to keep girls in school must be identified and implemented. Emphasis on female agency, gender egalitarian attitudes, and respect for women's reproductive rights and entitlements must be imparted in school curricula. At the same time, findings call for greater attention on promoting life skill education programmes for young women, both unmarried and married, that will not only raise their awareness of new ideas and the world around them, but also enable them to put new information into practice, encourage them to question gender stereotypes, develop self-esteem and strengthen their skills in problem-solving, decision-making, communication and inter-personal relations and negotiation. In the restrictive socio-cultural environment in which girls grow up, it is important that programmes provide girls safe spaces in which they can build social networks and find social support among their peers, gain a livelihood skill and a savings orientation, and develop self-efficacy and self-confidence. There are already programmes for girls, for example, the KSY/SABLA programme, and for both girls and boys, for example, the AEP and the University Talk AIDS programme, that offer opportunities through which to promote a much stronger gender component, and investment in such programmes and opportunities is much needed. At the same time, an increasing number of intervention models to build agency and promote egalitarian gender role attitudes among young people have been tested in India, and these models should be reviewed and replicated or scaled up as appropriate. Other programmes intended to empower girls, such as conditional cash transfer schemes that target the girl child, need to be reviewed to remove a number of obstacles to participation, such as, a multiplicity of eligibility criteria and conditions, cumbersome procedures for registering under the scheme, lack of coordination across sectors, lack of clarity about the guidelines for implementation, and limited involvement of panchayat raj institutions (PRIs).

There exist, likewise, programmes intended to empower adult women-skill building opportunities, self-help groups, credit facilities, awareness building programmes, for example, yet the opportunities these provide have not been fully exploited. Skill building programmes for women must focus on training women in market driven rather than traditional skills. Opportunities to establish social networks and build solidarity need to be provided through available public sector programmes. Programmes are needed, likewise, that support women who experience harmful practices like early marriage and violence. Finally, there is a need for efficient utilisation of resources allocated for various programmes for women which are thus far severely under-utilised. Multipronged programmes and upscaling of promising approaches that address issues of gender equity and harmful practices are needed. A number of civil society groups have piloted programmes that provide an opportunity to document lessons and challenges, as well as potentials for scaling up, and these opportunities need to be supported.

Efforts to empower women and girls, and to break down gender stereotypes, must pay special attention to the training needs of providers or facilitators of various services—teachers, health care providers, PRIs and so on. Promoting gender equitable norms and practices requires active engagement with the community. It is essential that programmes work with key community members, such as political and religious leaders, to critically examine prevailing gender norms and forces that perpetuate such norms.

In short, a greater commitment to making available programmes work for women is needed. It is not enough to make programmes available, efforts are needed to connect women to these opportunities. At the same time, far more attention must be paid to respecting women's rights, including their reproductive rights, and other rights such as right to inheritance, control over financial resources, including property, assets and financial products.

Engage Men and Boys

Men are also vulnerable, albeit in different ways than women, and in ways that influence not only their own sexual and reproductive health outcomes but also the health outcomes of their wife or partner and the progress in promoting female empowerment. However, men and boys remain relatively neglected in efforts to change norms and improve health outcomes.

Programmes must recognise these vulnerabilities and be more inclusive of boys and men. Boys and men can no longer be neglected in efforts to bring about gender equity and high standards of sexual and reproductive health. Education system changes are needed so that life skill programmes within and outside the schools system include boys and inculcate in them new notions of masculinity. Health system level changes are needed that provide men space to seek information, counselling, care, and contraceptive supplies. There is evidence that interventions intended to reverse traditional notions of masculinity and entitlement have succeeded in promoting gender equitable attitudes and behaviours among men, for example, reducing marital violence, increasing condom use, and reducing reported symptoms of infection among men. There is a need to expand and upscale such promising interventions among men, but at the same time, initiate programmes intended to change norms from an early age.

Address Emerging Issues in the Population and Sexual and Reproductive Health Arenas

Our review has highlighted concerns about such issues as food availability and employment generation that have a significant influence, directly and/or indirectly, on the pace at which improvements in population and sexual and reproductive health will take place. While food production has kept pace with population growth, the situation is far from comfortable. The availability of food grains has remained nearly stagnant, per capita food availability has not really improved and remains at a relatively low level, and nutritional conditions remain poor. Major initiatives are necessary to boost agricultural production and ensure the nutritional needs of the growing population. As far as employment is concerned, while open unemployment has not been large, underemployment is widespread and a serious concern. Given the seasonal nature of Indian agriculture, and the domination of the agricultural sector in the work force (albeit not in production), many are not engaged in work for large parts of the year. Female work participation remains low but is likely to increase.

Demand for year-round employment, including among women, suggests that India's labour force is likely to grow considerably in the foreseeable future, and concerted efforts towards employment generation are urgently required.

Address Social and Regional Inequities

Huge disparities have been documented in many development indicators like educational attainment, access to health care, fertility, neonatal mortality, child marriage, with the poor, the socially excluded including those belonging to scheduled castes and scheduled tribes, the poorly educated and those from lesser developed states far worse off than others. These inequalities are evident both at national level, and at the individual states, and in many instances, differences were starker for women than men. Programmes need to narrow these inequities, recognise that specific strategies need to be devised to address the needs of those left behind, and ensure that service providers including government officials, health service providers, teachers and so on, are oriented to focus on the most vulnerable and the marginalised, as well as states and regions that services have been left behind.

Meet the Needs of the Urban Poor

Thus far, the level of urbanisation has been low and the pace of increase in urbanization has been slow, but projections suggest that its pace is bound to increase. The 2011 census has shown, for example, that urbanization increased from 28 per cent in the previous decade (1991–2001) to 31 per cent in the 2001–2011 decade. Efforts must be made to accommodate the inflow of the population into urban areas, and meet the likely demands this will entail with regard to infrastructure, institutions and service provision. Also of concern is the fact that many urban areas contain large slum populations, and in many cities, very large sections of the urban population live in slums. If the tempo of urbanization increases, especially with rapid growth in the tertiary and secondary sectors, this segment of the population may increase. Accommodating the needs of the populations residing in slums calls for major investments in infrastructure and access to basic services like housing, water supply, sanitation, and other amenities for the urban poor, without which the quality of life for this large urban population will be severely and adversely affected. Linkages must be made, in order to address concerns about urban health, with the Ministry of Urban Development and urban local bodies.

Put Programmes in Place to Meet the Needs of an Ageing Population

Thus far, the age distribution of the population has contained a small segment in the elderly ages, and the pace of increase in this proportion has been marginal. At the same time, population projections emphasise that the share of the population aged above 60 (or 65) will increase far more rapidly than before, and, by the middle of the century, will have doubled. Efforts must be made with regard to the health system, social security nets and so on, to address the needs of the elderly and to ensure for them access to health, social security, comfort and dignity. With declining fertility, smaller numbers of children, and globalisation trends that may geographically separate parents from children, elderly parents will have fewer grown up children on whom they can depend than in the past. In such circumstances, as in other countries, the state will need to intervene to ensure the wellbeing of the elderly. There is a need to anticipate such changes, and develop mechanisms to provide old age support. Such mechanisms need to be put into place very soon in some states, that is, those leading the demographic transition, and later, in the rest of the country as well. The need for programmes for the elderly has been recognized and the National Policy for Older Persons (NPOP) and schemes to support the elderly must be implemented, and greater inputs from the Ministry of Social Justice and Empowerment (and, at state level, Departments of Social Welfare) must be sought.

Use the Media and New Technologies More Creatively to Raise Awareness and Promote Gender Equitable Norms

Although television, radio, and new information technologies offer a huge opportunity whereby to shape and transmit new ideas and attitudes, advocate for behaviour change, and provide sexual and reproductive health information, these opportunities have not been well exploited. Access to television and mobile phones has increased considerably, including in rural areas and among the urban poor, and the opportunities that this access provides for raising awareness and attitudes are considerable. Although popular media in India tends to uphold and reinforce, rather than question, traditional notions of masculinity, there are increasingly sophisticated efforts to use television to change norms, and greater investments are required in using the media such as radio, TV, and the internet more effectively and sensitively. NRHM's and NACO's current efforts to deliver key information through TV need to be sustained and expanded, and the reach of messages conveyed needs to be evaluated. More imaginative use of soap operas and serials for conveying messages must be encouraged. Together with investments in the mass media, there is a need to make better use of new ways of encouraging interpersonal contacts. Mobile phones are a powerful means through which messages can be conveyed, and in view of the fact they are widely accessed by rural women and men, they may be a useful technology through which to transmit messages on reproductive health and rights. At the same time, there is a need for more attention to pictorial and written information suitable for moderately educated women and men, and targeting, aside from adult women, special groups such as newlyweds and the unmarried, as well as men and family elders.

* * *

We have come a long way, but the agenda for the future is daunting. Our review clearly shows that many key features of policies and programmes remain unimplemented, inequities persist and the needs of the marginalised remain unmet. Of note, however, is that the policy environment, be it related to women and child development, health and family welfare, HIV/AIDS or youth development, has recognised the importance of redressing these shortcomings as the key to shaping India's future. Efforts have been initiated to translate this commitment into practice. What is needed is a similar level of commitment to ensuring that programmes do indeed reach the most excluded, that the scope and content of programmes are regularly reviewed for effectiveness and acceptability, and promising lessons are assimilated and scaled up. Meeting this agenda requires not only careful planning and programme implementation on the part of the government, but also recognition of the role that other sectors can play.

References

Jegeebhoy, S.J., S. Kalyamala, A.J.F. Zavier, R. Kumar, S. Mundle et al. 2011. Can Nurses Perform Manual Vaccum Aspiration (MVA) as safely and Effectively as Physicians, Evidence from India, *Contraception*. 84: 615–21.

Jegeebhoy, S.J., S. Kalyanmala, S. Mundle, J. Tank, A.J.F. Zavier, R. Kumar et al. 2012 'feasibility of Expanding the Medication Abortion, Provider Base in India to include Aurved Physicians and Nurses, *International Persefectives on Sexual and Reproductive Health*. 38(3): 133–42.

Ministry of Health and Family Welfare (MOHFW). 2009. *National Rural Health Mission Reproductive & Child Health Program Phase II,* 6th *Joint Review Mission*. New Delhi: Donor Coordination Division, MOHFW, Government of India.

———. 2010. *National Rural Health Mission, State-wise Progress as on 30.09.2010*. New Delhi: Department of Family Welfare, MOHFW, Government of India.

MOHFW, Expert Group on Amendments to the MTP Act. 2010. Draft Proposed Amendments to the MTP Act. New Delhi: MOHFW, unpublished draft

Planning Commission. 2011. *Mid-term Appraisal: Eleventh Five Year Plan 2007–2012*. New Delhi: Planning Commission.

World Health Organization. 2012. *Trends in Maternal Mortality: 1990 to 2010, WHO, UNICEF, UNFPA and The World Bank Estimates*. Geneva: World Health Organisation. Accessed on 25 March 2012 at http://whqlibdoc.who.int/publications/2012/9789241503631_eng.pdf

Index

About the Authors

Shireen J. Jejeebhoy is Senior Associate, Population Council, India, where she directs research activities related to young people's health and development, gender based violence, and prevention of unsafe abortion. Her research has focused on areas of gender, adolescent health and development, and sexual and reproductive matters both in India and other parts of the world. Earlier, she was Scientist in the Reproductive Health and Research Department, World Health Organisation, Geneva. She has written extensively on women's education and empowerment, violence, maternal health, abortion, and the sexual and reproductive health and rights of young people. Dr Jejeebhoy holds Ph.D. and M.A. degrees in demography from the University of Pennsylvania.

P. M. Kulkarni is Professor of Demography, Centre for the Study of Regional Development, School of Social Sciences, Jawaharlal Nehru University, New Delhi. Earlier, he worked in the Department of Population Studies at the Bharathiar University, Coimbatore, the Population Research Centre at the Institute for Social and Economic Change, Bangalore, the Population Research Centre at the J.S.S. Institute of Economic Research, Dharwad, and the Population Centre, Bangalore. He has authored two monographs and published research papers in the areas of fertility, family planning, population policy and programmes, health, social disparities, and mathematical demography. He holds a Ph.D. degree in statistics from the Colorado State University, and was Post Doctoral Fellow at the Population Studies and Training Centre, Brown University.

K.G. Santhya is Associate II, Population Council, and an economist and demographer with thirteen years of experience in designing and conducting rigorous qualitative and quantitative studies on rights of youth, gender equity and women's empowerment, reproductive health, and gender based violence. Dr Santhya has been the principal investigator of a number of large, complicated state and national level research initiatives. She has extensive experience in implementing and evaluating intervention models to empower married and unmarried adolescent girls and young women. She has authored forty book chapters, peer reviewed journal articles, and study reports on child marriage, the needs of married adolescents, violence against women, maternal health, and the sexual and reproductive health of young people. She is currently a member of the Scientific Panel on Reproductive Health, the International Union for the Scientific Study of Population and an elected member of the Asian Population Association Council.

Firoza Mehrotra is a former officer of the Indian Administration Service with forty years of experience of working both at the policy formulation and field levels. She has worked extensively in the areas of gender equality, women's empowerment, child development, adolescents, and population and development. She retired as Special Consultant in the Planning Commission of India where she looked after the women and child development, handlooms and handicrafts, north-eastern Indian states, and voluntary sectors. She played a key role in developing policies and new schemes for these sectors. During her stint with UNIFEM (now UNWomen) South Asia as the Deputy Regional Programme Director, she worked on policy and advocacy issues with governments of the region, civil society, especially women's groups and research institutions in Afghanistan, Bangladesh, Bhutan, India, Maldives, Nepal, Pakistan, and Sri Lanka. She also worked in UNFPA as the Gender Specialist, for four years.